PHARMACOLOGICAL CONTROL OF LIPID METABOLISM

ADVANCES IN EXPERIMENTAL MEDICINE AND BIOLOGY

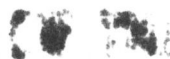

PHARMACOLOGICAL CONTROL OF LIPID METABOLISM

Proceedings of the Fourth International Symposium on
Drugs Affecting Lipid Metabolism held in Philadelphia,
Pennsylvania, September 8-11, 1971

Edited by
William L. Holmes

Director, Division of Research
Lankenau Hospital
Philadelphia, Pennsylvania

Rodolfo Paoletti

Director, Institute of Pharmacology and Pharmacognosy
University of Milan
Milan, Italy

and
David Kritchevsky

Member, The Wistar Institute of Anatomy and Biology
Philadelphia, Pennsylvania

⅏ PLENUM PRESS · NEW YORK · LONDON · 1972

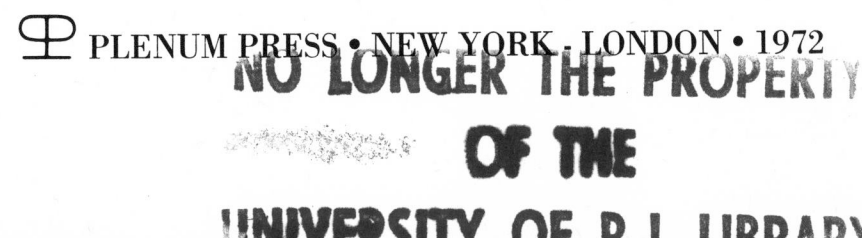

Symposium sponsored by

American Heart Association
  Council on Arteriosclerosis
International Society of Cardiology
  Scientific Council on Arteriosclerosis and Ischemic Heart Disease
International Society for Biochemical Pharmacology
The Heart Association of Southeastern Pennsylvania

Library of Congress Catalog Card Number 72-82746

ISBN 0-306-39026-4

© 1972 Plenum Press, New York
A Division of Plenum Publishing Corporation
227 West 17th Street, New York, N. Y. 10011

United Kingdom edition published by Plenum Press, London
A Division of Plenum Publishing Company, Ltd.
Davis House (4th Floor), 8 Scrubs Lane, Harlesden, London,
NW10 6SE, England

Printed in the United States of America

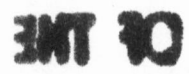

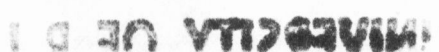

INTERNATIONAL ORGANIZING COMMITTEE:

S. Bergstrom - Sweden
L. A. Carlson - Sweden
S. Garattini - Italy
W. L. Holmes - U.S.A.
D. Kritchevsky - U.S.A.
M. F. Oliver - U.K.
R. Paoletti - Italy
G. Schettler - Germany
D. Steinberg - U.S.A.

LOCAL ORGANIZING COMMITTEE:

G. A. Braun
N. W. Di Tullio
W. L. Holmes
D. Kritchevsky
G. A. Reichard, Jr.
J. J. Spitzer

SCIENTIFIC SECRETARIES:

W. L. Holmes, Philadelphia, Pa. (U.S.A.)
R. Paoletti, Milan (Italy)

PROGRAM CHAIRMAN:

D. Kritchevsky, Philadelphia, Pa. (U.S.A.)

ACKNOWLEDGMENTS

The Organizing Committee gratefully acknowledges the contributions of the following organizations:

Ayerst Laboratories	New York, New York
Baxter Laboratories	Morton Grove, Illinois
Best Foods Research Center	Union, New Jersey
Bristol Laboratories	Syracuse, New York
CIBA Pharmaceutical Company	Summit, New Jersey
Dow Chemical Company	Zionsville, Indiana
Geigy Pharmaceuticals	Ardsley, New York
Hoechst Pharmaceutical Company	Somerville, New Jersey
Hoffmann-LaRoche, Inc.	Nutley, New Jersey
Eli Lilly and Company	Indianapolis, Indiana
McNeil Laboratories, Inc.	Fort Washington, Pennsylvania
Mead Johnson Research Center	Evansville, Indiana
Merck Sharpe & Dohme	Rahway, New Jersey
Pfizer Pharmaceuticals	Groton, Connecticut
A. H. Robins Company	Richmond, Virginia
Sandoz Pharmaceuticals	Hanover, New Jersey
Schering Corporation	Bloomfield, New Jersey
G. D. Searle & Company	Chicago, Illinois
Smith Kline & French Laboratories	Philadelphia, Pennsylvania
Sumitomo Chemical Company, Ltd.	Osaka, Japan
The Upjohn Company	Kalamazoo, Michigan
Wallace Laboratories	Cranbury, New Jersey
Warner-Lambert Pharmaceutical Company	Morris Plains, New Jersey

The generosity of these organizations made it possible for us to arrange this Symposium, which was attended by more than four hundred scientists working on problems of lipid metabolism.

The Organizing Committee

PREFACE

This Symposium was the fourth in a series which began in Milan, Italy, in 1960. Each meeting has introduced or developed some new concepts in the areas of lipid metabolism and drugs. The meetings have served as a springboard for new ideas which have, between meetings, become accepted and exploited. This meeting has been no exception. Principal among the many new concepts discussed were lipoprotein synthesis and metabolism, apoprotein structure and function, whole body metabolism of cholesterol, and aspects of myocardial and aortic metabolism. The Symposium also included a summary of current thought on management of hyperlipemias and atherosclerosis. Data on more than 30 drugs were introduced and discussed. We have every expectation that the next Symposium will include material which is now only in the formative stage.

The Organizing Committee would like to acknowledge the invaluable assistance of Miss Mary Constant, Mr. Ralph H. Hollerorth, Mrs. Carolyn P. Hyatt and Miss Jane T. Kolimaga, whose efforts contributed significantly ($p < .001$) to the success of this Symposium.

W. L. Holmes
R. Paoletti
D. Kritchevsky

CONTENTS

NEWER ASPECTS OF DRUGS AFFECTING LIPID METABOLISM

CAN HEART DISEASE BE POSTPONED OR PREVENTED?

OPENING REMARKS

W. L. Holmes

Division of Research, Lankenau Hospital

Philadelphia, Pennsylvania

In opening this Symposium on Drugs Affecting Lipid Metabolism, I thought it might be of interest to reflect for a moment on some of the past developments in this field. It was in 1931, exactly 40 years ago, that Dr. Paul Dudley White published the first edition of his celebrated book entitled "Heart Disease." In discussing the treatment of arterial disease, Dr. White said the following concerning arteriosclerosis: "For arteriosclerosis itself there is as yet no known therapy; some believe that the age-long use of potassium iodide or other drug of traditional value may some day prove to have a scientific basis. If the condition is rapidly progressive or pronounced, it is probably wise to prevent overexertion, overeating, and overexposure to infections without restricting too much the activities of life which in themselves favor health and happiness." Since that time, and particularly during the past twenty years, we have witnessed a tremendous explosion in the development of new basic knowledge concerning many facets of atherosclerosis, which in turn have led to new approaches to its treatment and even to its prevention. Testimony to this is seen in the ever increasing literature devoted to either the nutritional-hygenic or pharmacological approaches to the control of atherosclerotic vascular disease.

The recognition of a possible causal relationship of elevated serum cholesterol to atherosclerosis together with the demonstration in the early 1950's that soy sterols could inhibit atherogenesis in rabbits led to an intensified search for hypocholesterolemic

1

agents.   Of necessity, many of these studies were quite emperical in nature; however, during the latter part of this decade, somewhat more rational approaches to the problem began to emerge.   These were based on an ever increasing knowledge of the biochemical pathways involved in cholesterol biosynthesis, and of the factors concerned with its absorption, degradation and excretion.   By 1960 a number of potential leads had been uncovered and formed a large portion of the subject matter for the first of these symposia.   Of the ten or so potential drugs discussed at that meeting, only two or three have survived the test of time.

During this period we were beginning to hear rumblings of the possible relationship of triglyceride to certain types of vascular disease.   Also, new knowledge of the chemistry and physical properties, and of the role of lipoprotein in lipid transport was unfolding.   The low density lipoproteins were recognized as the culprits which invade the aorta and deposit their lipid therein—we began to think in terms of hyperlipoproteinemia and of decreasing circulating low density- and very low density lipoproteins rather than cholesterol or triglyceride alone.

Another milestone was achieved in 1965, when Fredrickson, Levy and Lees classified hyperlipoproteinemias into five distinct phenotypes.   It soon was shown that the different phenotypes did not necessarily respond to the same type of therapy.   This technique has proved to be of immense value, not only to the physician in planning therapeutic regimens for his hyperlipoproteinemic patients, but also to the research scientist searching for new lipoprotein lowering drugs.

Now to say a few words about the present meeting.   When it was planned by the Organizing Committee, it was felt that the subject matter should be limited to two rather broad areas: (1) new basic information providing it is relevant, and (2) newer aspects of drugs affecting lipid metabolism.   The Program Committee has attempted to organize the program within these guidelines, and we hope that you will find the result intellectually stimulating and satisfying.

Finally, a cursory inspection of the program shows that the effect of some thirty pharmacologic agents on various aspects of lipid metabolism will be discussed, some for the first time.

Further, it can be seen that contributions have been received from researchers representing seventeen different countries, which attests to the fact that this Symposium truly has become the international forum for this new but important area of medical research.

NEWER DEVELOPMENTS IN LIPID BIOCHEMISTRY

SYNTHESIS AND SECRETION OF PLASMA LIPOPROTEINS

Robert L. Hamilton, Ph.D.

Cardiovascular Research Institute and Department of Anatomy
University of California School of Medicine
San Francisco, California   U.S.A.

Virtually nothing is known about the initial intracellular events that lead to the formation of a nascent lipoprotein particle. However, recent technical advances in electron microscopy, cell frationation, and the biochemistry of apolipoproteins are providing subcellular probes for identifying and characterizing both the plasma lipoprotein secretory mechanisms and the newly made secretory products. Evidence for an extremely close relationship between nascent plasma lipoproteins and the membrane lipoproteins constituting the secretory mechanism is beginning to emerge.

It is generally recognized that there are two different forms of lipoproteins: 1) those of cells which constitute the membrane lipoproteins of subcellular organelles; 2) the soluble lipoproteins of extracellular fluids (1). Membrane lipoproteins are probably formed chiefly by planar sheets of phospholipid bilayers. The long fatty acid chains of each phospholipid occupy the inner core of the sheet as a non-polar phase. Polar head groups of the phospholipids, spaced about 40–45 Å apart, provide a hydrophilic surface on each side of the sheet (2,3). The heterogeneous proteins of biological membranes associate with the phospholipid bilayer structure in different ways. Some proteins are extended on the surface, others penetrate partially and still others may penetrate the full thickness of the lipid bilayer (3).

The soluble lipoproteins of blood plasma and lymph serve transport functions and differ from membrane lipoproteins in that they are specialized products of only two cells: hepatic parenchymal cells and absorptive cells of the small intestine. One might expect soluble lipoproteins to differ greatly in structure from membranes since they occur as spheroidal particles measuring between

7

50-5000 Å in diameter. Although the structure of plasma lipoproteins is not
established, many probably exist as a miniature droplet of oil containing
triglycerides and cholesteryl esters surrounded by a thin surface film of
phospholipid, protein and free cholesterol. Recent studies give evidence that
this surface film is a monolayer of invariant thickness of about 21-22 Å, precise-
ly one-half the thickness of a phospholipid bilayer (4). This model suggests
the working hypothesis that plasma lipoproteins might originate from a phospholipid bilayer by expansion of the nonpolar core.

        In order to discuss subcellular mechanisms of origin of soluble lipoproteins,
it is first necessary to classify plasma lipoproteins into functional groups. Four
major groups of lipoproteins isolated from plasma are generally recognized on
the basis of their ultracentrifugal and electrophoretic properties. These include
1) chylomicrons; 2) very low density (VLDL) or pre-beta lipoproteins, 3) low
density (LDL) or beta lipoproteins; 4) high density (HDL) or alpha lipoproteins.
Each group can be isolated and characterized by measurements of the proportions
of the major lipid components and total protein (5).

SECRETION OF VLDL AND CHYLOMICRONS

        The formation of VLDL and chylomicrons may be discussed together. The
liver develops as an outgrowth of the primitive foregut and from the standpoint
of ultrastructure, hepatic parenchymal cells share many morphologic features
with absorptive cells of the small intestine (Fig. 1 and 2). Functionally, these
two cells are unique in their special capability to export triglycerides and
cholesteryl esters in soluble particles. Both liver and small intestine respond
to availability of extracellular free fatty acids (FFA) by increasing their uptake and esterification, and by increased release of triglycerides in particulate
form back into the extracellular spaces. The secretory products released by
these cells, VLDL and chylomicrons, are generally similar in gross chemical
composition:

Rat Lipoproteins	Trigly-cerides	Chol. Esters	Chol.	Phospho-lipids	Protein	Mean Diameter
Serum VLDL	70	6	3	11	10	400 Å
Lymph Chylomicrons	90	2	1	6	1	2000 Å
	"Core"			"Surface"		

The major apparent difference is that larger chylomicrons contain more non-polar or "core" material in proportion to "surface" constituents. This difference in size probably reflects expansion and shrinkage of the core in response to the demand placed on the individual cells to transport fat. Smaller particles of VLDL size and chemical composition are continuously produced in small amounts by the intestine even during fasting (6,7,8), while larger particles resembling chylomicrons in size and chemical composition can be produced by the liver under stress of high carbohydrate diet (9,10) or in response to excessive influx of free fatty acids (11,12,13,14).

The Secretory Mechanism

Electron microscopic studies of intestine (15, 16) and liver (11, 17, 18, 19, 20) have uncovered the subcellular pathway for formation of nascent lipoproteins. Osmiophilic particles of the same size, shape and staining properties as chylomicrons are visualized in absorptive cells of the intestine by electron microscopy (Fig. 1). They appear within cisternae of the membranous compartments of absorptive epithelium of the gut within minutes of feeding polyunsaturated fatty acids (15). Particles first appear in the apical region of the cell within vesicular and tubular cisternae of smooth surfaced endoplasmic reticulum (SER) and soon thereafter within cisternae with some ribosomes attached. Particles are not seen in the long flattened cisternae of the rough endoplasmic reticulum (RER) studded with ribosomes except at the dilated ends which have few or no ribosomes. The SER appears to proliferate from the RER (16), possibly at these dilated ends which represent the site of continuity between RER and SER.

The newly made chylomicrons appear to migrate from the SER in the apical cytoplasm into the Golgi apparatus which is consistently supranuclear in intestinal absorptive cells (Fig. 1). The usual electron microscopic image obtained during fat feeding is that of round lipid particles enclosed by a membrane which usually has been interpreted to be a vesicle. However, in fasting, clear images have been published indicating the tubular organization of the SER in the apical cytoplasm (7,8). Recent studies of Golgi apparatus recovered from absorptive cells gives additional morphologic evidence (21) that tubular systems more correctly describe the subcellular organization of these membranous compartments which often appear as vesicles in cross section. The often reported images of vesicles could also result from disorganization of membranes caused by inadequate fixation of fat-filled cells.

Newly made chylomicrons probably must pass through the Golgi apparatus before release into the extracellular space. The particles accumulate in secretory vesicles of the Golgi apparatus and appear only at the same level, or basal to, the Golgi apparatus in the lateral extracellular spaces between absorptive

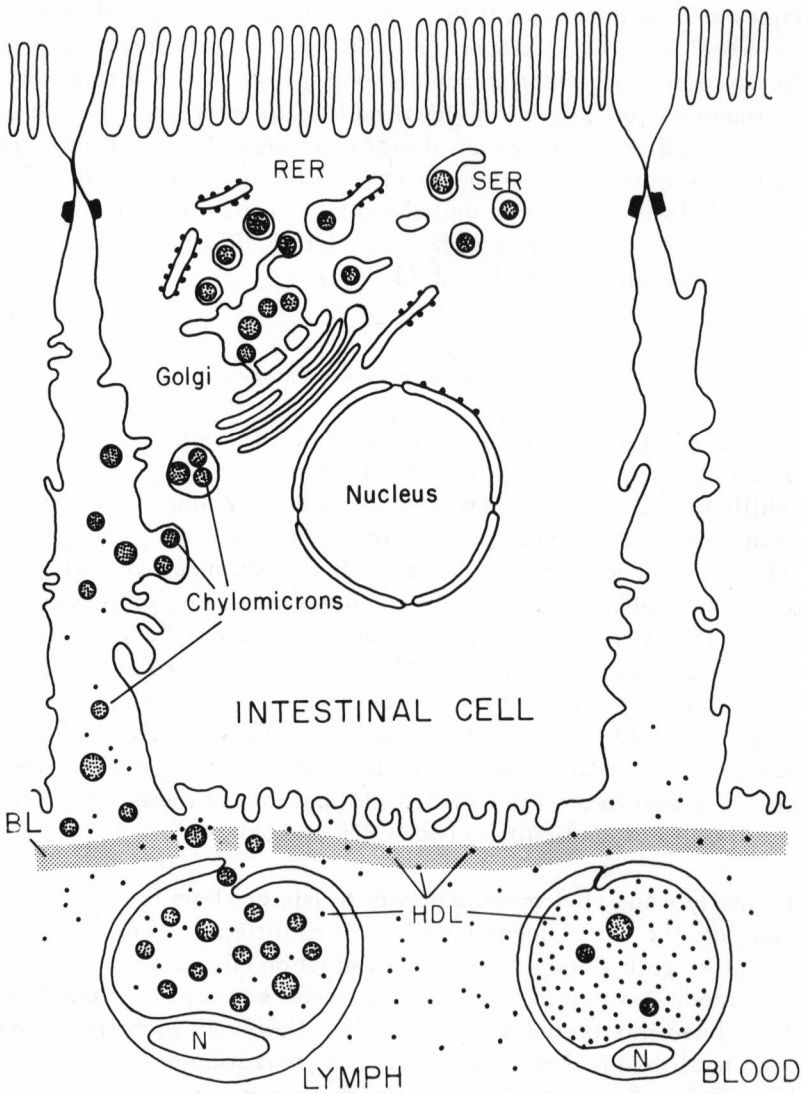

Fig. 1 and 2. These 2 diagrams outline the subcellular compartments that constitute the plasma lipoprotein secretory mechanism in liver and intestine.

Fig. 1. Formation and transport of chylomicrons occurs within membrane -
enclosed cisternae of rough endoplasmic reticulum (RER), smooth endoplasmic
reticulum (SER) and Golgi apparatus of intestinal cells. Nascent chylomicrons
are probably released by secretory vesicles of the Golgi apparatus and pass
through gaps in the basal lamina (BL). HDL leak from plasma into the extracellular spaces and mix with nascent chylomicrons there and in lymph vessels.
After reaching the blood (which has the highest concentration of HDL) transfer
of additional polypeptides to chylomicrons would be accelerated.

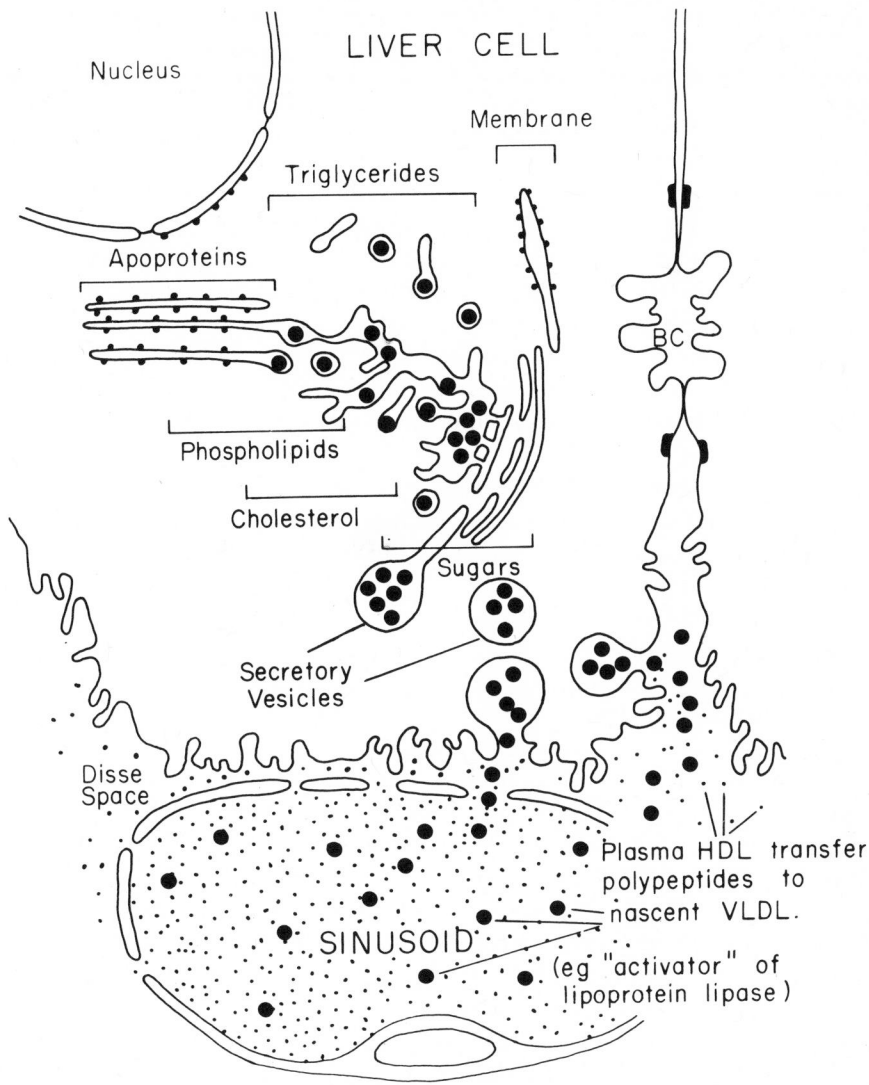

Fig. 2. The same subcellular compartments function in the synthesis and secretion of nascent VLDL in liver. Continuity of membrane compartments is indicated and the brackets imply functional regions some of which overlap in the synthesis of the various constituents of plasma lipoproteins. Also implied is the possible origin of the membrane synthesized for new secretory vesicles. Nascent VLDL are released by fusion of the membranes of secretory vesicles with the plasma membrane. Plasma HDL probably exist in the space of Disse at concentrations equal to that of plasma thereby facilitating the transfer of a specific group of polypeptides to nascent VLDL, one of which has the function of promoting the interaction of triglyceride-rich lipoproteins with lipoprotein lipase.

cells. Continued absorption of heavy fat loads diminishes the number of parallel flattened cisternae of the Golgi apparatus and puromycin virtually depletes the cell of recognizable Golgi membranes (22). These observations suggest that newly made secretory membranes of the Golgi apparatus must be replenished continously to carry nascent chylomicrons to the cell surface for discharge (22). During fasting the intestine continues to secrete triglycerides into mesenteric lymph as VLDL-sized particles. With the electron microscope intestinal VLDL, like chylomicrons, are found in both the ER and Golgi apparatus in rats and in man. Diversion of bile or administration of cholestyramine causes almost complete disappearance of these particles from both subcellular sites (7, 23). Thus, triglyceride-rich particles of VLDL and chylomicron size are formed and released by the intestinal cell by the same subcellular pathway. In fact, particles of both sizes appear together in single cells in the SER, in secretory vesicles, and in extracellular spaces in the absence of fat loading.

The subcellular pathway of synthesis and secretion of VLDL by liver shares many features with that of the intestine. Osmiophilic particles become visible with the electron microscope at the smooth-surfaced, terminal ends of the parallel flattened cisternae of RER (18, 20). They never are seen within the flattened cisternae of RER in normal liver. Only a few particles ordinarily appear within smooth surfaced cisternae but they become numerous after stimuli which increase production of VLDL such as partial hepatectomy (24), perfusion of liver with FFA (18, 19), administration of ethanol (17), infusion of norepinephrine (11), and injections of cortisone (13), anti-insulin serum or aminonucleoside (25, 26). Clusters of particles are always found in some of the Golgi apparatus in livers of both normal or treated experimental animals (11) and in man (27). The clustering of particles in this organelle appears to represent the formation of secretory vesicles developing from cisternae of the Golgi apparatus (11). Although the mechanism of formation of secretory vesicles is not fully understood, they show tubular continuities both in thin sections and in negatively stained fractions of Golgi apparatus isolated from rat liver (20, 28, 29). Some of these tubules contain nascent VLDL, and extend for distances of 1 to 2 microns in negative stains of isolated Golgi apparatus (11). Other tubules of the secretory vesicles form anastomoses which connect to the flattened cisternae of the Golgi apparatus (29). Recent observations of serial thin sections show that continuities exist not only between RER and SER, but also between the SER and membranes of the Golgi apparatus in rat liver. In this same study, a new "rigid" membrane was described which was: 1) always seen near the Golgi apparatus; 2) shaped like the flattened cisternae that make up the stacks of the Golgi apparatus; 3) continuous with RER (20). A similar observation has been made in intestinal cells and this mechanism has been postulated for the synthesis of new Golgi membranes (22). The synthesis of newly formed membrane proteins of secretory vesicles has been shown to accompany the synthesis of nascent proteins of zymogen granules in the parotid gland (30).

In the liver cell, secretory vesicles near the cell surface fuse with the plasma membrane resulting in the discharge of VLDL into the space of Disse (11, 18, 19). It is likely that "recognition proteins" exist in the membranes of secretory vesicles and in the plasma membranes which result in fusion of the two (31). Otherwise, discharge might be expected to occur randomly into other membranous compartments of the cell, into other secretory vesicles, or into the bile canaliculus. As does the intestine during fat absorption, the Golgi apparatus of hepatocytes becomes filled with particles during early phases of increased secretion of VLDL at the expense of flattened cisternae. The Golgi membranes virtually disappear as recognizable structures following continuous stimulation associated with uptake of FFA. The disappearance of this organelle is accompanied by accumulation of larger particles in cisternae of the SER and Golgi apparatus reflecting the early morphologic changes of fatty liver that accompany impaired release of VLDL by the liver cell (11, 13, 19). These observations suggest that continuous synthesis of new membrane of secretory vesicles must accompany secretion of VLDL (Fig. 2).

These morphological findings suggest several new concepts about the plasma lipoprotein secretory mechanism (Fig. 2). First, there appears to be a continuous membranous compartment within the hepatocyte (and probably the intestinal absorptive cell) extending from the RER, SER, and Golgi tubules into the forming secretory vesicles of the Golgi apparatus. This compartment contsitutes an intracellular transport pathway for nascent VLDL and it probably functions in the assembly of plasma lipoproteins as well (Fig. l and 2). Discharge from the cell appears to depend upon the synthesis of new membranes of secretory vesicles, the separation of secretory vesicles filled with clusters of nascent VLDL from the Golgi apparatus, movement of the free vesicle to the cell surface and fusion of the membrane of the secretory vesicle with the plasma membrane. These data suggest that passage of nascent VLDL through the Golgi apparatus in all likelihood is obligatory for the release of nascent VLDL into the plasma by both hepatic parenchymal cells and intestinal absorptive cells.

The mechanism of transport through the tubular system linking RER, SER and secretory vesicles of the Golgi apparatus in liver is not known. Transport of nascent proteins from RER to secretory vesicles and their subsequent discharge requires ATP in pancreatic acinar cells (32). Ethionine, which lowers ATP levels in liver cells, causes a rapid accumulation of VLDL-sized particles throughout SER cisternae (33). It has been postulated that a continuous production and flow of membrane from RER to SER to Golgi apparatus accompanies the synthesis of VLDL and accounts for the movement of particles through this system (20). Since the tubular membranes appear to be dilated by each VLDL particle, both in thin sections (11, 20) and in negative stains of isolated Golgi fractions (11, 28) a form of "peristalsis" at the subcellular level could be conceived to propel substances through these channels. Besides VLDL, other secretory proteins of liver such as albumin and glycoproteins of plasma traverse a similar subcellular pathway (34,35,36,37,38). It has not been shown that these different secretory products destined for plasma are mixed within these compartments. However, their production and release appear to be coupled in certain conditions. In choline deficiency there is a reduced flow of VLDL, albumin and glycoproteins to plasma (39,40), whereas in nephrosis the liver secretes both albumin and VLDL at an accelerated rate (41).

A precise localization of the subcellular sites of synthesis of the various components of plasma lipoproteins and the sequence of assembly of these components is crucial but lacking. Owing to the sparse and ambiguous data that is available on this point, the scheme shown in Fig. 2 should be interpreted only in a general sense.

Most information pertaining to localization of the enzymes of phospholipid, triglyceride and cholesterol synthesis are based on studies of microsomes. Microsomes represent vesicular fragments of cell membranes derived chiefly from the rupture of the endoplasmic reticulum. In all likelihood the SER in the intestine and liver is synthesized from the RER (16,42). Thus the proteins (enzymes) of the SER exist in the RER at some time but are not necessarily functional in the RER. SER and RER frequently are in continuity and, in the cells of liver and gut, lipid droplets interpreted as the initial formation of a lipoprotein appear to form within outpouchings of smooth surfaced membrane derived from RER. This might explain the difficulty of achieving a clear-cut separation of microsomes originating from RER and SER. No data are available which identify those enzymes specifically related to the formation of soluble lipoproteins. A second approach, which has had limited trial, is the use of electron microscopic radioautography to localize sites of lipid synthesis soon after intravascular injection of lipid precursors. Because of the complexity of RER-SER associations mentioned above, and the limited resolution of this technique, no conclusions can be drawn about the relative synthetic roles of RER and SER membranes (43).

Microsomes from intestinal epithelium and from liver contain enzymes for both phospholipids and triglyceride synthesis. Rough surfaced microsomes from cat intestine are reportedly more active in both phospholipid and glyceride synthetic enzymes than smooth microsomes (44). Lecithin synthesis is reportedly equally active in rough and smooth surfaced microsomes obtained from liver (45). Smooth surfaced membrane fractions isolated from fat absorbing intestine contain the bulk of the newly synthesized triglycerides (46). It has also been suggested that the rough and smooth surfaced microsomes obtained from liver participate to a similar degree in cholesterol synthesis (47).

A new approach to this important problem has been reported recently. Electron microscopic localization of acyltransferase activity by histochemical

techniques in intestinal absorptive cells suggests that monoglyceride acyltransferase, associated with triglyceride synthesis, is localized mainly in the SER and
to a lesser degree with one surface of the Golgi apparatus. The α-glycerophos-
phate pathway, associated chiefly with phospholipid synthesis, appears to be
localized in the RER (48). A localization of this α-glycerophosphate pathway
also occurs in certain regions of RER in liver cells (49). It is clear that more precise studies are needed to localize the sites of synthesis of plasma lipoprotein
lipid constituents.

Apoproteins of the plasma lipoproteins are no doubt synthesized by ribosomes
bound to membranes of the RER (50). Studies in vitro indicate that both free
ribosomes and microsomes with bound ribosomes incorporate labeled amino
acids into peptides which bind to added carrier LDL and HDL from plasma (51, 52).
Similarly, microsomes from intestinal cell homogenates synthesize new LDL apoproteins (53). A question often asked is whether or not apoprotein synthesis is
obligatory for secretion of lipoproteins. Apoprotein synthesis is probably necessary
for formation of VLDL since puromycin virtually eliminates particles from the SER
and Golgi apparatus of perfused livers as well as from the perfusate (18). Moreover, the increased production of VLDL which accompanies perfusion with FFA-
rich solutions increases synthesis of VLDL protein in rat liver (14). Secretion of
chylomicrons appears to be less sensitive to inhibition of protein synthesis although
lipoproteins in mesenteric lymph are greatly increased in size (54) and intracellular lipid particles accumulate and enlarge (16). This comparative insensitivity
could be related to the very small amounts of protein contained in newly formed
chylomicrons as contrasted to nascent VLDL from liver. As will be discussed
below, chylomicrons can be secreted which contain less than 1% protein by
weight (55). Their content of protein is subsequently increased several fold by
transfer of apoproteins from HDL. In contrast, the protein content of nascent
VLDL from liver increases only about one-third after they enter the blood.
It is probable that one apoprotein is necessary for formation of both VLDL and
chylomicrons in liver and intestine. In patients with abeta-lipoproteinemia, the
major LDL apoprotein is absent as are plasma LDL, VLDL and chylomicrons. HDL,
its major apolipoproteins and the other apolipoproteins which are shared by HDL,
VLDL and chylomicrons are present (56).

A functional role of the Golgi apparatus as a portal to the extracellular
environment has already been mentioned. The newly discovered synthetic activity of this organelle may be related to this function. Histochemical studies have
shown that the Golgi apparatus stains specifically for complex carbohydrates in
many cells. Moreover, this staining reportedly is increased in intensity in those
saccules of the mature face of the Golgi apparatus representing the development of
secretory vesicles which ultimately migrate to the cell surface (57). Methods of
isolating Golgi apparatus from liver (28, 58) have contributed to the discovery
that a group of enzymes, the nucleotide glycoprotein glycosyltransferases, which

add the terminal sugars to proteins to form glycoproteins, are localized in this organelle (36,37,58). This information has been applied to studies of rat lipoproteins which contain significant amounts of carbohydrate (59). Fractions of Golgi apparatus from liver incorporate labelled glucosamine into carrier lipoproteins from plasma to a much greater extent than do smooth microsomes. Both free and membrane-bound ribosomes are inactive (60). The scheme in Fig. 2 indicates that the terminal sugars are probably added to serum lipoproteins by enzymes of the Golgi apparatus but it should be recognized that the sugars which are covalently linked to apoprotein are presumably added in the RER (37).

Nascent VLDL and Chylomicrons

The observation that nascent VLDL are always present in highest concentration in secretory vesicles of the Golgi apparatus and the assumption that this represents the final stages of their assembly led to the isolation of this organelle from rat liver. The success of the isolation technique which was developed depends upon maintaining the structure of the Golgi apparatus as an intact organelle by gentle homogenization (28). Preservation of its structure proved important for its separation from the other cell components and for rapid identification of the Golgi fraction by negative staining electron microscopy (11, 28). Protection of the nascent VLDL within the membranous compartment from contamination by serum, lysosomal enzymes and floating fat is also achieved by isolating intact Golgi apparatus. In these early studies it was easily observed that particles with the same dimensions and staining properties of plasma VLDL are contained within secretory vesicles and tubular networks of the isolated cell fraction (11, 28). The next step, that of releasing and separating the nascent VLDL from the Golgi membranes without altering them, has proven to be a major problem.

In the first attempts, nascent VLDL were released from the membranes by repeated cycles of freezing, thawing and sonication. The chemical composition of these nascent VLDL, isolated by a single ultracentrifugal flotation, was similar to that of plasma VLDL. However, these nascent VLDL did not migrate as a band on paper electrophoresis and it was difficult to stain them with potassium phosphotungstate for electron microscopy (61). In subsequent studies, nascent VLDL which were released by gentle sonication were reported to contain the same major apoprotein moieties as VLDL from plasma (62).

Nascent VLDL have been studied in detail following their release from Golgi membranes by several different techniques (63). The use of ultrasound has been found to cause the appearance in nascent VLDL of additional peptide bands that are not present in plasma VLDL. These peptide bands can be introduced into plasma VLDL by sonication in the presence of Golgi membranes. Since these proteins are also present in the Golgi membranes, their presence in nascent

VLDL is interpreted as an artifact produced by ultrasound. Nascent VLDL obtained by sonication also contain substantially less protein than plasma VLDL and migrate more slowly than plasma VLDL during electrophoresis on agarose gel. Since the content of core constituents is almost identical to that of plasma VLDL it appears likely that only the surface constituents are altered by ultrasound.

Release of nascent VLDL from Golgi membranes by use of the pressure drop obtained with a French pressure cell has greatly improved the experimental results. The extra polypeptide bands do not appear in polyacrylamide gel patterns, and crushing plasma VLDL in the presence of Golgi membranes produces little detectable change. The total amount of protein recovered from washed, nascent VLDL released by pressure from Golgi apparatus of 15 pooled rat livers is remarkably constant (0.7 - 1.0 mg). Other properties of nascent VLDL released from Golgi membranes in the French pressure cell have been re-investigated in detail (63). Like those particles obtained by sonication, the core constituents are almost identical to plasma VLDL, but the nascent VLDL differ from plasma VLDL in their surface constituents. They contain about 25% less protein and proportionately more phospholipid than plasma VLDL. The ratio of surface to core constituents and the size (about 400 Å mean diameter (64)) are virtually the same for both nascent and plasma VLDL. On agarose electrophoresis, nascent VLDL migrate more slowly than plasma VLDL but the basis for this is now apparent. Polyacrylamide gels show the same general pattern of peptide bands but, when equal amounts of apoprotein are subjected to electrophoresis, nascent VLDL contain much less of each of the fast-migrating polypeptide bands. This same group of polypeptides is also present in HDL from rat plasma (63,65,66). This difference in surface polypeptides and phospholipid is probably of physiological significance. All of these differences betwen nascent and plasma VLDL are abolished by simply mixing sufficient plasma HDL with nascent VLDL (63). In addition, following reisolation, nascent VLDL promote the interaction of lipoprotein lipase with triglyceride emulsions to the same extent as do plasma VLDL whereas unmodified nascent VLDL contain this "activator" property to only a very limited degree. The polypeptide responsible for this property has been isolated from VLDL and HDL of rat plasma lipoproteins and has similar electrophoretic mobility on polyacrylamide gels (63) to the major active polypeptide of human plasma lipoproteins (67). Thus in the rat, as in man, the "activator" in plasma VLDL and HDL is one of the three major polypeptides which migrate rapidly as a group on polyacrylamide gels.

Supporting data for the functional significance of these observations is derived from other studies. The fast-migrating polypeptides of nascent VLDL from rat livers perfused with radioactive lysine contain less label than the other major polypeptides, indicating a comparatively lower rate of synthesis (68). Two of the fast-migrating polypeptides have been found to transfer rapidly between human VLDL and HDL in proportion to the concentrations of these lipoproteins.

They also persist in plasma longer than other apoproteins indicating a slower rate of turnover (69,70). In addition, studies in vivo have shown that heparin-induced catabolism of VLDL is accompanied by an increase in the quantity of one of these polypeptides in HDL of plasma (71).

A similar process probably occurs during secretion of chylomicrons and VLDL from the intestine. It has been found repeatedly that lymph chylomicrons contain less protein, but more phospholipid, than those isolated from plasma (55, 72). The same is true for lymph VLDL (73) and the electrophoretic mobility of each increases after they are mixed with plasma (6,72). Incubation of HDL from plasma with lymph chylomicrons results in more than a 3-fold increase in chylomicron protein (55).

Comparative studies of the apoprotein subunits of rat lipoproteins indicate that VLDL of intestinal lymph share with plasma HDL not only the fast-migrating polypeptides but, in addition, a group of slow-migrating polypeptides (74). In labeling experiments, the isolated perfused intestine does not appear to synthesize fast-migrating polypeptides . However, they are present in the VLDL of lymph (68), suggesting that they are transferred from plasma HDL leaking into the extracellular fluid (Fig. 2). This group of polypeptides appears to be missing from VLDL and chylomicrons obtained from Golgi apparatus isolated from the rat intestine (21). In man, the "activator" property of plasma HDL is diminished during alimentary lipemia but it increases in plasma chylomicrons (75), consistent with the concept that these polypeptides cycle between HDL and newly secreted triglyceride-rich lipoproteins (76)

The structural and functional relationship between plasma HDL and nascent VLDL and chylomicrons is presented in the diagrams of Fig. I and 2. In the liver (Fig. 2), plasma HDL permeate the space of Disse, into which nascent VLDL are released (the sinusoidal endothelium is penetrated by pores of sufficient size for the much larger VLDL to pass easily into the blood (77)). The number of HDL in plasma and presumably in this space greatly exceed that of nascent VLDL thus favoring rapid transfer of HDL-polypeptides to nascent VLDL. In the intestine, a progressive addition of HDL-polypeptides to nascent chylomicrons is presumed to continue from the extracellular space to the blood stream. Here, plasma HDL gain access to the extracellular space through the leaky fenestrated blood capillaries of the intestinal mucosa but less rapidly than into the space of Disse in liver. After intravascular injection, ferritin molecules, which are about the same diameter as HDL in the rat (110-120 Å) , enter the extracellular spaces from intestinal capillaries at an appreciably faster rate than into muscle capillaries (78). Nascent chylomicrons apparently pass through gaps of the basal lamina (Fig. 1) to gain access to the lamina propria (8). Both HDL from plasma and chylomicrons from intestinal epithelium enter lacteals between endothelial cells and mix during transit through the lymphatic system. Additional HDL from plasma might be expecte to enter the thoracic duct from other tissues, especially the liver, favoring additional exchange. Finally, more protein would be expected to be transferred to chylomicrons in the blood where HDL are far more numerous (Fig. I and 2).

SECRETION OF LDL

Available evidence suggests that LDL, as found in plasma, are not secreted directly into the blood by liver or intestine. Electron microscopic studies of thin sections of liver and intestine are not suitable to evaluate this question since LDL isolated from plasma are not clearly visualized by present methods of fixation and thin sectioning. Although occasional particles the size of LDL are seen in negatively stained fractions of Golgi apparatus, these few particles could simply represent small or incompletely formed VLDL. Antisera against preparations of LDL from rat plasma produce intense precipitin lines of identity between LDL and nascent VLDL isolated from the Golgi apparatus of rat liver (63). These antisera also produce the characteristic "B" immunoprecipitin arc with partially delipidated nascent VLDL from liver (63) or from intestinal lymph (79). The presence of the major "B" apoprotein has been shown in chylomicrons (72) and this apoprotein becomes heavily labeled from amino acid precursors during the synthesis of VLDL and chylomicrons by perfused liver and intestine (68). The "B" apoprotein does not transfer between VLDL and LDL in vitro. Thus the apoprotein of LDL is incorporated into newly made VLDL and chylomicrons within liver and intestinal cells.

The most compelling data on the mechanism of formation of plasma LDL comes from infusions of VLDL which contain labeled "B" apoprotein. These studies show a precursor-product relationship between VLDL and LDL which strongly indicates that LDL are formed during the catabolism of VLDL (80) and perhaps chylomicrons (76). Thus plasma LDL most probably originate indirectly from the liver and perhaps intestine through the transformation of triglyceride-rich lipoproteins in the plasma.

SECRETION OF HDL

There is good evidence that the liver secretes HDL. Patients with abetalipoproteinemia have HDL in their plasma (56), and rats fed orotic acid, whose livers cannot form VLDL, continue to release lipoproteins with electrophoretic and immunoelectrophoretic properties of HDL (81). An inhibitor of protein synthesis, actinomycin D, inhibits the secretion of HDL by perfused rat livers but to a much lesser degree than it inhibits secretion of VLDL (82). An HDL fraction obtained from sonicated Golgi apparatus from rat liver contains a lipoprotein which has alpha mobility on agarose gel electrophoresis and reacts with immunochemical identity with the major apoprotein of plasma HDL (83,84).

Nascent HDL

Although the evidence described above suggests that the liver secretes HDL independently of VLDL, the isolation and characterization of these newly made lipoproteins has not been documented previously. Preliminary studies (84) of nascent HDL fractions from isolated liver cells, perfused rat liver, and Golgi apparatus isolated from rat liver indicate that newly secreted HDL: 1) contain mostly phospholipid, protein and free cholesterol; 2) appear in negative stains as discs about 45 Å thick by 150-250 Å across; 3) show in thin sections the image and dimensions of a lipid bilayer (that is, two dark lines spaced about 45 Å apart and representing the region of the polar head groups of the phospholipids are separated by an unstained central region corresponding to the non-polar acyl chains (85)). A plasma lipoprotein with the structure of a lipid bilayer not un-like that of a cell membrane has been shown to exist in the blood plasma of patients with cholestasis 86). Furthermore, an HDL fraction of subjects lacking the enzyme lecithin-cholesterol acyltransferase (LCAT) is remarkably similar in structure and composition to nascent HDL from rat liver. These HDL appear as discs about 45 Å thick by 150-200 Å across in negative stains and contain many times the normal amounts of phospholipid and free cholesterol (87,88). LCAT normally forms cholesteryl esters in the plasma by catalyzing the transfer of a fatty acyl group from the lecithin to the free cholesterol of HDL (89). In the plasma of patients lacking LCAT, the existing HDL could represent the accumu-lation of nascent HDL which have not undergone transformation to the usual spheroidal structure because of the enzyme deficiency. A lipid bilayer composed chiefly of phospholipid and free cholesterol could be the appropriate substrate for LCAT (90) in the plasma compartment provided that the specific "activator" polypeptide of this enzyme were present (91). Such a transformation of discs to spheroidal particles occurs in vitro when LCAT converts free cholesterol to cholesteryl esters (92). Thus, the conversion of free cholesterol to cholesteryl ester in the lipid bilayer of a nascent HDL could cause this new molecule to move into the central non-polar phase occupied by the acyl chains of the phospholipids. This movement could cause the non-polar phase to expand by pushing apart the phospholipids, thereby generating the oily core and producing a spheroidal lipo-protein molecule. The enzymatic transformation of a bilayer structure in plasma might also have its counterpart in cells. Perhaps an initial event in the formation of VLDL and chylomicrons in hepatic parenchymal and intestinal absorptive cells is the formation of a lipid bilayer associated with the "B" apoprotein which subse-quently becomes transformed, by enzymatic expansion of its non-polar core, into a spherical plasma lipoprotein.

CONCLUSION

Progress is being made in identifying and characterizing the subcellular components of liver and intestine which constitute the plasma lipoprotein secretory mechanism. The functional roles of some of these compartments in the formation, intracellular transport and discharge of nascent VLDL and chylomicrons have been partially defined but critical information is still lacking. There are many similarities between the processes of lipoprotein secretion by hepatic parenchymal cells and absorptive cells of the intestine. Nascent VLDL and chylomicrons contain some apoproteins but others are added after they reach the extracellular spaces. Chylomicrons apparently gain most of their protein extracellularly whereas VLDL from liver gain most of their protein intracellularly. A specific group of polypeptides is transferred to nascent VLDL and chylomicrons from plasma HDL. One of these polypeptides promotes the interaction of lipoprotein lipase with triglyceride emulsions. LDL are probably not directly secreted by liver and intestine but are generated during the intravascular catabolism of VLDL and perhaps chylomicrons. HDL are secreted by liver independently. Their nascent form may be that of a lipid bilayer structure not unlike a cell membrane.

The personal research cited was supported
by grants HL-13684, HL-24187, HL-06285 and
HL-04237 from the U.S. Public Health Service.

REFERENCES

1. Oncley, J.L. in Structural and Functional Aspects of Lipoproteins in Living Systems. (Eds.) E. Tria and A.M. Scanu. Academic Press, New York (1969) p. vii.

2. Wilkins, M.H.F., A.E. Blaurock and D.M. Engelman. Nature New Biol. 230: 72 (1971)

3. Singer, S.J. and G.L. Nicolson. Science 175:720 (1972)

4. Sata, T., R.J. Havel and A.L. Jones. J. Clin. Invest. In press.

5. Havel, R.J., H.A. Eder and J.H. Bragdon. J. Clin. Invest. 34:1345 (1955)

6. Ockner, R.K., F.B. Hughes and K.J. Isselbacher. J. Clin. Invest. 48:2079 (1969)

7. Jones, A.L. and R.K. Ockner. J. Lipid Res. 12:580 (1971)

8. Tytgat, G.N., C.E. Rubin and D.R. Saunders. J. Clin. Invest. 50:2065 (1971)

9. Windmueller, H.G. and H.E. Spaeth. Arch. Biochem. Biophys. 122:362 (1967)

10. Ruderman, N.B., A.L. Jones, R.M. Krauss and E. Shafrir. J. Clin. Invest. 50:1355 (1971)
11. Hamilton, R.L. Proc. 1968 Deuel Conf. on Lipids, G. Cowgill, D.L. Estrich, P.D.S. Wood, Eds. (Govt. Printing Office, Wash. D.C. 1969) P.1
12. Böhmer, T., R. J. Havel and J. Long. J. Lipid Res. In press.
13. Mahley, R.W., M.E. Gray, R.L. Hamilton and V.S. LeQuire. Lab Invest. 19:358 (1968)
14. Ruderman, N.B., K.C. Richards, V. Valles de Bourges, and A.L. Jones. J. Lipid Res. 9:613 (1968)
15. Strauss, E. W. in Handbook of Physiology (Ed.) J. Field. American Physiological Society, Washington (1968) p. 1377.
16. Cardell, R.R., S. Badenhausen and K.R. Porter. J. Cell Biol. 34:123 (1967)
17. Stein, O. and Y. Stein. J. Cell Biol. 33:319 (1967)
18. Jones. A.L., N.B. Ruderman and M. G. Herrera. J. Lipid Res. 8:429 (1967)
19. Hamilton, R.L., D.M. Regen, M.E. Gray and V.S. LeQuire. Lab. Invest. 16:305 ' 1967)
20. Claude, A.J. Cell Biol. 47:745 (1970)
21. Mahley, R.W., B.D. Bennett, D.J. Morré, M.E. Gray, W. Thistlethwaite and V.S. LeQuire. Lab Invest. 25:435 (1971)
22. Friedman, H.I. and R.R. Cardell. J. Cell Biol. 52:15 (1972)
23. Porter, H.P., D.R. Saunders, G. Tytgat, O. Brunser and C.E. Rubin. Gastroenterology 60:1008 (1971)
24. Trotter, N.L. J. Cell Biol. 25:41 (1965)
25. Jones, A.L., N.B. Ruderman, J.B. Emans. Gastroenterology 56:402a (1969)
26. Jones, A.L. Personal communication.
27. Ma, M.H. and L. Biempica. Am. J. Pathol 62:353 (1971)
28. Morré, D.J., R.L. Hamilton, H.H. Mollenhauer, R.W. Mahley, W.P. Cunningham, R.D. Cheetham and V.S. LeQuire. J. Cell Biol. 44:484 (1970)
29. Morré, D.J., T.W. Keenan, and H.H. Mollenhauer in Advances in Cytopharmacology First Internat. Symp. on Cell Biol. and Cytopharmacol. (Eds) F. Clementi and B. Ceccarelli. Raven Press, N.Y. (1971) V.1 P.159
30. Amsterdam, A., M. Schramm, I. Ohad, Y. Salomon and Z. Selinger. J. Cell Biol. 50:187 (1971)
31. Satir, B., C. Schooley and P. Satir. Nature 235:53 (1972)
32. Jamieson, J.D. and G.E. Palade. J. Cell Biol. 39:589 (1968)
33. Baglio, C.M. and E. Farber. J. Cell Biol. 27:59 (1965)
34. Glaumann, H. and J.L.E. Ericsson. J. Cell Biol. 47:555 (1970)
35. Peters, T., B. Fleischer and S. Fleischer. J. Biol. Chem. 246:240 (1971)
36. Schachter, H., I. Jabbal, R.L. Hudgin and L. Pinteric. J. Biol. Chem. 245:1090 (1970)
37. Wagner, R.R. and M.A. Cynkin. J. Biol. Chem. 246:143 (1971)
38. Redman, C.M. and M.G. Cherian. J. Cell Biol. 52:231 (1972)
39. Oler, A. and B. Lombardi. J. Biol. Chem. 245:1282 (1970)

40. Mookerjea, S. Can. J. Biochem. 47:125 (1969)
41. Marsh, J.B. in Structural and Functional Aspects of Lipoproteins in Living Systems (Eds.) E.Tria and A.M.Scanu. Academic Press, New York (1969) p. 447
42. Dallner, G., P. Siekevitz and G.E. Palade. J.Cell Biol. 30:73 (1966)
43. Stein, O. and Y. Stein. in Advances in Lipid Research (Eds.) R. Paoletti and D. Kritchevsky. Academic Press, New York (1971) V. 9, p. 1
44. Brindley, D.N. and G. Hubscher. Biochim. Biophys. Acta 106:495 (1965)
45. Schneider, W.C. J. Biol. Chem. 238:3472 (1963)
46. Sjostrand, F.S. and B. Borgstrom. J. Ultrastruct. Res. 20:140 (1967)
47. Chesterton, C.J. J. Biol. Chem. 243:1147 (1968)
48. Higgins, J.A. and R. Barrnett. J. Cell Biol. 50:102 (1971)
49. Benes, F.M., J.H. Higgins and R.J. Barrnett. Anat. Rec. 169:276 (1971)
50. Stein, Y. and O. Stein. Atherosclerosis. Proc. II Internat. Symp. (Ed.) R.J. Jones. Springer Verlag, New York (1970) p. 151.
51. Marsh, J.B. J. Biol. Chem. 238:1752 (1963)
52. Bungenberg de Jong, J.J. and J.B. Marsh. J. Biol. Chem. 243:192 (1968)
53. Kessler, J.I., J. Stein, D. Dannacker and P. Narcessian. J. Biol. Chem. 245:5281 (1970)
54. Glickman, R.M., K. Kirsch and K.J. Isselbacher. J. Clin. Invest. 51: 356 (1971)
55. Lossow, W.J., F.T. Lindgren and L.C. Jensen. Biochim. Biophys. Acta 144:670 (1967)   234:813 (1971)
56. Gotto, A.M., R.I. Levy, K. John and D.S. Fredrickson. N.E.J.M ed.
57. Rambourg, A., W. Hernandez and C. P. Leblond. J. Cell Biol. 40:395 (1969)
58. Fleischer, B., S. Fleischer and H. Ozawa. J. Cell Biol. 43:59 (1969)
59. Marsh, J.B. and Fritz, R. Proc. Soc. Exp. Biol. Med. 133:9 (1970)
60. Lo, C.-H. and J.B. Marsh. J. Biol. Chem. 245:5001 (1970)
61. Mahley, R.W., R.L. Hamilton and V.S. LeQuire. J. Lipid Res. 10:433 (1969)
62. Mahley, R.W., T.P. Bersot, V.S. LeQuire, R.I. Levy, H.G. Windmueller and W.V. Brown. Science 168:380 (1970)
63. Hamilton, R.L., R.J. Havel and A.L. Jones. Unpublished observations.
64. Quan, J., A.L. Jones and R.L. Hamilton. Unpublished observation.
65. Bersot, T.P., W.V. Brown, R.I. Levy, H.G. Windmueller, D.S. Fredrickson and V.S. LeQuire. Biochem. 9:3427 (1970)
66. Koga, S., L. Bolis and A.M. Scanu. Biochim. Biophys. Acta 236:416 (1971)
67. Havel, R.J., V.G. Shore, B. Shore and D.M. Bier. Circl. Res. 27:595 (1970)
68. Windmueller, H.G., P.N. Herbert and R.I. Levy. Circulation 42:II-10 (1971)
69. Eisenberg, S., D.W. Bilheimer, F.T. Lindgren, and R.I. Levy. Circulation 42:II-9 (1971)
70. Bilheimer, D., S. Eisenberg and R.I. Levy. J. Clin. Invest. 50:8a (1971)
71. LaRosa, J.C., R.I. Levy, W.V. Brown and D.S. Fredrickson. Am. J. Physiol. 220:785 (1971)

72. Zilversmit, D.B. in Structural and Functional Aspects of Lipoproteins in Living Systems. (Eds.) E. Tria and A.M. Scanu. Academic Press, New York (1969) p. 229.
73. Windmueller, H.G., F.T. Lindgren, W.J. Lossow and R.I. Levy. Biochim. Biophys. Acta 202:507 (1970)
74. Herbert, P.N., H.G. Windmueller and R.I. Levy. Circulation 42:II-177 (1971)
75. Havel, R.J., M.L. Kashyap and J.P. Kane. Circulation 42:II-9 (1971)
76. R.J. Havel. This symposium. Fig. 1.
77. Wisse, E. J. Ultrastruct. Res. 31:125 (1970)
78. Williams, M. Doctoral dissertation. University of California at San Francisco. (1971)
79. Windmueller, H.G. and R.I. Levy. J. Biol. Chem. 242:4878 (1968)
80. Langer, T., W. Strober and R.I. Levy. J. Clin. Invest. 48:49a (1969)
81. Windmueller, H.G. and R.I. Levy. J. Biol. Chem. 242:2246 (1967)
82. Faloona, G.R., B.N. Steward and M. Fried. Biochemistry 7:720(1968)
83. Mahley, R.W., T.P. Bersot, R.I. Levy, H.G. Windmueller and V.S. LeQuire. Federation Proc. Abstracts 29:629 (1970)
84. Hamilton, R.L. and Havel, R.J. Unpublished observation.
85. Miyamoto, V.K. and W. Stoeckenius. J. Membrane Biol. 4:252 (1971)
86. Hamilton, R.L., R.J. Havel, J.P. Kane, A.E. Blaurock and T. Sata. Science. 172:475 (1971)
87. Forte, T., K.R. Norum, J.A. Glomset and A.V. Nichols. J. Clin. Invest. 50:1141 (1971)
88. Norum, K.R., J.A. Glomset, A.V. Nichols and T. Forte. J. Clin. Invest. 50:1131 (1971)
89. Glomset, J.A. Am. J. Clin. Nutr. 23:1129 (1970)
90. Fielding, P.E. and C.J. Fielding. Circulation 42:II-5 (1971)
91. Fielding, C.J., V.G. Shore and P.E. Fielding. Biochem. Biophys. Res. Comm. In press.
92. Forte, T.M., A.V. Nichols, E.L. Gong, S. Lux and R.I. Levy. Biochim. Biophys. Acta. 248:381 (1971)

THE APOLIPOPROTEINS

Donald S. Fredrickson, Samuel E. Lux, and

Peter N. Herbert

Molecular Disease Branch, National Heart and Lung

Institute, Bethesda, Maryland

As the circulatory system evolved in higher organisms, one of the problems that had to be overcome was the transport of fats and other apolar substances having low affinity for water. At least in mammals, binding to albumin became the vehicle for carrying out the exceedingly rapid movement of unesterified fatty acids that exist in extracellular fluid as anions (FFA). Different proteins were selected to transport the esterified fatty acids and sterols that make up the bulk of lipids in plasma, as well as acyclic alcohols and traces of hydrocarbons. These proteins combined with the lipids to form macromolecular complexes which today we call lipoproteins.

The structure of lipoproteins is poorly understood. Available models have none of the three-dimensional elegance or accuracy now possible for hemoglobin or the cytochromes (1,2). Instead we must rely mainly on more surrealistic schema to suggest certain features of lipoproteins that emerge from existing data. In Fig. 1 is depicted no particular lipoprotein but rather a few features that may be common to all. The least polar lipids, such as triglycerides and cholesteryl esters, are shown in the center (C/TG). The wavy lines at the surface providing interface with water, represent protein. A coupling of sorts between protein and nonpolar lipids by phospholipid molecules (PL) is suggested. From this minimum of lipoprotein ingredients we will select only the protein as the subject of this short review.

We will refer here to the lipoproteins in the language of the ultracentrifuge. Plasma lipoproteins fall into four major families: chylomicrons (CHYLOS), very low density lipoproteins (VLDL), low density lipoproteins (LDL), and high density lipoproteins (HDL)

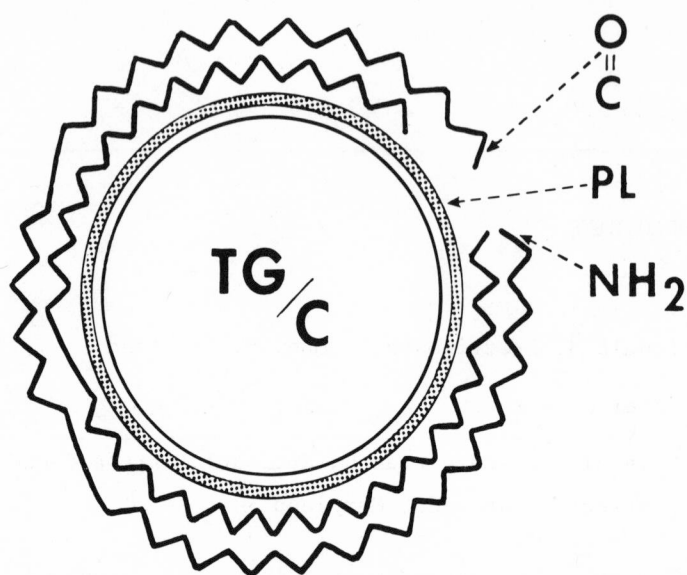

Fig. 1. Schematic model of a hypothetical lipoprotein.

(see Fig. 2). There exists a possible fifth lipoprotein family,
the Lp(a) lipoprotein (3). Although Lp(a) is usually considered a
polymorphic form of LDL (having a density of 1.050-1.080) that can
be detected only in some persons by specific antisera, these facts
are not yet incontrovertible. Schultz, Shreffler, and Harvie (4)
suggest that at least small amounts of Lp(a) may exist in all plasma
samples. Simons et al. (5) have reported that the protein and sialic
acid content of LDL and Lp(a) are different. Lp(a) has also been
defined by a combination of ultracentrifugation and electrophoresis
as "sinking pre-beta lipoprotein" (6). Lp(a) will not be dealt
with further in this review.

It is now the convention to refer to the protein parts of lipoproteins as *apolipoproteins* (7) or simply *apoproteins*. To obtain
them, the lipoproteins are "delipidated," usually by exposing them
to organic solvents. Polar solvents, such as mixtures of chloroform-
methanol or ethanol-diethyl ether, are required to remove all of the
lipids, the most tenaciously bound being the phospholipids. Only
traces of lipids are so tightly linked to the protein that they cannot be extracted by solvents (8).

With the exception of the apoproteins of LDL (apoLDL), the delipidated lipoprotein proteins are soluble in aqueous buffers at or
near neutral pH. After preparation, the apoproteins are further separated and can be characterized by use of the wide variety of techniques

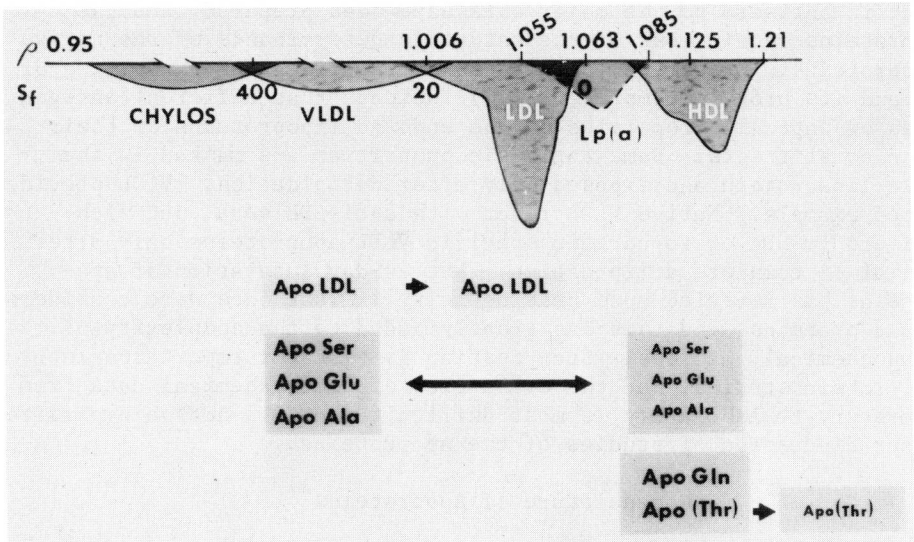

Fig. 2. The plasma lipoprotein spectrum as segregated by the ultracentrifuge (top). The apolipoproteins in VLDL, LDL, and HDL are shown below their respective lipoprotein families. The arrows indicate metabolic interrelationships between apolipoproteins in different density classes. The Lp(a) lipoprotein family has been enlarged for the purpose of illustration.

that are applicable to other proteins. Presently there is heavy emphasis upon gel filtration and ion exchange chromatography for separation, and there is increased use of preparative polyacrylamide gel electrophoresis and isoelectric focussing. Nearly all of the apoproteins that can be reproducibly isolated have been examined for their content of total and terminal amino acid residues, and their secondary structure has been examined by optical measurements. None of the apoproteins have been obtained in crystalline form and hence none have yielded meaningful x-ray diffraction patterns.

Most of the apoproteins are glycoproteins and some information about their content of sugars, hexosamine, and sialic acid is available. None of the glycosidic chains have been fully characterized. Such data are not far away. It is noteworthy that at this meeting the first complete covalent sequence of one of the apoproteins is being reported (9). We may expect that in this decade the sequences of many others will be determined and perhaps one or more will soon be synthesized in the laboratory.

It is worth entering a comment here about the power, and the hazards, of immunological techniques in the pursuit of apoproteins.

Specific antisera to the major ones have been prepared, and the
apoproteins retain most of the antigenic determinants of the native
lipoproteins. Extensive comparisons of immunological properties of
LDL and its protein complement (10) indicate that different antigenic
sites or haptenic properties may be endowed lipoproteins by their
lipid constituents. Some antigenic properties are masked in the
whole lipoprotein and exposed only after delipidation. VLDL provide
a good example. Native VLDL react with anti-LDL sera, but with
antisera to HDL or to certain specific VLDL apoproteins only after
partial or complete delipidation. Latter-day separation of apoproteins has revealed much heterogeneity in what once were considered
single proteins, and this has greatly added to the complexity of
immunochemical analyses. Such testing is of major importance in
lipoprotein studies, but the evaluation of immunochemical data from
laboratory to laboratory is most difficult and will not be emphasized
in our discussion of studies of the apoproteins.

Nomenclature of Apoproteins

The naming of something that is new but whose individuality
emerges slowly is always a problem. Sometimes a trivial name is born
of early inspiration and survives well. With complex chemical substances, the idiom often evolves parallel with technique, and usually
multiple designations arise, each with its champion. Even after
conventions are settled by common consent among experts, evolution
continues. The apoproteins are currently in a disordered stage of
development. Neither their number, functions, nor most distinctive
qualities are known. New personalities seem to be arriving with
such frequency that it is probably too early to settle upon a durable
system of nomenclature. The apolipoproteins today are most commonly
identified in one of two ways. The systems are not mutually
exclusive.

ABC nomenclature. One way, advocated by Alaupovic and his
colleagues (11,12), is to consider apoproteins in three groups: A,
B, and C, letters referring initially to the lipoprotein density
classes in which they predominate and where they were first discovered. For a time this terminology was used as though there were
only three proteins despite evidence of greater heterogeneity. This
discrepancy has been reconciled by adoption of a more pluralistic
approach in which it is suggested that different polypeptides be
designated A-I, A-II, or C-I, C-II, C-III, etc. (13).

By the ABC convention apoprotein A, or apoA, and apoprotein B,
or apoB, refer to the major apoprotein or apoproteins found in HDL
and LDL, respectively. ApoC refers to apoproteins first discovered
in VLDL. ApoB is also an important contributor to the apoproteins
of VLDL. The apoproteins C are perhaps even more gregarious. They
are also found in HDL and in some preparations of LDL. This cross-
contamination of A, B, and C in different lipoprotein density classes

reveals interrelationships between them that are believed to be of
great significance in the metabolic processes by which lipoproteins
carry out fat transport. There are one or two assumptions that
underlie use of the ABC system. One is an assumption that each of
the polypeptides belongs in one of three (or more) corporate groups
of different proteins that have some functional relationships and
presumably common origin. A second assumption is that either each
such group of apoproteins (A, B, and C) or even single polypeptides
(A-I, C-II, etc.) form lipoproteins that exist independent of the
other lipoproteins that may have the same density or electrophoretic
mobility (13,14). Thus in the HDL family as conventionally defined,
there might coexist many separate lipoproteins (LP-A-I, LP-A-II,
LP-C-I, LP-C-II, LP-C-III, etc.). These assumptions have neither
been proved nor disproved.

   C-terminal nomenclature. Another system of nomenclature for
apoproteins that perhaps is even more widely used at present has
been favored in our laboratory and was particularly useful during
the period when "apoprotein C" (15,16) was being dissected into
three or more distinctly different polypeptides (17-20). It is more
chemically oriented and employs the C-terminal residue as the
principal name tag for each protein. The minimum appelations that
have been used are "R-ala," "R-gln," etc., but the proteins are
usually referred to in the generic sense as "apoLP-ala," "apoLP-
gln," etc. This may be changed, for example, to "apoVLDL-ala" or
"apoHDL-ala" when one wishes to indicate the lipoprotein family
from which the apoprotein is obtained. The system is open-ended;
it is used to refer to proteins that are chemically identical regardless of the lipoproteins in which they are found and without
presumption of their functional relationships to other apolipoproteins that may be isolated along with them.

   The weakest feature of the naming of apoproteins according to
their C-terminal residues is the determination of the residues themselves and the possible occurrence of the same terminal residue in
different proteins. Significant errors have already been made in
C-terminal analysis of apoproteins. We have found that, at birth,
apoLP-val (17) should instead have been named apoLP-ser (21). It
has also been reported that "apoLP-thr" actually contains C-terminal
glutamine (22), a transformation that, if confirmed, will place two
apoLP-gln's (apoLP-gln-I and -gln-II) in the registry. The C-
terminal residue of the LDL apoproteins (apoB) is quite uncertain,
and we prefer to call this protein simply apoLDL (see below). The
finding of polymorphism or micro-heterogeneity of apoproteins having
the same C-terminal residue, whether they shall be called, for
example, apoA-I-2 or apoLP-gln-I-2, forecasts greater confusion in
the apoprotein season now underway. From inertia we will cling to
the C-terminal nomenclature in this review, but each figure describing
an apoprotein will also bear the most recently suggested ABC convention (13) or others that may be in use. All are summarized in
Table I.

TABLE I

APOLIPOPROTEIN NOMENCLATURE

C-terminal	Other
ApoLP-ser	C-I (13)
	D1 (17)
	"ApoLP-val"(19)
	"R-val"
	Fraction V (86)
ApoLP-glu	C-II (13)
	D2 (18)
	R-glu
	Fraction V (86)
	? d (88)
ApoLP-ala	C-III (13)
	D3, D4 (17)
	R-ala (20)
	Fraction V (86)
	? e (88)
ApoLDL	B (16)
	ApoLP-ser
	R-ser
"ApoLP-thr"	A-I (22)
	R_1-thr, R_2-thr, R_3-thr (20)
	Fraction III (86)
	Fraction II (87)
	b (88)
ApoLP-gln	A-II (22)
	R-gln (20)
	Fraction IV (86)
	Fraction III (87)
	c (88)

We now turn to a fuller description of the apoproteins, with some assurance that they shall someday be spoken of in other terms. This need not detract from the opportunity to describe a group of molecular transport proteins whose interesting properties are no doubt of importance to many aspects of this symposium. They also represent a topic of future fascination in regard to the evolution and comparative biochemistry of proteins. As far as the apolipo-proteins are concerned, this study has barely begun.

The VLDL Apoproteins

Perspectives. There are reasons why the last-discovered among
the apoproteins, those of the VLDL, should be discussed first. The
triglyceride-bearing lipoproteins, VLDL and chylomicrons, are present
in concentrations that, if integrated over a 24-hour period, are
much less than the concentrations of LDL and HDL, the first studied
and better characterized of the lipoproteins. Yet the functions of
chylomicrons and of the VLDL are of greater immediate consequence
to caloric economy than are those of either of the other lipoprotein
families. Chylomicrons must carry into the circulation tidal increments that total upwards of 100 grams of ingested fatty acids per
day. The role of VLDL is presently understood to be mainly that of
an "escape path," for return of excess fatty acids from liver and
other tissues to the adipose tissue where they can be more economically stored. The shipment of fat from the adipose tissue to muscle
and other sites of utilization is accomplished primarily by transport of FFA. The FFA pathway has great capacity, its high turnover
rate compensating for relatively low plasma concentrations of anionic
fatty acids. It is controlled in part by carbohydrate availability,
and by insulin which balances a host of other hormonal influences.
Yet delivery of FFA is not so delicately regulated that quantities
of "fat calories" are not infrequently dispatched in excess of
actual utilization. The liver promptly returns excessive FFA to
the storage sites as newly synthesized "endogenous" triglycerides.
VLDL provide the carrier for this reshipment.

Glucose is also converted to glycerides in the liver and when
hepatic glycogen stores are replenished, glucose in excess of oxidative demand is discharged in the form of glycerides, again contained in VLDL. VLDL are also made in the intestine (23,24) and
possibly arise in other organs as well.

There is another reason why VLDL should command some primacy of
consideration. Their metabolism--and possibly that of chylomicrons--
may be the source of LDL and HDL, the more conspicuous plasma lipoproteins. This is an old idea, given new credence by recent turnover data (25,26). As long ago as 1956, it was proposed that large
triglyceride-rich particles containing HDL might be sequentially
degraded to lipoproteins of decreasing size and increasing density
by the action of lipoprotein lipase (27). In those days the little
available information about apoproteins (28) did not provide much
support for a close interrelationship among lipoprotein families.
Now it seems that VLDL apoproteins almost certainly do become part
of both LDL and HDL as triglyceride catabolism proceeds (25,26,29,30).

Discovery of the VLDL apoproteins. Until about 15 years ago,
there was very little chemical information about any of the apoproteins. It consisted only of a known difference between the
amino-terminal residues of proteins isolated from LDL and HDL. The

former contained N-terminal glutamic acid, the latter N-terminal aspartic acid (31,32). In 1957 Shore reported the first chemical analyses of the proteins in VLDL; he found both N-terminal glutamic and aspartic acid and also N-terminal threonine, the latter suggesting another apoprotein. A year later Rodbell added evidence that an additional protein containing N-terminal serine was present among the VLDL proteins (33). This finding was confirmed by Shore and Shore in 1962 (34), who also found C-terminal alanine in the VLDL apoproteins. This was seven years before apoLP-ala, a new VLDL apoprotein, was definitely uncovered (17).

It was not until 1964 that new attempts to fractionate VLDL apoproteins were reported by Gustafson, Alaupovic, and Furman (15,16). They extracted the neutral lipids from VLDL with heptane and separated the resulting phospholipid-protein complexes by zonal electrophoresis. Fractions with N-terminal glutamic and aspartic acid were present, along with a "zone II" which contained proteins having N-terminal serine and threonine. They digested their several fractions with pepsin and trypsin, subjected the peptide fragments to high voltage electrophoresis and paper chromatography, and concluded that the resulting fingerprints formed three distinct patterns, one similar to LDL, one similar to HDL, and a third they called "apolipoprotein C."

In 1969 "apoprotein C" was resolved into more than one protein. Brown, Levy, and Fredrickson (17) confirmed what Gustafson et al. had achieved with heptane delipidation, including the detection of an immunochemical reactant differing from the major proteins of LDL and HDL. They then delipidated VLDL completely with ethanol-ether and isolated two new proteins. The first, as it has turned out (21), was named incorrectly. The product of hydrazinolysis, carboxyl-terminal serine, was mistaken for valine, its contiguous companion in the chromatographic system employed (17). The second protein was identified as apoLP-ala and its appearance in two polymorphic forms observed (17). The presence of apoLP-ala was confirmed independently at about the same time by Shore and Shore (20) who also presented evidence for even greater heterogeneity of VLDL apoproteins.

Brown et al. (18,19) then identified a third VLDL apoprotein containing carboxyl-terminal glutamic acid, further characterized all three new VLDL apoproteins, and described differences in sialic acid content as the explanation for the polymorphism of apoLP-ala. The identity of apoLP-glu has been recently confirmed (35).

At this time the cumulative efforts of several laboratories all point to a minimum of four different apoproteins in VLDL isolated from human plasma. These are: apoLDL, apoLP-ser, apoLP-glu, and apoLP-ala. The reader will note the omission of apoHDL, protein or proteins that have been considered to be in VLDL. That omission, as well as the suggestion of greater complexity in apoVLDL, will be dealt with later. Let us first examine what is currently known about the more certain constituents of the VLDL apoproteins.

Fractionation of VLDL apoproteins. In the usual procedure, delipidated VLDL proteins are dissolved in a buffer of pH about 8. Detergent is added (0.1 M sodium decyl sulfate) to facilitate solubilization of apoLDL, which is insoluble at this pH in the absence of detergent. The mixture can then be separated into several fractions by gel filtration (Sephadex G-100 or G-150) (17-19) (Fig. 3). The first fraction eluted contains protein immuno-chemically identical to apoLDL (17,36). The second fraction, representing only a small amount of protein, contains albumin, a protein designated "R-X$_1$" by Shore and Shore (37), and other uncharacterized proteins (38). The third fraction (Fraction III) (Fig. 3) contains the low-molecular weight polypeptides isolated by Brown et al.from "apoprotein C" (17-19).

Ion exchange chromatography on DEAE-cellulose is then used to separate Fraction III (17-20). If the delipidated mixture of all

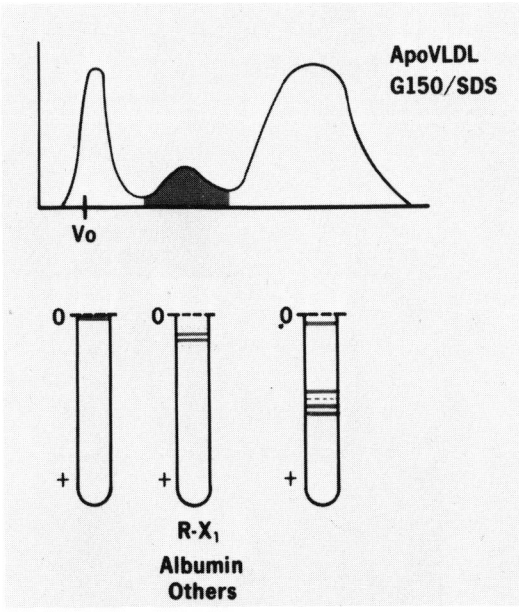

Fig. 3. Chromatography of apoVLDL on Sephadex G-150. Depicted are the three major peaks and a schematization of their alkaline polyacrylamide gel patterns.

VLDL apoproteins is applied directly to DEAE, the first two fractions obtained by gel-filtration are not reproducibly recovered (38). Optimal separation of Fraction III on DEAE is obtained in the presence of 6 M urea. Five major peaks are obtained. The proteins in these peaks can best be described sequentially.

ApoLP-ser (Fig. 4). The first peak eluted from DEAE [at one time called D1 (17)] contains a protein with a molecular weight of approximately 7000 daltons (19). It has N-terminal threonine and C-terminal serine (21) (Fig. 5). As noted above, this protein was initially described as containing C-terminal valine; hence repeated references to it as "R-val" or "apoLP-val" have appeared in the literature (12,19,35,37). ApoLP-ser represents approximately 10 per cent of the VLDL apoproteins, and, like the other three "C proteins," also appears in HDL and possibly LDL (Fig. 5). It contains no carbohydrate (39), histidine, tyrosine, or cysteine (17). It has a relatively high content of lysine and, probably for this reason, is unusually soluble at acid pH (38). At pH 7.5, this protein appears to contain a relatively large amount of helical conformation as deduced from its circular dichroic spectrum (CD) and optical rotatory dispersion (ORD) (19) (Fig. 5).

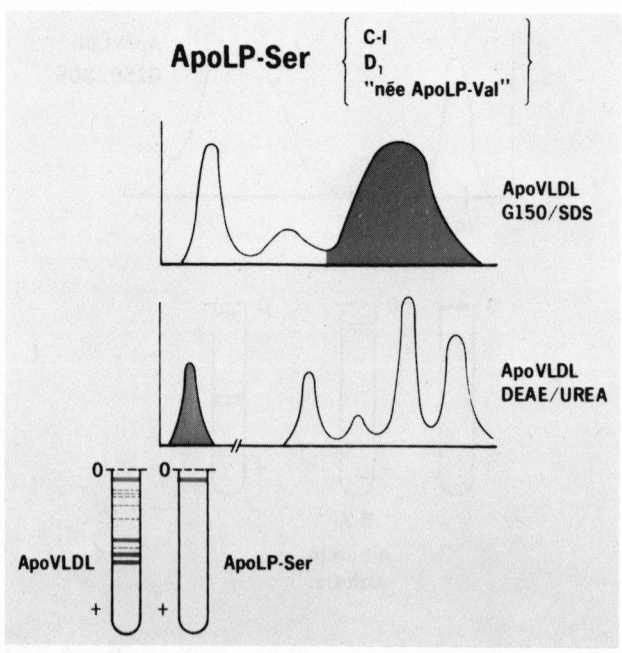

Fig. 4. Isolation of apoLP-ser by chromatography of Fraction III from Sephadex G-150 on DEAE cellulose.

ApoLP-Ser

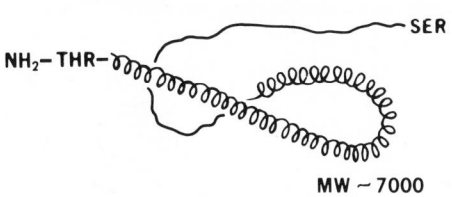

MW ~ 7000

	% of proteins
VLDL	8-10
LDL	+
HDL	2-4

Fig. 5. Schematic model of apoLP-ser. In this and subsequent
figures the relative proportions of α-helical (𝕩𝕩𝕩𝕩𝕩𝕩), beta
(ᐯᐯᐯᐯ) and disordered (～ ～) structure estimated from circular
dichroism experiments are shown. The "+" indicates that apoLP-ser
is present as a minor, poorly quantified component of LDL.

ApoLP-glu. The second DEAE peak (Fig. 6) contains apoLP-glu
(18) and possibly other proteins (38). Brown et al. initially
reported the N-terminal residues to include "equimolar amounts of
serine, threonine, and aspartic acid" (17), and later concluded
that threonine was the principal residue (18). By the hydrazinolysis
technique, glutamic acid is the principal C-terminal residue (18)
(Fig. 7), but significant amounts of valine are also obtained (21).
Carboxypeptidase A does not consistently release any amino acid
from this protein at pH 8. If apoLP-glu is considered as a single
protein--a conclusion that seems increasingly hazardous--its amino
acid composition is distinguished by the absence of histidine and
cysteine and the highest content of tyrosine of the VLDL apoproteins
(19). The conformation is primarily disordered structure (37)
(Fig. 7). ApoLP-glu appears to have little, if any, carbohydrate
(40). ApoLP-glu accounts for about 10 per cent of VLDL apoproteins.

The small peak immediately following apoLP-glu on DEAE
chromatography (Fig. 6) is consistently present but has not been
completely characterized. The amino acid composition suggests that
it contains a mixture of apoLP-glu and apoLP-ala. The protein
migrates as a single band on polyacrylamide gel electrophoresis and
reacts with antisera made against either apoLP-glu or apoLP-ala (38).

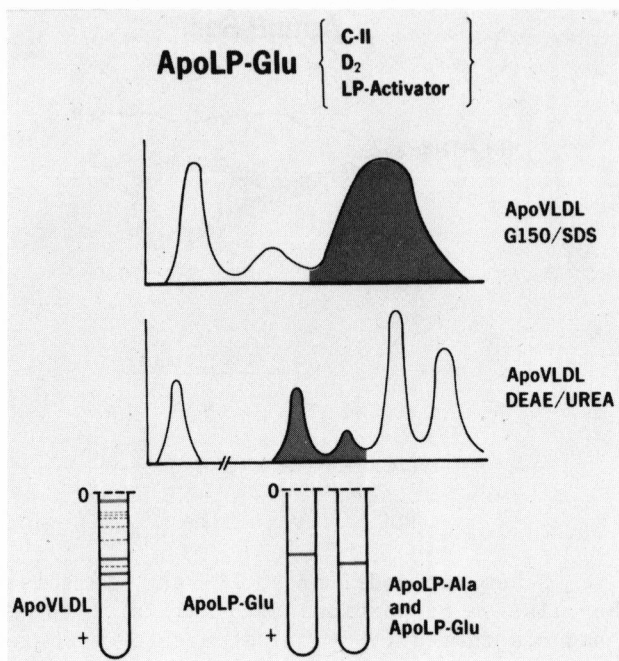

Fig. 6. Isolation of apoLP-glu by chromatography of Fraction III from Sephadex G-150 on DEAE cellulose.

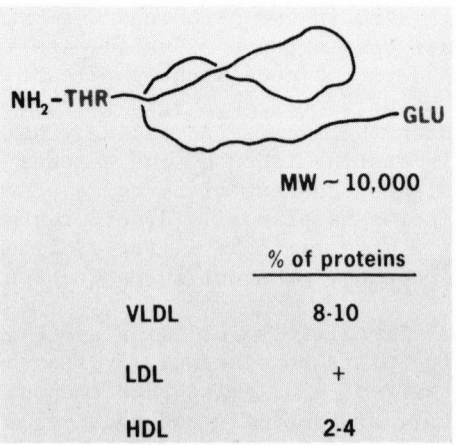

Fig. 7. Schematic model of apoLP-glu.

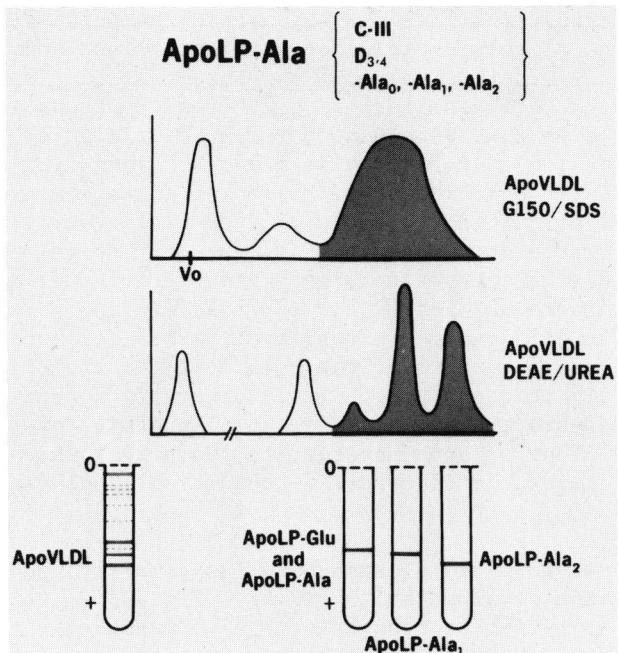

Fig. 8. Isolation of apoLP-ala by chromatography of raction III from Sephadex G-150 on DEAE cellulose.

ApoLP-ala. The last two DEAE peaks (Fig. 8) represent two forms of the same protein. It has N-terminal serine and C-terminal alanine (Fig. 9) (17) and contains no cysteine or isoleucine.

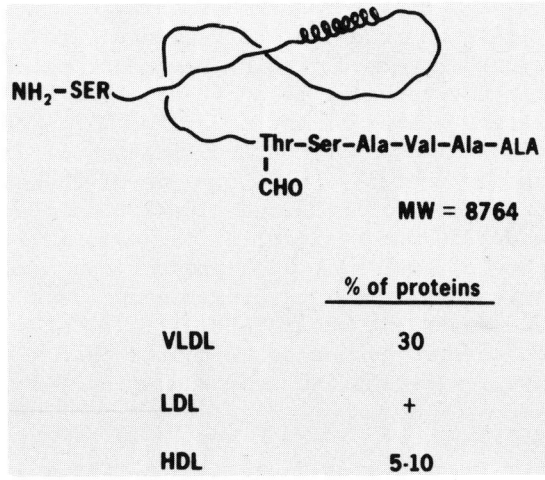

Fig. 9. Schematic model of apoLP-ala.

Fig. 9 indicates only the last six amino acid residues, but the
complete sequence of this protein has been determined and is briefly
described elsewhere in this volume (9). Note that the carbohydrate
moiety is attached to threonine, the sixth residue shown in Fig. 9.
This glycosidic side chain includes terminal sialic acid, galactose,
and galactosamine (40). Polymorphism of apoLP-ala is related to
the number of sialic acid residues (19). Two forms are present in
plasma VLDL, one containing a single mole of sialic acid. The
other, which migrates more rapidly on polyacrylamide gel electrophoresis (Fig. 8), contains two moles of sialic acid per mole of
protein (19). Albers and Scanu have reported finding a sialo apoLP-
ala in plasma VLDL (35). Preliminary experiments (41) suggest that
the sialic acid greatly enhances the solubility of apoLP-ala at
neutral and mildly acid pH. Since it is generally recognized that
glycosidic residues are covalently linked to proteins by the Golgi
apparatus, it will be of some interest to learn what may be the
intracellular role of the lipoprotein-bound sialic acid and other
carbohydrates.

The secondary structure of apoLP-ala is primarily random coil
with a small amount of alpha helix (19,42) (Fig. 9). Its anhydrous
protein molecular weight is 8764 daltons (9). ApoLP-ala makes up
about 30 per cent of VLDL apoproteins. It was also early recognized
in HDL (20) and has rapidly become one of the best known of the
apoproteins. Revelation of its primary structure (9) offers the
first real opportunity to glimpse characteristics that may help to
explain the ability of apolipoproteins to bind lipids.

Further heterogeneity. There are undoubtedly more than three
components of the so-called C group of apoproteins in VLDL. Shore
and Shore usually have directly chromatographed the delipidated
VLDL proteins on DEAE, without preliminary separation by gel
filtration. They have recently reported finding as many as 13
fractions in VLDL isolated from various patients with hyperlipidemia
(43). Earlier they had reported finding six major peaks in apoVLDL;
two of these clearly corresponded to apoLP-ala, but the others did
not obviously represent either of the other two VLDL apoproteins
described above. In their most recent publications (37,43), the
Shores describe two new proteins in VLDL. One of these, "R-X$_1$,"
has a very high content of arginine and glutamic acid and a remarkable amount (about 70 per cent) of alpha helix (37). The
second, "R-X$_2$," contains extremely high proportions of serine,
glycine, and glutamic acid. It lacks tryptophan (37). They believe
that R-X$_1$, R-X$_2$, and apoLP-ala occur in "multiple, or polymorphic,
forms" (37). These workers have also suggested that a form of
apoLP-ala which contains isoleucine can be obtained from sera of
normal subjects (43).

ApoLDL in VLDL. The proteins dealt with so far account for 55-
60 per cent of all the apoproteins of VLDL. The remaining 40-45

per cent consists of the protein or proteins known as apo-LDL
(sometimes called apoLP-ser) or apoprotein B. The apoLDL found in
VLDL appears to be indistinguishable from the apoLDL in LDL. The
amino acid composition, immunochemical properties, and CD are the
same (36). These comparisons have been made in VLDL obtained from
patients with Types II-V hyperlipoproteinemia (36).

What of the HDL proteins in VLDL? In the many analyses of the
N-terminal amino acids carried out on VLDL apoproteins, one residue
has often appeared and been attributed to apoHDL. This is aspartic
acid, repeatedly detected along with glutamic acid, serine, and
threonine in whole or delipidated VLDL (16,17,32-34,44). While the
latter three residues are those of apoproteins now well characterized
in VLDL, the terminal aspartic acid residue has not been accounted
for. The vagaries of the principal methods for terminal analyses
are considerable. Aspartic acid is also the N-terminal residue on
albumin and doubtless many other proteins. It is therefore not
necessarily surprising that the purified VLDL apoproteins have not
included the major HDL proteins. Yet it will be recalled that
peptide fingerprints identified as "apoA" (HDL) have been found in
the VLDL proteins (16). Significant quantities of HDL, identified
by density, electrophoretic migration, and reaction with anti-HDL
sera,have also been observed in partially delipidated VLDL (45,46).

There are possible explanations for the discrepancies evident
in the available data. It is now known that some antisera excited
by HDL contain reactants to the apoLP-ser, apoLP-glu, and particularly, apoLP-ala that are also present in HDL. Alternatively, the
fractionation experiments performed to date have not excluded
significant loss of protein during purification of VLDL apoproteins.
All in all, however, "the case of the missing HDL in VLDL" has not
been solved.

Chylomicron Apoproteins

This is an untimely review from the standpoint of the chylomicrons. Their complement of apoproteins remains undetermined.
No doubt, techniques that have proved quite effective when applied
to other lipoprotein families, especially VLDL, will soon prove as
useful for chylomicrons.

Not much more is known about the small amounts of protein in
chylomicrons (about 1 per cent of the total mass) than was known in
1958 (28). This included some evidence that the protein in lymph
chylomicrons probably changes somewhat upon entrance of the particles
into plasma. In 1958 Rodbell found that the proteins in chylomicrons from human chyle contained N-terminal aspartic acid,
threonine, and serine residues (33). Rodbell and Fredrickson (47)

isolated three protein fractions from human and dog lymph chylomicrons. In both species, they found a fraction "A" that was
soluble in Veronal buffer and appeared identical by peptide finger-
printing to the protein isolated from HDL. Both fraction A and
the HDL proteins contained N-terminal aspartic acid. The Veronal-
insoluble material was electrophoretically separated into "B" and
"C" proteins. These proteins from human chylomicrons yielded N-
terminal serine and those from dogs contained N-terminal glutamic
acid. No N-terminal threonine was found. The fingerprints of A
and B did not resemble those obtained from plasma apoLDL. They
suggested that "apoHDL" was present in the chylomicron apoproteins
and that apoLDL was not. Scanu and Page (48) also reported finding
apoHDL in chylomicrons. Later, Wathen and Levy (49) concluded that
all of the Veronal-soluble protein in dog lymph chylomicrons was
not identical to apoHDL, perhaps due to the presence of additional
protein(s). Rodbell, Fredrickson, and Ono also provided evidence
that the "apoHDL" in chylomicrons did not come from the plasma HDL
and that chylomicron apoproteins probably were synthesized in the
intestinal mucosa (50). A few other studies of chylomicron proteins
have since appeared but protein fractionation techniques have not
been applied to determine how much of the major apoHDL proteins may
be present, whether the N-terminal serine is due to apoLP-ala,
whether others of the VLDL apoproteins are present, and whether
apoLDL is there at all.

The Apoprotein(s) of LDL

The LDL family of lipoproteins is conventionally isolated between the densities of 1.006 to 1.063 (Fig. 2). This rather broad
cut includes two subclasses according to the Gofman definition,
S_f 0-12 (D 1.063-1.019) and S_f 12-20 (D 1.019-1.006). Hammond and
Fisher have failed to find evidence of any protein other than apoLDL
in LDL isolated over the whole S_f 0-20 range (51). Lee and Alaupovic
(52) find that LDL of S_f 12-20 usually reacts with antisera against
some of the C apoproteins and that the S_f 0-12 fraction may also
produce precipitin lines with antisera made to C apoproteins. One
of two apoA antigens also was detected in LDL. It is possible to
prepare LDL which seems to be immunochemically free of HDL and the
"C" proteins but inherent immunochemical heterogeneity of apoLDL
itself (B apoprotein) has not been excluded (52,53).

Preparation of ApoLDL. Delipidated LDL protein is relatively
insoluble. The methods of preparation fall into several groups.
Most often detergents are used to facilitate solubilization.
Initially, dodecyl sulfate (44), and then decyl sulfate, which is
more easily removed by dialysis (54), were used. It has been reported more recently that LDL can be completely delipidated by
using any of a variety of detergents in combination with gel filtration (55) or density gradient ultracentrifugation (56). It is

noteworthy that apoLDL prepared with bile salts and non-ionic detergent retains immunochemical identity with LDL, while apoLDL prepared with sodium dodecyl sulfate or a cationic detergent has altered immunochemical properties (55). ApoLDL prepared with decyl sulfate is closer immunochemically to LDL than is apoLDL prepared by succinylation (10,57). All of the above methods require the presence of some detergent to maintain the apoLDL in solution. This effect of detergents can be facilitated by dissociating agents such as urea or guanidine HCl (58,59,60).

A second group of techniques for preparing apoLDL are based on altering the surface charge of the protein and facilitating solubilization through charge-charge repulsion. These methods include succinylation (61), maleation (62), and basic buffers (pH 11.5) (63). Finally, Shore and Shore have found it possible to extract soluble proteins from LDL without using detergents or derivatization by employing sequential extractions with ether to which is added gradually increasing amounts of ethanol (20).

Heterogeneity of LDL apoprotein(s). The relative insolubility of apoLDL and its tendency to aggregate are major reasons why these apoproteins are the least well characterized of the apolipoproteins. LDL proteins solubilized by detergents are aggregated, appear in or near the void volume when subjected to gel filtration (Fig. 10)

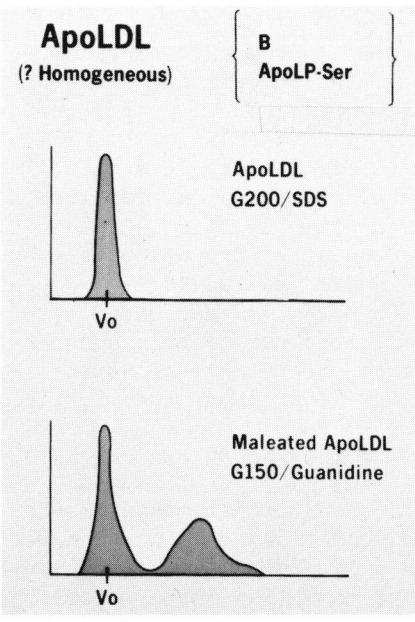

Fig. 10. Gel filtration chromatography of apoLDL (64) and maleated apoLDL (62).

(55,64), and bind irreversibly to DEAE-cellulose (64). Scanu,
Pollard, and Reader (61) obtained two fractions when succinylated
apoLDL was filtered through agarose, but both fractions had an amino
acid composition comparable to the parent LDL fraction. Both had
C-terminal serine. They concluded they were dealing with an
associating system, i.e., monomer-polymers of the same basic subunit. Shore and Shore, however, have reported isolation from DEAE
chromatography of two components of LDL apoproteins that are not
identical and are different from any of the other known apoproteins
(20). About one-third of the apoLDL applied to the column was
represented by these proteins. More recently the Shores have found
even greater heterogeneity in apoLDL (43). Day and Levy (65) also
observed an assymmetrical peak when apoLDL was chromatographed on
Sephadex G-200 and two components after electrophoresis on cellulose acetate.

The major evidence for heterogeneity of apoLDL has been presented by Kane, Richards, and Havel (62). They chromatographed
maleated apoLDL in 6 M guanidine HD1 on Sephadex G-150. Two peaks
with different acid compositions were obtained (Fig. 10). One was
in the void volume (Fr I); the second peak (Fr II) comprised not
more than 25 per cent of the total protein recovered. It had a
molecular weight of 26,000 daltons. The composition of Fr I
resembled whole LDL protein more closely than did Fr II. They
concluded that the two fractions represented different proteins and
that Fr II did not resemble any of the known HDL or VLDL apoproteins.

The properties of ApoLDL. From the foregoing it is obvious
that we take considerable risk in defining the properties of apoLDL
as though it is a single protein species. For the present, however,
we have represented apoLDL as though it were one apoprotein (Fig. 11).
The principal or sole N-terminal amino acid in LDL protein has remained glutamic acid since this was first reported by Avigan,
Redfield, and Steinberg in 1956 (31,32,33,44,66). C-terminal serine
in apoLDL was first reported after hydrazinolysis by Shore in 1957
(32). More recently the Shores failed to find any end group in
C-terminal analyses of LDL of S_f 4-8 performed by both hydrazinolysis
and carboxypeptidase (20). Because of this and the absence of any
other published confirmation of C-terminal serine in apoLDL, we
have indicated that residue in a tenuous way in Fig. 11.

The molecular weight of the apoLDL monomer is still quite uncertain. It has been extremely difficult to overcome the problem
of aggregation in the ultracentrifugal measurements. Molecular
weights estimated by sedimentation equilibrium have ranged from
64,000 to 42,000, depending on the value chosen for the partial
specific volume (58), to 27,500 (59). The latter measurement was
made on material remaining at the top of the ultracentrifuge cell,
however, and represents a minimum, rather than an average, molecular
weight. If apoLDL is indeed homogeneous, 27,500 is probably the

ApoLDL

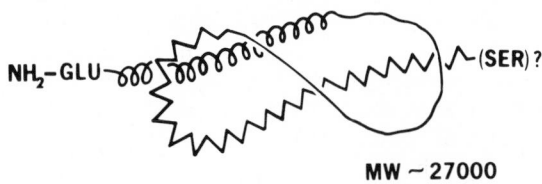

NH$_2$-GLU

(SER)?

MW ~ 27000

	% of proteins
VLDL	40-45
LDL	90+
HDL	0

Fig. 11.   Schematic model of apoLDL.

best current estimate of the minimum particle weight. If it is heterogeneous, this lower molecular weight is similar to that estimated from gel filtration for the minor fraction from apoLDL prepared by Kane et al. (62).

Using information derived from ultracentrifugal and electron microscopic studies of LDL, Pollard, Scanu, and Taylor (59) and Pollard and Devi (67) have concluded that LDL is composed of 20 protein subunits arranged in a dodecahedral pattern. In this model the protein subunits, together with cholesterol and phospholipid, are arranged on the surface of the LDL particle. The neutral lipids (cholesteryl esters and triglycerides) are confined to the core of the molecule.

ApoLDL is a glycoprotein (68) containing about 5 per cent carbohydrate by weight (39). It contains sialic acid, hexose, and hexosamine (39). The location, sequence, and number of possible glycoside chains are still undetermined. Half-cystine is present in apoLDL but the total amino acid composition does not appear to be remarkable (68,69).

ApoLDL has a significant content of beta and disordered structure, and probably also contains some α-helical conformation (63,70) (Fig. 11). The protein conformation varies substantially as a function of lipid composition and temperature (63,71). There is evidence that lipid in the lipoprotein stabilizes the structure of the apoprotein (63).

The HDL Apoproteins

The high density lipoproteins contain about half of the total apolipoproteins in plasma in the normal state. At birth, and in some women, they contain a clear majority of the apoproteins. HDL is conventionally isolated between the densities of 1.063 to 1.21. Two major subclasses of HDL have long been defined in the ultracentrifuge (72) and are represented by asymmetry in the Schlieren peak for HDL shown in Fig. 2. The major peak is HDL_3, which has a mean hydrated density of about 1.15 (73). HDL_2 has a mean density of about 1.09 (73). A third small fraction, HDL_1, corresponds to an S_f 0-3 subclass (73). The apoproteins in HDL_2 and HDL_3 appear to be very similar, although there is some evidence that HDL_2 may contain some minor apoproteins that are not present in HDL_3 (20,43). We will confine this description mainly to HDL as though it were a single family.

Historical. Until relatively recently it was considered that apoHDL was a single subunit of molecular weight 21,000 to 31,000, having N-terminal aspartic acid and C-terminal threonine (32,74,75). Heterogeneity of apoHDL had been suggested earlier by immunochemical studies (76-79) and partial fractionation (79-81); but the inhomogeneity of the lipoprotein was mainly attributed to differences in lipid content. In 1966 (82) Cohen used starch gel electrophoresis in urea to separate apoHDL into two protein fractions. The lesser fraction contained reactive disulfide groups and the major one did not (83). This is probably the first report of chemical evidence that more than one major apoprotein existed in HDL.

The Shores in 1968 (84,85) were the first to purify and characterize partially the two principal apoHDL components. Using carboxypeptidase, they found one had C-terminal threonine and the other C-terminal glutamine. Earlier failure to detect C-terminal glutamine can be attributed to the technique of hydrazinolysis that was employed. In this method all amino acids except the C-terminal one are converted to their hydrazides and are removed. Glutamine, even when in the C-terminal position, also forms a hydrazide and therefore will go undetected (84). Scanu et al. (86), Rudman, Garcia, and Howard (87), and Camejo, Suarez, and Munoz (88) have subsequently confirmed the presence of two major apoproteins in HDL. Ironically, the C-terminal threonine, accepted as a marker of apoHDL since 1957, now is in question. Kostner and Alaupovic have recently reported that both major apoHDL proteins contain C-terminal glutamine (22). We will in this review refer to the two major HDL apoproteins as "apoLP-thr" and apoLP-gln. Alternative designations for these used by different workers are shown in Table 1.

The presence in HDL of smaller amounts of the lower molecular weight polypeptides more recently discovered in the VLDL (particularly apoLP-ala and apoLP-glu) became obvious after 1968 (20,29,43,86,88-90).

In retrospect, N- and C-terminal analyses of apoHDL by Shore made as long ago as 1957 were consonant with the presence of some of these polypeptides. About 5-10 per cent of the apoHDL is represented by the "C" or VLDL apoproteins. These apoproteins appear to be in equilibrium between VLDL and HDL (25).

Fractionation of HDL apoproteins. There are now at least five different methods for separating delipidated HDL apoproteins on a preparative scale: (1) chromatography on DEAE-cellulose in Tris buffer and urea (20,43,84,85); (2) gel filtration on Sephadex G-200 in Tris buffer and urea (86); (3) gel filtration in G-200 in 1 N acetic acid following delipidation with 2-butanol:acetic acid:water (4:1:5) and separation of lipids from proteins on Sephadex LH-20 (87); (4) preparative polyacrylamide gel electrophoresis in Tris buffer and urea (88); and (5) isoelectric focussing in urea (91).

At present none of these techniques alone is adequate for complete fractionation of apoHDL (92). By gel filtration it is difficult to obtain apoLP-gln completely free of "apoLP-thr" even when small protein loads are used. In addition, apoLP-ser, apoLP-glu, and apoLP-ala and the various polymorphic forms of "apoLP-thr" (see below) are not resolved. ApoLP-ser, apoLP-glu, and apoLP-ala are separated by DEAE chromatography alone; and the various polymorphic forms of apoLP-ala and "apoLP-thr" are resolved, but the different forms of "apoLP-thr" are frequently contaminated with apoLP-gln or apoLP-glu (93). Satisfactory separation of all components is best achieved by the combined use of gel filtration and ion-exchange chromatography.

"ApoLP-thr." As shown in Fig. 12, "apoLP-thr" is eluted as the first major peak on gel-filtration (Sephadex G-200) of apoHDL. This fraction is free of contamination with apoLP-gln and the other minor apoHDL constituents. On polyacrylamide gel electrophoresis, it gives a single broad band at pH 9.4 (86,87), pH 4.4 and pH 2.9 (93). Rechromatography on DEAE cellulose (Fig. 12) permits separation of 3-5 polymorphic forms of "apoLP-thr" (20,43,92). Similar findings are obtained with isoelectric focussing of the first G-200 peak (86, 91). We, as well as Albers, Albers, and Aladjem, find that these polymorphic forms all have the same amino acid composition; none contain significant amounts of isoleucine. Shore and Shore, however, have reported that "R-thr$_2$" and "R-thr$_3$" (Fig. 12) contain one isoleucine per mole of protein (43). All of these forms of "apoLP-thr" migrate identically on polyacrylamide gel electrophoresis; all are identical immunochemically (92). They have the same molecular weight by sedimentation equilibrium (20) and by SDS gel electrophoresis (93); and all have N-terminal aspartic acid (93) and reportedly the same C-terminal residue (20). The reason for this polymorphism is unclear. The more likely possibilities include differences in content of carbohydrate or amides. The proportion of the different polymorphic forms varies from subject to subject (20). A question remains as to

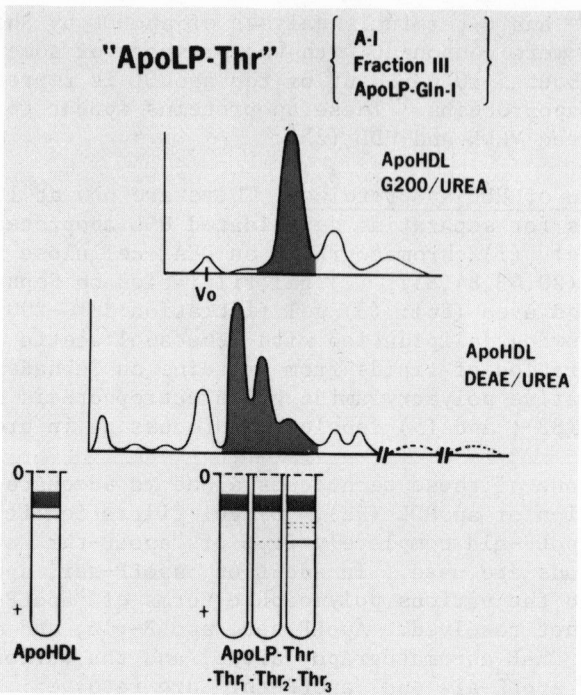

Fig. 12. Isolation of "apoLP-thr" by chromatography of apoHDL
on Sephadex G-200 or DEAE cellulose. (The polyacrylamide gels
refer to fractions obtained on DEAE.)

whether the various forms of "apoLP-thr" exist in vivo or are an
artefact of preparation.

The possibility that the C-terminal residue of "apoLP-thr" is
glutamine, and not threonine, has already been mentioned. The N-
terminal residue is aspartic acid (22) (Fig. 13). Missing amino
acids are isoleucine, cystine, and cysteine (20). A partial sequence (the first 39 amino acids) of "apoLP-thr" has been reported
by Shore and Shore (37). "ApoLP-thr" contains carbohydrate, but
there are no published data as to its composition.

The monomeric molecular weight has been estimated to be 15,500
to 17,000 (85,86). CD spectra indicate that "apoLP-thr" has a high
content of α-helix (estimated to be about 55 per cent) (86,94,95).
The remainder is mainly disordered structure, little or no β-
structure being present (95) (Fig. 13). "ApoLP-thr" is present in
HDL_1, HDL_2, and HDL_3 (37) and represents 65-75 per cent of all HDL
apoproteins (86,87) (Fig. 13).

ApoLP-gln. The second major fraction of apoHDL eluted from
Sephadex G-200 (Fig. 14) is apoLP-gln. Contamination with "apoLP-

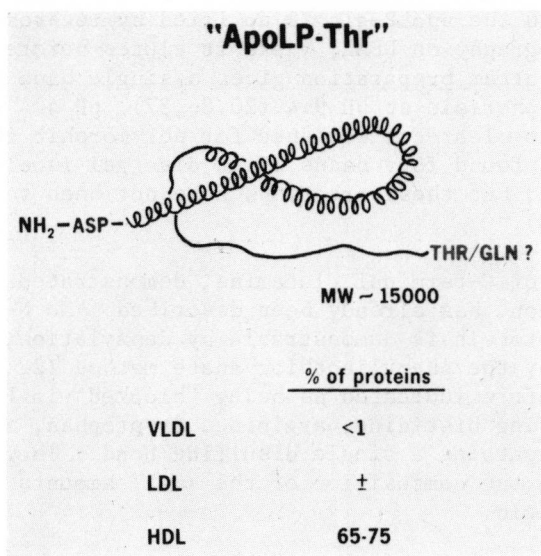

Fig. 13.   Schematic model of "apoLP-thr."

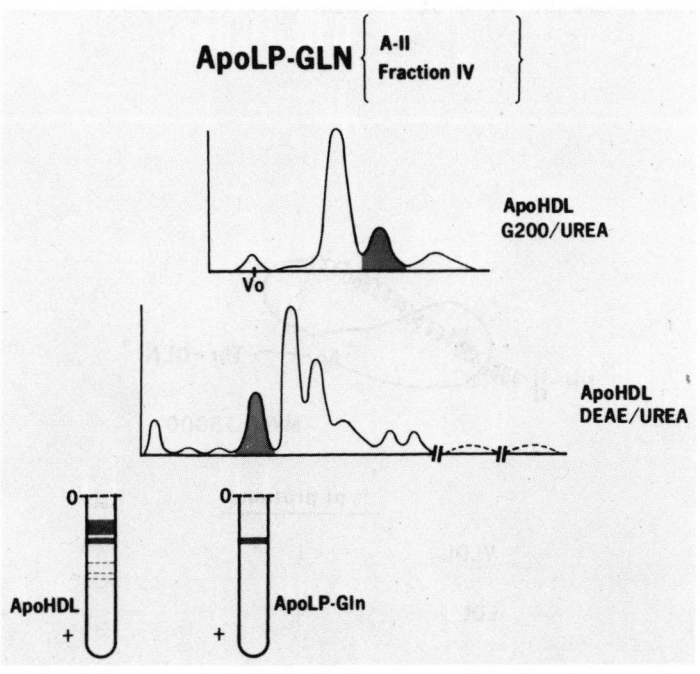

Fig. 14.   Isolation of apoLP-gln by chromatography of apoHDL on Sephadex G-200 or DEAE cellulose.

thr" is common and the apoLP-gln is purified by rechromatography on
G-200 or chromatography on DEAE, where it elutes before "apoLP-thr"
(Fig. 14). The latter preparation gives a single band on polyacrylamide gel electrophoresis at pH 9.4 (20,86,87), pH 4.4 and pH 2.9
(93). There is no clear-cut evidence for polymorphic forms of apoLP-
gln. Scanu et al found four bands after disc gel isoelectric
focussing in urea, but these fractions have not been separately
characterized (86).

    The presence of C-terminal glutamine, demonstrated by carboxy-
peptidase digestion, has already been described. No N-terminal
residue in this protein is demonstrable by dansylation, dinitro-
phenylation, or by the phenylisothiocyanate method (22,37,92). This
terminus is therefore indicated as being "blocked" in Fig. 15.
ApoLP-gln is missing histidine, arginine, tryptophan, and cysteine
(20,86,87). It contains a single disulfide bond. There are no
published data on the composition of the small amounts of carbohydrate in apoLP-gln.

    The CD spectra of apoLP-gln contain about 35 per cent α-helix,
less than that in "apoLP-thr" (86,94,95). Scanu has shown that the
helical content is further decreased by reduction and alkylation
(96). The remaining secondary structure is mainly disordered with
perhaps a small amount of β-structure (95) (Fig. 15).

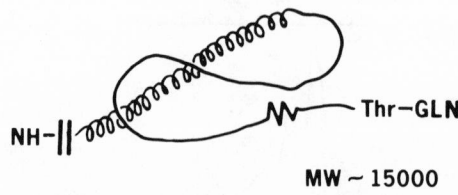

NH–‖   Thr–GLN

MW ~ 15000

	% of proteins
VLDL	<1
LDL	±
HDL	20·25

Fig. 15.   Schematic model of apoLP-gln.

Monomeric molecular weights have been reported from 14,900 (85) to 17,600 (86). ApoLP-gln is present in HDL_1, HDL_2, and HDL_3 (37). It constitutes 20 to 25 per cent of the HDL apoproteins (87,88) (Fig. 15).

Other HDL apoproteins. Other minor components of HDL obtained by DEAE chromatography are shown in Fig. 16, as described by Shore and Shore (20,43). These include the hydrophilic polypeptide, "R-X_2," described above under VLDL apoproteins. Another, "R-Y_1," is incompletely characterized, but samples obtained from different subjects have varying tyrosine content (20). The protein designated "R-gly-gln" (Fig. 16) is found only in HDL (20). In our experience these three poorly characterized apoproteins account for less than 5 per cent of the total HDL apoproteins. Because we have not been able to confirm the presence of "R-gly-gln" and the neighboring form of R-X_2 in apoHDL, these apoproteins are represented by a dotted line in Figs. 12 and 14. In the DEAE chromatogram (Fig. 11), there also appear apoLP-ser (the peak preceding R-X_2) and two polymorphic forms of apoLP-ala (the two peaks preceding R-gly-gln). ApoLP-glu co-elutes with "apoLP-thr_2" and "apoLP-thr_3" (92). These three

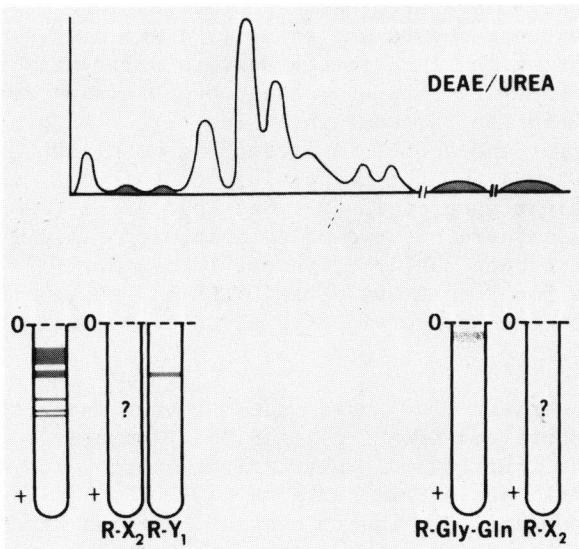

Fig. 16. Other apoproteins isolated from apoHDL by chromatography on DEAE cellulose.

apoproteins first discovered in VLDL (17,18,20) account for 5-10
per cent of the total proteins in HDL.

There is currently much speculation about whether all of these
apoproteins are part of the same macromolecular complex. Albers
and Aladjem have recently presented immunochemical evidence for the
existence of at least two types of HDL molecules, with respect to
the major HDL apoproteins (97). The predominant form contains both
"apoLP-thr" and apoLP-gln; the minor form contains only "apoLP-thr."
These correspond, respectively, to immunochemical forms of HDL previously designated "αLP_A" and "αLP_B" by Levy and Fredrickson (79).
Since, in the latter studies, significant amounts of "αLP_B" were
found only in stored plasma or after ultracentrifugation, it may be
that only HDL complexes containing both "apoLP-thr" and apoLP-gln
are present in the circulation. There is no published evidence of
whether the minor apoproteins found in HDL are associated in an
integral way with the HDL complexes formed by "apoLP-thr" and
apoLP-gln or represent independent lipoproteins.

                        Apoproteins in the Rat

The more complete of the few available studies of apolipoproteins
in species other than man have been made in the rat. Koga, Horwitz,
and Scanu were the first to publish polyacrylamide gel electrophoresis fractionation of rat plasma apoproteins into numerous bands
(98). This was expanded by Bersot et al.(99) who also used gel
filtration and ion exchange chromatography to purify the apoproteins.
There is great similarity between rat and human plasma apoproteins.
Both HDL and VLDL in the rat contain at least four apoproteins of
low molecular weight and apoLDL is present in both VLDL and LDL.
Initially, rat HDL was thought to possibly contain only one major
high molecular weight apoprotein (99) but Koga et al.(100) have
presented data that there are two major apoproteins similar to human
HDL. This has also been confirmed in our laboratory (101) and,
moreover, we have found that rat plasma VLDL and HDL, unlike man,
may share at least one apoprotein of high molecular weight (ca.
50,000).

Mahley and coworkers (102) have made the very interesting observation that VLDL obtained from rat liver Golgi apparatus contain at
least three of the four low molecular weight apoproteins and the
apoLDL, that are all present in rat plasma VLDL. This has been confirmed by Pottenger and Getz in "liposomes" from rat liver (103).
There is also evidence of a difference in apoprotein composition of
VLDL from liver and intestine (101). Thus, as earlier evidence had
suggested, the search for plasma apoproteins will require separate
characterization of lipoproteins contributed by different organs.

The Functions of the Apolipoproteins

The most obvious function of the apoproteins is to bind lipids in a manner that affords the latter solubility in extracellular fluids and at the same time permits their transfer to and from cellular sites with a minimum expenditure of energy. How the apoproteins do this is not yet established, but some details are beginning to emerge. Recently a technique has been presented for recombining HDL apoproteins and lipids to form lipoprotein complexes resembling the parent HDL in structure and lipid composition (104, 105). When purified "apoLP-thr" or apoLP-gln are recombined with sonified phospholipid ("liposomes"), there is an increase in the α-helical content and decrease in the disordered structure of the apoprotein (106). The phospholipid liposomes are transformed into discoid lipoprotein complexes (107). The introduction of cholesteryl ester into these complexes produces an additional increase in helical content (106) and generates spherical lipoprotein complexes indistinguishable from HDL (107). Thus specific alterations in both the lipid and protein moieties accompany their interaction.

Undoubtedly variations in the primary structure of an apoprotein will be found which will affect the efficiency of lipid-binding by changing the character of hydrophobic or hydrophilic regions or the conformation of the protein. The search for such abnormalities will proceed hand-in-hand with clarification of the chemistry of the apoproteins. Indeed, mutations may provide the best available proof of the essentiality of certain apoproteins and of critical portions of their structures. Already a suggestion has been derived from study of abetalipoproteinemia that apoLDL may have a primal role in enabling glyceride transport from cells (90). The available evidence also suggests that the severe deficiency of HDL that is inherited in Tangier disease may particularly involve "apoLP-thr" synthesis or utilization (108).

ApoLP-glu may have a special function. In the test tube it has proved to be an effective activator of lipoprotein lipase (109-111). This enzyme, functioning at some intracellular loci, is almost certainly of the utmost importance in the removal and catabolism of triglycerides from the blood. Early evidence that apoLP-ala might also activate lipoprotein lipase (109,110) has not been substantiated in further studies (112). The contention that apoLP-ser (the old "apoLP-val") is also an activator (111) cannot be supported in our studies (112).

Coda

Much of the more solid knowledge about the structure of plasma apolipoproteins has been touched upon in this paper. There are, however, many reports that have received little mention, and some no attention at all, that should have been dealt with were this

meant to have been a complete review. Among the latter are some
imaginative explorations, employing electron spin probes, nuclear
magnetic resonance and other techniques designed to illuminate the
interactions of lipids and proteins in lipoproteins, the increasing
wealth of turnover data, and many of the theories of particular
roles played by lipoproteins in physiology and in disease.

What we have compiled is a handy guidebook for those to whom
the terrain of the apoproteins may be new and confusing. We have
summarized how the apoproteins have been obtained and characterized
thus far and the chemical features of six major proteins
that are recognized as constant constituents of lipoproteins. This
has included a gathering together of the various code-names by which
the apoproteins, both the established and the possible ones, are
known.

Some reasons have been given why it seems to us too early to
choose an entirely satisfactory single convention for naming apoproteins. Such a convention will depend particularly upon agreement
that all of the important apoproteins have been discovered and their
interrelations elucidated. When this has all been done, it may be
that our way of looking at lipoproteins, including the familiar
density bench-marks, could radically change. There is promise of
much intellectual excitement to come.

REFERENCES

1. Perutz, M. F. J. Mol. Biol. $\underline{13}$:646 (1965).
2. Dickerson, R. E., T. Takano, D. Eisenberg, O. B. Kallai,
    L. Samson, A. Cooper, and E. Margoliash. J. Biol. Chem.
    $\underline{246}$:1511 (1971).
3. Berg, K. Acta Path. Microbiol. Scand. $\underline{59}$:369 (1963).
4. Schultz, J. S., D. C. Shreffler, and N. R. Harvie. Proc. Nat.
    Acad. Sci. $\underline{61}$:963 (1968).
5. Simons, K., C. Ehnholm, O. Renkonen, and B. Bloth. Acta Path.
    Microbiol. Scand. $\underline{78}$:459 (1970).
6. Rider, A. K., R. I. Levy, and D. S. Fredrickson. Circulation
    $\underline{42}$:III-10 (1970).
7. Oncley, J. L., in Brain Lipids and Lipoproteins, and the
    Leucodystrophies. (Eds.) J. Folch-Pi and H. Bauer, Elsevier,
    Amsterdam (1963) p. 1.
8. Fisher, W. R., and S. Gurin. Science $\underline{143}$:362 (1964).
9. Brewer, H. B. Jr., R. Shulman, P. Herbert, R. Ronan, and K.
    Wehrly. Advances in Experimental Medicine and Biology. In
    press (1972).
10. Gotto, A. M., R. I. Levy, M. E. Birnbaumer, and D. S.
    Fredrickson. In preparation.
11. Alaupovic, P. Progr. Biochem. Pharmacol. $\underline{4}$:91 (1968).
12. Alaupovic, P. Atherosclerosis $\underline{13}$:141 (1971).

13. Alaupovic, P., in Proceedings of the XIX Annual Colloquium on Protides of the Biological Fluids (Bruges), Pergamon Press, New York. In press (1972).
14. Alaupovic, P. Personal communication.
15. Gustafson, A., P. Alaupovic, and R. H. Furman. Biochim. Biophys. Acta 84:767 (1964).
16. Gustafson, A., P. Alaupovic, and R. H. Furman. Biochemistry 5:632 (1966).
17. Brown, W. V., R. I. Levy, and D. S. Fredrickson. J. Biol. Chem. 244:5687 (1969).
18. Brown, W. V., R. I. Levy, and D. S. Fredrickson. Biochim. Biophys. Acta 200:573 (1970).
19. Brown, W. V., R. I. Levy, and D. S. Fredrickson. J. Biol. Chem. 245:6588 (1970).
20. Shore, B., and V. Shore. Biochemistry 8:4510 (1969).
21. Herbert, P., R. I. Levy, and D. S. Fredrickson. J. Biol. Chem. In press (1971).
22. Kostner, G., and P. Alaupovic. FEBS Letters 15:320, (1971).
23. Windmueller, H. G. J. Biol. Chem. 243:4878 (1968).
24. Ockner, R. K., F. B. Hughes, and K. J. Isselbacher. J. Clin. Invest. 48:2079 (1969).
25. Bilheimer, D., S. Eisenberg, and R. I. Levy. J. Clin. Invest. 50:8a (1971).
26. Langer, T., D. Bilheimer, and R. I. Levy. Circulation 42: III-7, (1970).
27. Lindgren, F. T., N. K. Freeman, A. V. Nichols, and J. W. Gofman, in Blood Lipids and the Clearing Factor (Third Internat. Conf. on Biochemical Problems of Lipids, July 1956). Koninkl. Vlaam. Acad. Wetenschappen, Brussels (1956) p. 224.
28. Fredrickson, D. S., and R. S. Gordon, Jr. Physiol. Reviews 38:585 (1958).
29. LaRosa, J. C., R. I. Levy, W. V. Brown, and D. S. Fredrickson Am. J. Physiol. 220:785 (1971).
30. Windmueller, H. G., P. Herbert, and R. I. Levy. Circulation. In press (1971).
31. Avigan, J., R. Redfield, and D. Steinberg. Biochim. Biophys. Acta 20:557 (1956).
32. Shore, B. Arch. Biochem. Biophys. 71:1 (1957).
33. Rodbell, M. Science 127:701 (1958).
34. Shore, B., and V. Shore. J. Atheroscler. Res. 2:104 (1962).
35. Albers, J. J., and A. M. Scanu. Biochim. Biophys. Acta 236: 29 (1971).
36. Gotto, A. M., W. V. Brown, R. I. Levy, M. E. Birnbaumer, and D. S. Fredrickson. In preparation.
37. Shore, B., and V. Shore. Preceedings of European Society of Atherosclerosis. Masson and Cie, Paris, France, In press (1972).
38. Herbert, P., R. I. Levy, and D. S. Fredrickson. In preparation.
39. Sloan, H. R., P. O. Kwiterovich, R. I. Levy, and D. S. Fredrickson. Circulation 42:III-8 (1970).

54

D. S. FREDRICKSON, S. E. LUX, AND P. N. HERBERT

40. Herbert, P., P. O. Kwiterovich, H. R. Sloan, R. I. Levy, and D. S. Fredrickson. In preparation.
41. Herbert, P. N. Unpublished observation.
42. Shulman, R., P. Herbert, and H. B. Brewer. Fed. Proc. 30:1187 (1971).
43. Shore, B., and V. Shore, in Atherosclerosis: Proceedings of the Second International Symposium. (Ed.) R. J. Jones, Springer-Verlag, Berlin (1970), p. 144.
44. Granda, J. L., and A. Scanu. Biochemistry 5:3301 (1966).
45. Levy, R. I., R. S. Lees, and D. S. Fredrickson. J. Clin. Invest. 45:63 (1966).
46. Kook, A. I., A. S. Eckhaus, and D. Rubinstein. Can. J. Biochem. 48:649 (1970).
47. Rodbell, M., and D. S. Fredrickson. J. Biol. Chem. 234:562 (1959).
48. Scanu, A., and I. H. Page. J. Exptl. Med. 109:239 (1959).
49. Wathen, J. D., and R. S. Levy. Biochemistry 5:1099 (1966).
50. Rodbell, M., D. S. Fredrickson, and K. Ono. J. Biol. Chem. 234:567 (1959).
51. Hammond, M. G., and W. R. Fisher. J. Biol. Chem. 246:5454 (1971).
52. Lee, D. M., and P. Alaupovic. Biochemistry 9:2244 (1970).
53. Simons, K., and A. Helenius. Ann. Med. Exp. Biol. Fenn. 47:48 (1969).
54. Gotto, A. M., R. I. Levy, and D. S. Fredrickson. Biochem. Biophys. Res. Commun. 31:151 (1968).
55. Helenius, A., and K. Simons. Biochemistry 10:2542 (1971).
56. Muesing, R. A., and T. Nishida. Biochemistry 10:2952 (1971).
57. Gotto, A. M., R. I. Levy, M. E. Birnbaumer, and D. S. Fredrickson. Nature 223:835 (1969).
58. Shore, B., and V. Shore. Biochem. Biophys. Res. Commun. 28:1003 (1967).
59. Pollard, H., A. M. Scanu, and E. W. Taylor. Proc. Nat. Acad. Sci. 64:304 (1969).
60. Kane, J. P. Biophysical J. 9:146a (1969).
61. Scanu, A., H. Pollard, and W. Reader. J. Lipid Res. 9:342 (1968).
62. Kane, J. P., E. G. Richards, and R. J. Havel. Proc. Nat. Acad. Sci. 66:1075 (1970).
63. Scanu, A., H. Pollard, R. Hirz, and K. Kothary. Proc. Nat. Acad. Sci. 62:171 (1969).
64. Shulman, R. S. Personal communication.
65. Day, C. E., and R. S. Levy. J. Lipid Res. 9:789 (1968).
66. Bobbitt, J. L., and R. S. Levy. Biochemistry 4:1282 (1965).
67. Pollard, H. B., and S. K. Devi. Biochem. Biophys. Res. Commun. 44:593 (1971).
68. Margolis, S., and R. G. Langdon. J. Biol. Chem. 241:469 (1966).
69. Levy, R. S., and A. C. Lynch. Fed. Proc. 21:75 (1962).
70. Gotto, A. M., R. I. Levy, and D. S. Fredrickson. Proc. Nat. Acad. Sci. 60:1436 (1968).

71. Dearborn, D. G., and D. B. Wetlaufer. Proc. Nat. Acad. Sci. 62:179 (1969).
72. deLalla, O. F., and J. W. Gofman. Methods Biochem. Anal. 1: 459 (1959).
73. Nichols, A. V. Advances Biol. Med. Phys. 11:109 (1967).
74. Scanu, A. J. Lipid Res. 7:295 (1966).
75. Shore, V., and B. Shore. Biochemistry 6:1962 (1967).
76. Aladjem, F., M. Lieberman, and J. W. Gofman. J. Exptl. Med. 105:49 (1957).
77. Ayrault-Jarrier, M., G. Lévy, and J. Polonovski. Bull. Soc. Chim. Biol. 45:703 (1963).
78. Burstein, M., and J.-M. Fine. Rev. Franc. Études Clin. Biol. 9:105 (1964).
79. Levy, R. I., and D. S. Fredrickson. J. Clin. Invest. 44:426 (1965).
80. Scanu, A. Nature 207:528 (1965).
81. Scanu, A., and J. L. Granda. Biochemistry 5:446 (1966).
82. Cohen, L., and J. Djordjevich. J. Clin. Invest. 45:996 (1966).
83. Cohen, L., and J. Djordjevich. Proc. Soc. Exptl. Biol. Med. 129:788 (1968).
84. Shore, B., and V. Shore. Biochemistry 7:2773 (1968).
85. Shore, V., and B. Shore. Biochemistry 7:3396 (1968).
86. Scanu, A., J. Toth, C. Edelstein, S. Koga, and E. Stiller. Biochemistry 8:3309 (1969).
87. Rudman, D., L. A. Garcia, and C. H. Howard. J. Clin. Invest. 49:365 (1970).
88. Camejo, G., Z. M. Suárez, and V. Muñoz. Biochim. Biophys. Acta 218:155 (1970).
89. LaRosa, J. C., W. V. Brown, R. I. Levy, and D. S. Fredrickson. Circulation 40:III-15 (1969).
90. Gotto, A. M., R. I. Levy, K. John, and D. S. Fredrickson. New Engl. J. Med. 284:813 (1971).
91. Albers, J. J., L. V. Albers, and F. Aladjem. Biochem. Med. 5:48 (1971).
92. Lux, S. E., R. I. Levy, A. M. Gotto, and D. S. Fredrickson. In preparation.
93. Lux, S. E., and K. M. John. Unpublished observations.
94. Gotto, A. M., and B. Shore. Nature 224:69 (1969).
95. Lux, S. E., R. Hirz, R. I. Shrager, and A. M. Gotto. In preparation.
96. Scanu, A. M. Biochim. Biophys. Acta 200:570 (1970).
97. Albers, J. J., and F. Aladjem. Biochemistry 10:3436 (1971).
98. Koga, S., D. L. Horwitz, and A. M. Scanu. J. Lipid Res. 10: 577 (1969).
99. Bersot, T. P., W. V. Brown, R. I. Levy, H. G. Windmueller, D. S. Fredrickson, and V. S. LeQuire. Biochemistry 9:3427 (1970).
100. Koga, S., L. Bolis, and A. M. Scanu. Biochim. Biophys. Acta 236:416 (1971).

101. Herbert, P. N., H. G. Windmueller, and R. I. Levy.
      Circulation In press (1971).
102. Mahley, R. W., T. P. Bersot, V. S. LeQuire, R. I. Levy,
      H. G. Windmueller, and W. V. Brown. Science 168:380 (1970).
103. Pottenger, L. A., and G. S. Getz. J. Lipid Res. 12:450
      (1971).
104. Hirz, R., and A. M. Scanu. Biochim. Biophys. Acta. 207:364
      (1970).
105. Scanu, A., E. Cump, J. Toth, S. Koga, E. Stiller, and
      L. Albers. Biochemistry 9:1327 (1970).
106. Lux, S. E., R. Hirz, R. I. Shrager, and A. M. Gotto.
      Biophysical J. 11:181a (1971).
107. Forte, T. M., A. V. Nichols, E. L. Gong, S. E. Lux, and
      R. I. Levy. In preparation.
108. Lux, S. E., R. I. Levy, A. M. Gotto, and D. S. Fredrickson.
      Pediat. Res. 4:439 (1970).
109. LaRosa, J. C., R. I. Levy, P. Herbert, S. E. Lux, and D. S.
      Fredrickson. Biochem. Biophys. Res. Commun. 41:57 (1970).
110. Havel, R. J., V. G. Shore, B. Shore, and D. M. Bier. Circ.
      Res. 27:595 (1970).
111. Ganesan, D., R. H. Bradford, P. Alaupovic, and W. J.
      McConathy. FEBS Letters 15:205 (1971).
112. Krauss, R. M., P. N. Herbert, R. I. Levy, and D. S.
      Fredrickson. In preparation.

MECHANISMS OF HYPERLIPOPROTEINEMIA

Richard J. Havel, M.D.

Cardiovascular Research Institute and Department of Medicine
University of California School of Medicine
San Francisco, California U.S.A.

Our understanding of the pathogenesis of hyperlipoproteinemia stems from knowledge of the synthesis, secretion and metabolism of plasma lipoproteins and the regulation of these processes. Application of this knowledge in recent years has provided an explanation of several secondary hyperlipoproteinemias in terms of altered regulation of fat transport. This paper will review current knowledge of fat transport in lipoproteins and the increasing evidence that all major lipoprotein classes are involved in this process. The pathogenesis of certain secondary hyperlipoproteinemias will be discussed in the context of this review. Finally, a speculative assessment of the pathogenesis of the primary hyperlipoproteinemias will be attempted with particular reference to possible mechanisms of defective catabolism.

FAT TRANSPORT IN LIPOPROTEINS

Lipoprotein Secretion

Quantitatively, triglycerides (TG) are by far the most important class of lipids transported in lipoproteins (1). During active absorption of dietary fat, the small intestine secretes TG into the intestinal lymph, mainly in large particles which we recognize as chylomicrons from their size ($>$ 1000 Å diameter) and chemical composition (more than 80 % TG by weight). Small amounts of fat are also transported in smaller particles (300–800 Å diameter) which we recognize as very low density lipoproteins (VLDL). At all times, the liver secretes VLDL into hepatic venous blood. Although the intestine continues to secrete TG in VLDL in the post-absorptive state, current evidence suggests that the liver accounts for more than 80% of VLDL transport in man after an overnight fast. From rates of flow and TG content of thoracic duct lymph (2) and from maximal rates of entry of biliary lipid into the duodenum (3), it appears that entry of VLDL-TG from the thoracic duct does not exceed 0.2 g/hr in the post-absorptive state, while secretion of VLDL-TG from the liver is on the order of 1 g/hr.

The role of the liver and intestine in the formation of other plasma lipoproteins is less well understood. Morphological and biochemical studies of rat liver have provided no evidence that the liver can secrete low density lipoproteins (LDL) as such, although the apoprotein of LDL is well represented in nascent VLDL isolated from a Golgi apparatus-rich fraction of the liver cell (4). Because of its slower turnover rate in the blood, a relatively small amount of LDL would have to be present in the liver at any given time, however, for it to represent a significant independent pathway of formation of LDL in blood plasma. The absence of both VLDL and LDL from blood plasma in abetalipo-proteinemia does not exclude the possibility that such an independent pathway exists, since the absence of TG-rich lipoprotein in abetalipoproteinemia can be explained by an obligatory requirement for the B-apoprotein of LDL in their formation. In contrast, high density lipoproteins (HDL) that are apparently nor-mal in all respects circulate in the blood in this disorder (5), indicating that their synthesis and secretion in all likelihood occur normally, presumably from both liver and intestine. HDL may, however, be secreted in a "primordial" form, as a particle of density >1.2 ("VHDL") containing one of the major HDL apoprotein subunits together with lecithin and free cholesterol. Evidence for such a concept has been supported by the recent studies of the abnormal HDL of subjects with genetically determined deficiency of lecithin-cholesterol acyl transferase (LCAT) (6). Normally, LCAT, by esterifying cholesterol in HDL with a fatty acid derived from the beta-carbon of lecithin, causes the accumulation of nonpolar cholesteryl esters which are carried in the hydrophobic interior of HDL as well as others of the lipoproteins.

Lipoprotein Interconversions and Catabolism

The catabolism of VLDL and, probably, of chylomicrons, is closely coupled to the formation of LDL. It also involves participation of certain com-ponents of HDL. As indicated in Figure 1, VLDL secreted from the liver appear to contain less of certain small polypeptides that are protein components of plasma VLDL (4) (C apoprotein group in man). HDL apparently supply these polypeptides to the TG-rich particles. In man at least one of the peptide sub-units ("R-glu") of this group of proteins ("activator" polypeptide) promotes the interaction of TG-rich lipoproteins with lipoprotein lipase in extrahepatic tissues (7,8). This reaction constitutes the first step in the catabolism of TG-rich lipoproteins. No function can presently be assigned to the other subunits,

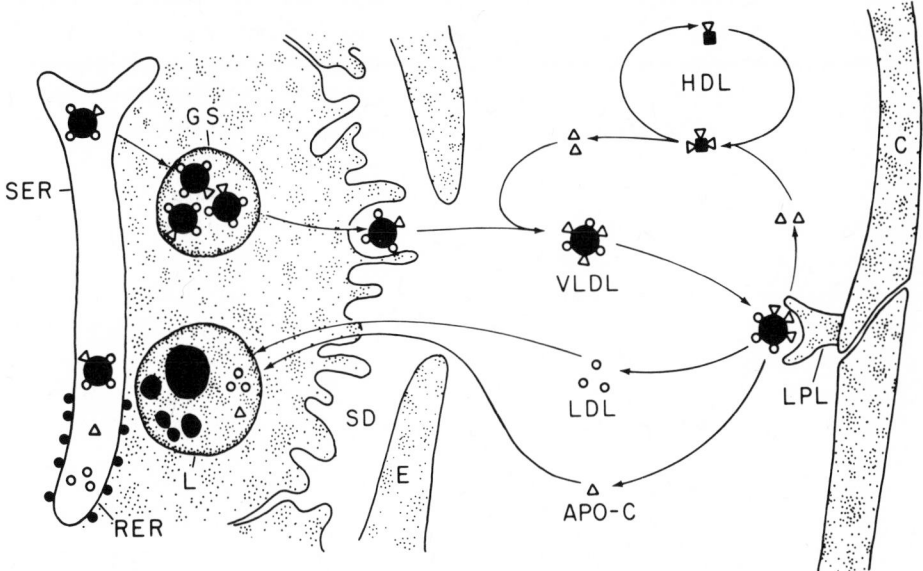

Fig. 1. This diagram indicates some of the steps involved in the synthesis, secretion and catabolism of VLDL and emphasizes postulated participation of specific apoproteins in these processes. The sequence and interactions shown here
may apply to the metabolism of chylomicrons as well (see text). Newly secreted VLDL are deficient in certain apoprotein subunits (apo-C) which are transferred from HDL after the VLDL have been secreted from the cell. One or more
of these subunits promotes the interaction of VLDL with lipoprotein lipase (LPL)
at a capillary surface. Following removal of the VLDL-TG, at least some of
the apo-C is transferred back to HDL. Eventually, LDL containing their
specific apoprotein are produced also. This process is accompanied by formation
of intermediate species ("remnants") which may be metabolized further in the
liver (not shown). Presumably, LDL are eventually removed in liver and are
not re-utilized in the formation of new VLDL. Other abbreviations: RER =
rough endoplasmic reticulum; SER = smooth endoplasmic reticulum; GS = Golgi
saccule; L = lysosome; SD = space of Disse; E = endothelial cell; C= capillary.

although one of them ("R-ala") can inhibit the enzyme-substrate interaction in
some in vitro systems (7). In the rat, the role of HDL can be shown by mixing
nascent VLDL obtained from liver with HDL obtained from plasma. Peptides can
be shown to transfer from HDL to the nascent VLDL which thereupon have considerably enhanced ability to promote the hydrolysis of triglyceride in an artificial fat emulsion by lipoprotein lipase from cows' milk (4). Indirect evidence
suggests that newly secreted chylomicrons in man may also contain less of the

C apoproteins than do chylomicrons in blood plasma. During alimentary lipemia, the content of activator peptide in whole plasma does not change, but the fraction contained in HDL falls dramatically while that in TG-rich lipoproteins rises (9). Thus, HDL may furnish one or more apoprotein subunits both to newly secreted VLDL and chylomicrons. This concept is supported by studies with radioiodine-labeled VLDL which indicate that certain small polypeptide components turn over more slowly in plasma than the B apoprotein and which confirm the transfer of C apoprotein subunits between VLDL and HDL in vitro (10). Since it is known that HDL_2 subfraction of HDL (density 1.063-1.125) contains relatively more of these small polypeptides (collectively referred to as C apoprotein) than does HDL_3 (density 1.125-1.21) (11), it is possible that their transfer to TG-rich lipoproteins is accompanied by conversion of HDL_2 to HDL_3. Thus, the various molecular forms of HDL could be related to their functions as substrate for LCAT and as a reservoir of polypeptides that influence the catabolism of VLDL.

The removal of TG from TG-rich lipoproteins in extrahepatic tissues very likely represents an essential step in their metabolism. Less is known about the steps that follow. In the case of chylomicrons, "skeletons" or "remnants" produced by the action of lipoprotein lipase are further metabolized by the liver (12, 13). The liver removes cholesterol from these partially degraded particles (14). Presumably, at least some of the C apoprotein is returned to HDL either before or after this occurs. The fate of the remainder of the particle has not been determined, but any B apoprotein present may be returned to the plasma as described below for VLDL. Studies in rabbits indicate that VLDL may also be partially degraded in the course of their metabolism. When subfractions of VLDL of differing particle size, one of which has been labeled endogenously with palmitate-^{14}C and the other with palmitate-^{3}H, are infused into recipient rabbits, the larger particles can be shown to become smaller in the course of a few minutes, while the size of the smaller particles does not change appreciably (15). During clearance of radioiodine-labeled VLDL from human plasma, the label appears in a fraction of intermediate density (1.006-1.019) before it appears in LDL (10). Analogy with the process shown to occur with chylomicrons suggests that remnants have been produced which are metabolized further in the liver. Whatever intermediate processes occur, including transfer of C apoprotein back to HDL, LDL appear to be a major product of the metabolic sequence. This has been shown from studies in man in which radioiodinated VLDL are infused intravenously (10, 16). As label disappears from protein of VLDL, it appears in LDL-protein in a manner consistent with a precursor-product relationship. When radioiodine-labeled LDL are infused, no accumulation of label in VLDL can be demonstrated. Further studies are required to demonstrate whether all steps occurring during metabolism of chylomicrons and VLDL are identical in a qualitative sense. If formation of LDL occurs similarly from both, much more will be formed per unit weight of TG transported for VLDL than for chylomicrons. However, so much more TG is normally transported in chylomicrons that its contribution to formation of LDL may be substantial. Understanding of the pathogenesis of hyperlipoproteinemias accompanied by increased concentration of LDL will be greatly advanced by determination of the relative contributions of chylomicrons, VLDL, and independent secretion of LDL to the plasma pool.

SECONDARY HYPERLIPOPROTEINEMIAS

Regulation of Lipoprotein Secretion

Most secondary hyperlipoproteinemias are accompanied by increased levels of VLDL (endogenous hyperlipemia). Their pathogenesis can be studied in man under ordinary conditions with the aid of radioisotopes and strategically placed intravascular catheters. The various methods that have been used have been reviewed elsewhere (17). Here we will emphasize results obtained with a method which employs continuous infusion of labeled precursor of VLDL-lipid and periodic sampling of arterial and hepatic venous blood to quantify the splanchnic uptake of the precursor and its fractional conversion to lipid in VLDL and to other products.

In the post-absorptive state and in healthy subjects on ordinary diets, free fatty acids (FFA) derived from adipose tissue are virtually the only precursor of VLDL-triglyceride fatty acids (TGFA) and the secretion of these TGFA is a linear function of the transport of FFA (18). The details of the regulation of fat mobilization are beyond the scope of this discussion and it suffices for our purpose to emphasize the central antilipolytic role of insulin. Insulin, together with the sympathetic nervous system and hormonal activators of lipolysis, regulates the rate at which FFA enter the blood. In resting subjects, hepatic uptake of FFA is proportional to the supply of FFA and accounts for about two-fifths of FFA transport. The supply of FFA to the liver is a major determinant of the rate of hepatic TG synthesis and this, in turn, regulates the synthesis and secretion of VLDL. When this rate is increased by the intravenous injection of norepinephrine into dogs, the liver responds with an approximately proportional increase in rate of secretion of VLDL into hepatic venous blood (19). Similarly, when anti-insulin serum is injected intravenously so as to produce a state of insulin deficiency abruptly, a similar sequence occurs (20). This increased supply of fatty acid is an important cause of the hyperlipemia that frequently accompanies insulinopenic diabetes mellitus, but as discussed below, it is by no means the sole explanation. A similar increase in rate of fat mobilization occurs with exercise of large muscle groups. However, in this situation, there is an absolute decrease in splanchnic blood flow, while flow to the working muscles increases many-fold. This interrupts the sequence by diverting FFA from the liver to the working muscles (21) so that production of VLDL may actually decrease. After

ingestion of carbohydrate, secretion of insulin rapidly inhibits fat mobilization
and the resulting fall in hepatic TG synthesis may contribute to the reduction in
VLDL levels that frequently occurs during the ensuing few hours (22).

The rate of hepatic synthesis of TG depends not only upon the supply of
FFA but also upon the extent to which these FFA are used as an energy source
for synthesis of glucose and protein and for other energy-utilizing processes. In
the post-absorptive state in man, FFA are the chief fuel of hepatic oxidative
metabolism (18). To some extent an increased supply of FFA seems to drive oxidative metabolism in liver, but the FFA that are not oxidized to form ketone
bodies or completely to form CO_2 and water are inevitably esterified to form TG,
and, to some extent, other lipid esters. This can be observed when healthy human subjects are fasted for three days. Splanchnic uptake of FFA approximately doubles as compared with the early post-absorptive state (about 15 hours after
the last meal), oxidation of FFA nearly doubles and synthesis of TG increases
almost three-fold (23). Under these circumstances, secretion of VLDL appears
not to keep pace with TG synthesis. After an overnight fast, about 18% of the
FFA entering the splanchnic region is secreted as VLDL-TGFA (18); this value
falls to about 8% after a three-day fast and the absolute rate of conversion of
FFA to VLDL-TGFA remains nearly constant (23). In long-standing severe deficiency of insulin, the situation may be altered to a greater extent. In chronically depancreatized dogs withdrawn from insulin for two days, conversion of
FFA to VLDL-TGFA falls to only about 1-3% of hepatic uptake of FFA (19).
There is evidence that the precursor-pool of newly synthesized hepatic TGFA
may be derived to a substantial extent from stored TG which are continually
hydrolyzed to yield unlabeled fatty acids. However, the observations in these
dogs strongly suggest that secretion of VLDL is not increased; thus, the hyperlipemia observed at this stage of insulin-deficiency cannot be ascribed to increased secretion of VLDL resulting from increased fat mobilization. The basis
for the moderate fall in fractional conversion of FFA to VLDL-TGFA in fasting
man and the marked fail in chronically diabetic dogs is unknown. In both states,
synthesis of glucose from amino acids and other carbohydrates is increased. The
energy requirements for this process may preempt the supply of high energy phosphate needed for the various steps involved in the synthesis and secretion of
VLDL. This includes a requirement for synthesis of protein.

As mentioned earlier, mobilization of FFA from adipose tissue falls in
the post-prandial state and this may decrease the rate of hepatic TG synthesis.
However, concomitant alterations in metabolism of FFA and other energy-rich
substrates within the liver may also influence this rate. First, ingested carbohydrate may be oxidized preferentially in the liver so that a larger fraction of
FFA entering from the blood is esterified to form TG. Second, carbohydrate
entering the liver may be converted directly to fatty acid. The former process
has been demonstrated directly only in experimental animals (24), but the latter

has recently been shown to occur in man when fed diets very high in carbohydrate for two days or more (25). This has been shown in two ways: first, by demonstrating that the asymptotic specific activity of VLDL-TGFA reached during prolonged infusion of palmitate-^{14}C is substantially lower than that of plasma FFA; second, by demonstrating appreciable conversion of infused glucose-^{14}C to VLDL-TGFA. It should be emphasized that evidence for such conversion has not been obtained except by prolonged feeding of large amounts of carbohydrate and it is not known whether lipogenesis from carbohydrate is a quantitatively important source of VLDL-TGFA in man under less stringent conditions. Simple administration of glucose-^{14}C together with substrate amounts of glucose for several hours is not followed by appreciable labeling of plasma TGFA (26).

The importance of hepatic oxidative metabolism in determining synthesis of triglycerides and VLDL in human liver has been shown in two situations, one rare (glycogenosis type I – von Gierke's disease) and the other quite common (ingestion of ethanol). Hyperlipemia is a constant feature of glycogenosis type I. The genetic defect, glucose-6-phosphatase deficiency, leads to fasting hypoglycemia, hypoinsulinemia, and increased mobilization of fat from adipose tissue. The expected increased splanchnic uptake of FFA and TG synthesis ensue, but unlike the situation in insulinopenic diabetes mellitus, hepatic oxidation of FFA is suppressed and synthesis and secretion of VLDL-TGFA are greatly increased (27). Because of the basic enzymatic defect, glycogen is not degraded efficiently to glucose in the post-absorptive state, but rather to lactate, apparently frustrating the gluconeogenic drive that normally accompanies insulinopenia. How this situation leads to depressed oxidation of fatty acids is uncertain, but it can be appreciated that the continuing glycolysis occurring in these livers resembles the post-prandial rather than the post-absorptive state. Evidently, the fasted peripheral tissues deliver substantial quantities of fuels and normal precursors of gluconeogenesis to a liver which deals with them as it would in the fed state. The resulting traffic jam leads to active TG and, perhaps, protein synthesis, with adequate high-energy phosphate available for the packaging and secretion of VLDL.

Provision of ethanol to the liver provides it with a food that results in a rather similar alteration in hepatic metabolism (23). When the liver burns ethanol to acetaldehyde and then to acetate, its oxygen consumption does not change but oxidation of fatty acids decreases in direct proportion to the rate of oxidation of ethanol. When small amounts of ethanol are given to healthy subjects in the post-absorptive state, this amounts to a fall of about 50%. Hepatic TG synthesis and secretion of VLDL tend to increase, although this is modified by the inhibiting effect of acetate produced during oxidation of ethanol on fat mobilization from adipose tissue. When subjects fasted three days are given similar amounts of ethanol, fat mobilization does not fall, for reasons as yet undetermined, but actually tends to rise further. The result of the inhibition of hepatic fatty acid oxidation in this situation is a substantial increase in TG synthesis and secretion of VLDL. The occurrence of alcoholic lipemia in poorly nourished subjects may thus be explained. When alcoholic lipemia occurs in well-nourished subjects, it may be ascribed in part to the extra caloric load imposed by the ethanol and in part to its preferential oxidation. Frequently, in this situation, the ethanol appears to aggravate a pre-existing primary hyperlipemia rather than produce it in an otherwise normolipemic individual. Hepatic oxidation of ethanol increases the ratio of reduced to oxidized pyridine nucleotides; this, in turn, impairs hepatic utilization of lactate and increases the concentration of alpha-glycerophosphate. The latter may promote triglyceride synthesis, thus providing one explanation for the inhibition of fatty acid oxidation. Such an alteration in redox state does not appear to be present in glycogenosis type I, but interruption of the Cori cycle in both diseases extends their general metabolic similarity.

Synthesis and secretion of VLDL depend upon active protein synthesis. Numerous studies in experimental animals indicate that inhibition of hepatic protein synthesis causes virtual cessation of secretion of VLDL (28). Investigations of experimental nephrotic hyperlipemia suggest that the augmented protein synthesis may be accompanied by increased synthesis and secretion of VLDL (29). Apparently, the leak of protein through the renal glomerulus leads to some signal that results indiscriminately in increased synthesis of a number of plasma proteins produced in the liver (30). With relatively small rates of urinary protein loss in human nephrotic syndrome, the hyperlipoproteinemia is confined mainly to LDL, but with increasing hypoalbuminemia, endogenous hyperlipemia predominates and levels of LDL tend to fall (31). Possibly, efficient conversion of VLDL to LDL prevents their accumulation until rates of secretion approach saturation of catabolic mechanisms. The increased rate of catabolism of VLDL would account for accumulation of LDL in mild nephrosis, but the fall in concentration of LDL in severe nephrosis would appear to require an additional catabolic defect. This explanation of course implies acceptance of the hypothesis that LDL are not secreted from liver as independent entities. As emphasized earlier, quantitative estimates of such a process are not available.

Regulation of Lipoprotein Catabolism

Impaired catabolism contributes to accumulation of VLDL and, frequently, chylomicrons as well in a number of hyperlipoproteinemic disorders. Possible mechanisms include impaired functioning of the lipoprotein lipase system in extrahepatic tissues. This could involve impaired activity of the enzyme or abnormalities of the substrate, such as might be produced by deficiency of normal activator polypeptides. Impaired uptake of products of the action of lipo-

protein lipase, mainly FFA, could also result in retention of VLDL and chylomicrons. Finally, abnormalities of the metabolism of "remnants" of lipolysis
of lipoprotein-TG could lead to hyperlipemia. It is reasonable to suppose
that retention of VLDL and chylomicrons of normal composition and structure
results from abnormalities of the initial lipolytic step, while retention of abnormal particles represents failure of subsequent catabolic steps.

Several acquired hyperlipemias are accompanied by impaired catabolism
of VLDL and, to a lesser extent, of chylomicrons with apparently normal composition and structure. In uncontrolled diabetes, impaired functioning of the
lipoprotein lipase system is suggested by decreased lipolytic activity in plasma
obtained after intravenous injection of heparin (PHLA) (32). A similar situation
exists in von Gierke's disease (27). Presumably, long-standing insulinopenia
is responsible for these abnormalities. Impaired esterification of FFA released
by the action of lipoprotein lipase may contribute to impaired lipolysis in
these conditions. In diabetes, abnormal retention of TG-rich lipoproteins in
the blood may contribute to, or be mainly responsible for, the hyperlipemia,
depending upon the duration of the insulinopenia. In von Gierke's disease,
both increased secretion of VLDL from liver and retention in the blood contribute to hyperlipemia. In several conditions accompanied by insulin resistance
and hyperinsulinism, endogenous hyperlipemia occurs frequently. These conditions include partial and "total" lipodystrophy, chronic renal failure, late-
onset (frequently "centripetal") obesity and the altered hormonal state induced
by administration of contraceptive steroids (33). The mechanism of hyperlipemia
in these states is not understood, although abnormality of the lipoprotein lipase
system has been suspected. This general situation will be discussed further in
relation to primary endogenous hyperlipemia. Impaired PHLA has also been
described in endogenous or mixed hyperlipemia accompanying myxedema (34).
Exogenous hyperlipemia occurs in certain gammopathies in which binding of
heparin to gamma globulins has been demonstrated (35). PHLA is reduced but
it is not known how this heparin-binding leads to decreased function of the
enzyme system at its normal site of action. Highly purified lipoprotein lipase
from rat post-heparin plasma contains none of the injected heparin (36), but
heparin may act as an allosteric modifier of enzyme activity (37).

Whether mechanisms other than impaired activity of lipoprotein lipase
per se contribute to defective catabolism of VLDL in secondary hyperlipemias
is uncertain. As mentioned earlier, catabolism of TG-rich lipoproteins may be
impaired in severe nephrosis. With profound hypoalbuminemia, a substantial
fraction of FFA is transported by lipoproteins (38). Possibly, these FFA interfere with one or more of the steps in the catabolism of VLDL.

A few secondary hyperlipoproteinemias are accompanied primarily by
increased concentration of LDL. This occurs in "mild" nephrotic syndrome as

noted earlier and it is the most characteristic alteration in hypothyroidism. Presumably, the latter results from impaired catabolism of LDL. Recent studies suggest that removal of several plasma proteins from the blood depends upon cleavage of the terminal sialic acid residue of associated carbohydrate moieties (39). Since the apoprotein of LDL contains carbohydrate, including sialic acid (40), impairment of this reaction may contribute to retention of LDL. However, rates of formation of LDL from VLDL and chylomicrons in hypothyroidism are not known.

PRIMARY HYPERLIPOPROTEINEMIAS

Impaired catabolism of TG-rich lipoproteins or of LDL probably contributes to all of the primary varieties of hyperlipoproteinemia. Given a defect in catabolism, the several influences discussed above that promote lipoprotein biosynthesis may, however, have substantial influence on the magnitude of the hyperlipoproteinemia at any given time. In the best understood primary hyperlipoproteinemia - the exogenous hyperlipemia (type I) associated with genetic deficiency of lipoprotein lipase - chylomicronemia is a direct function of the quantity of dietary fat. Likewise, caloric excess and ethanol may have a major role in the severity of primary endogenous (type IV) and mixed (type V) hyperlipemias. Many apparently mixed hyperlipemias revert to endogenous hyperlipemias when diet and intake of ethanol are controlled. However, some mixed hyperlipemias occurring mainly in nonobese individuals appear to be separate entities. PHLA is often reduced in clearly defined mixed hyperlipemias, but usually to a lesser extent than in primary exogenous hyperlipemia (41). In contrast to earlier reports (42, 43), a careful recent study indicates that PHLA also tends to be reduced in primary endogenous hyperlipemia (44) and activity of lipoprotein lipase extracted from subcutaneous adipose tissue has been shown to be inversely related to the concentration of triglycerides in plasma (45). Thus, there is some evidence for defective lipolysis in all of the primary hyperlipemic states.

The high prevalence of insulin resistance in both endogenous and mixed hyperlipemias, with or without carbohydrate intolerance, suggests an intimate connection between the abnormal metabolism of fat and carbohydrate (I). However, the nature of the association is not known. The nearly constant occurrence of abnormal carbohydrate metabolism in all of the primary endogenous and mixed hyperlipemias, including dysbetalipoproteinemia (type III) and in several secondary hyperlipemias, raises the possibility that hyperlipemia in some way leads to an insulin-resistant state. Some studies have shown an association between measures of insulin secretion and severity of hypertriglyceridemia in primary hyperlipemias, leading to the suggestion that the insulin stimulates processes such as hepatic fatty acid and TG synthesis which produce hyperlipemia by increasing secretion of VLDL (46). Measurements of net splanchnic secretion of VLDL-TGFA by both radiochemical and direct chemical methods do not support this concept (18, 44). Rather, they suggest that catabolism of VLDL is impaired. It is possible, therefore, that the hyperinsulinism reflects an abnormal state of tissues accompanied by insulin resistance and that ineffective action of insulin leads to impaired functioning of one or more steps in the catabolism of VLDL. Because of the common occurrence of obesity in these hyperlipemias, however, it is not at all certain that the insensititivy to insulin is an intrinsic component of the individual genotypes.

The relationship between concentration of VLDL and LDL in primary endogenous hyperlipemias may also be relevant to the nature of the metabolic defect. If hypersecretion of VLDL were the major abnormality, this would be expected to lead to increased content of LDL as a result of increased formation from VLDL (the hyperlipoproteinemia of the nephrotic syndrome may be prototypic of such a situation). In contrast, absolutely low levels of LDL occur commonly in endogenous hyperlipemia (41). Concurrently increased levels of LDL and VLDL do occur in the absence of other diseases. This produces another "mixed" state, now commonly called type "II-B" hyperlipoproteinemia. Possibily, in such situations, both increased secretion and impaired catabolism of VLDL coexist. Why chylomicrons do not accumulate in endogenous hyperlipemia of mild to moderate severity is unknown. Possibly, chylomicrons interact more readily with the enzyme and effectively compete with VLDL. Evidently many questions remain to be resolved about the primary endogenous and mixed hyperlipemias. A number of abnormalities may be uncovered by further studies of the lipolytic system or systems involved.

In primary dysbetalipoproteinemia the VLDL that accumulate are abnormally rich in cholesterol and have lower electrophoretic mobility than normal VLDL (41). Recent studies suggest that this disorder results from retention in the blood of partially degraded chylomicrons and VLDL (47, 48). It could, therefore, reflect abnormality in hepatic metabolism of partially degraded TG-rich lipoproteins.

It has been suggested that primary hyperbetalipoproteinemia (type II) is accompanied by impaired catabolism of LDL-apoprotein (49). This accords with the concept that LDL are exclusively a product of catabolism of TG-rich lipoproteins. It would be difficult to explain the striking hyperbetalipoproteinemia and low normal levels of VLDL that may be present in this disorder (type II-A) on the basis of hypersecretion of VLDL. This phenotype could, of course, result from an abnormality leading to appreciable direct secretion of LDL from liver or intestine. As discussed earlier, no clear evidence for such a process exists, either in normal or hyperlipoproteinemic individuals.

CONCLUSION

Determination of the role of plasma lipoproteins in the transport of fat has provided important insights into the pathogenesis of many hyperlipidemic disorders. Advances in this field have been promoted by studies of fat transport in health and in several disease states, including some resulting from rare mutations. Many details of the processes involved in fat transport remain to be clarified and some major gaps remain. We still know little about the function of lipoproteins in the transport of cholesterol although a promising start has been made. Factors influencing the amount of fat and cholesterol transported in the blood have important effects on lipoprotein levels in health. The inefficient transport system that exists in many hyperlipoproteinemic states is particularly susceptible to such factors and their regulation can contribute substantially to the control of hyperlipidemia even though it does not directly influence the step, genetically determined or acquired, that is defective.

The personal research cited was supported
by a grant(HL06285) from the U.S.P.H.S.

REFERENCES

1. Havel, R.J. New Engl. J. Med. In press.
2. Werner, Bengt. Acta Chir. Scand. 132:63 (1966)
3. Scherstén, T., S. Nilsson, E. Cahlin,M. Filipson and G. Brodin-Persson. Europ. J. Clin. Invest. 1: 242 (1971)
4. Hamilton, R.L. This symposium.
5. Gotto, A.M., R.I. Levy, K. John, and D. S. Fredrickson. New Engl. J. Med. 284:813 (1971)
6. Glomset, J.A., K.R. Norum, and W. King. J. Clin. Invest. 49:1827 (1970)
7. Havel, R.J., V.G. Shore, B. Shore, and D. M. Bier. Circ. Res. 27: 595 (1970)
8. LaRosa, J.C., R.I. Levy, P. Herbert, S.E. Lux, and D. S. Fredrickson. Biochem. Biophys. Res. Comm. 41:57 (1970)
9. Havel, R.J., M.L. Kashyap, and J. P. Kane. Circulation 42:II-9 (1971)
10. Bilheimer, D., S. Eisenberg, and R. I. Levy. J. Clin. Invest. 50:8a (1971)
11. Shore, B. and V. Shore. Biochem. 8:4510 (1969)
12. Nestel, P.J., R. J. Havel and A. Bezman. J. Clin. Invest. 42:1313 (1963).
13. Redgrave, T.G. J. Clin. Invest. 49:465 (1970)
14. Bergman, E.N., R. J. Havel, B. M. Wolfe, and T. Bøhmer. J. Clin. Invest. 50:1831 (1971)
15. Sata, T. and R. J. Havel. Unpublished observations.
16. Gitlin, D., D.G. Cornwell, D. Nakasato, J.L. Oncley, W.L. Hughes, Jr., and C. A. Janeway. J. Clin. Invest. 37:172 (1958)

17. Havel, R.J. Atherosclerosis, Proc. II Internat. Symp. (Ed.) R.J. Jones, Springer Verlag, New York (1970) p. 210
18. Havel, R.J., J.P. Kane, E.O. Balasse, N. Segel, and L. V. Basso. J. Clin. Invest. 49:2017 (1970)
19. Basso, L.V. and R. J. Havel. J. Clin. Invest. 49:537 (1970).
20. Balasse, E.O., D. M. Bier, and R. J. Havel. Diabetologia 6:618(1970)
21. Havel, R.J., in Muscle Metabolism During Exercise. (Eds.) B. Pernow and B. Saltin, Plenum Press, New York (1971) p. 315.
22. Havel, R.J. J. Clin. Invest. 36:855 (1957)
23. Wolfe, B.M., R.J. Havel, E.B. Marliss, J.P. Kane, and J. Seymour. J. Clin. Invest. 49:104a (1970)
24. Mayes, P.A. and J. M. Felts. Nature 215:716 (1967)
25. Barter, P.J. and P.J. Nestel. Metabolism. In press.
26. Sandhofer, F., K. Bolzano, S. Sailer. and H. Braunsteiner. Klin. Wschr. 47: 1086 (1969)
27. Havel, R.J., E.O. Balasse, H.E. Williams, J.P. Kane, and N. Segel. Trans. Assoc. Amer. Physicians 82:305 (1969)
28. Farber, E. Adv. Lipid Res. 5:119 (1967)
29. Havel, R.J. Calif. Med. 115:23 (1971)
30. Marsh, J.B. and D.L. Drabkin. Metabolism 9:946 (1960)
31. Baxter, J.H., H.C. Goodman, and R.J. Havel. J. Clin. Invest. 39: 455 (1960)
32. Bagdade, J.D., D. Porte, Jr., and E. L. Bierman. New Engl. J. Med. 276:427 (1967)
33. Havel, R.J. Adv. Int. Med. 15:117 (1969)
34. Porte, D., Jr., D.D. O'Hara, and R.H. Williams. Metabolism 15:107 (1966)
35. Glueck, C.J., A.P. Kaplan, R.I. Levy, H. Greten, H. Gralnick, and D.S. Fredrickson. Ann. Int. Med. 71:1051 (1969).
36. Fielding, C.J. Personal communication
37. Whayne, T.F. and J.M. Felts. Circulation 62:III-6 (1970)
38. Shafrir, E. J. Clin. Invest. 37:1775 (1958)
39. Morell, A.G., G. Gregoriadis, I.H. Scheinberg, J. Hickman and G. Ashwell. J. Biol. Chem. 246:1461 (1971)
40. Margolis, S. and R.G. Langdon. J. Biol. Chem. 241:469 (1966)
41. Fredrickson, D.S., R.I. Levy, and R.S. Lees. New Engl. J. Med. 276: 32 (1967)
42. Fredrickson, D., K. Ono, and L.L. Davis. J. Lipid Res. 4:24 (1963)
43. Sandhofer, F., S. Sailer, M. Herbst, and H. Braunsteiner. Dtsch. Med. Wschr. 90:755 (1965)
44. Boberg, J. Acta Univ. Upsaliensis. 105:1 (1971)
45. Persson, B., P. Björntorp, and B. Hood. Metabolism 15:730 (1966).
46. Reaven, G.M., R.L. Lerner, M. P. Stern, and J.W. Farquhar. J. Clin. Invest. 46:1756 (1967)

47. Quarfordt, S., R.I. Levy, and D.S. Fredrickson. J. Clin. Invest.
    50:75 (1971)
48. Hazzard, W.R. and E. L. Bierman. Clin. Res. 19:476 (1971)
49. Langer, T., W. Strober and R.I. Levy. J. Clin. Invest. 48:49a (1969)

CLEARING FACTOR LIPASE AND ITS ROLE IN THE REGULATION OF TRIGLYCERIDE UTILIZATION. STUDIES ON THE ENZYME IN ADIPOSE TISSUE.

D. S. Robinson and D. R. Wing

Department of Biochemistry, University of Leeds

England

It is now generally accepted that the main physiological function of the enzyme clearing factor lipase, or lipoprotein lipase, is to facilitate the uptake of triglyceride fatty acids (TGFA) from the blood by the extrahepatic tissues (1). This function is thought to be exercised through the initiation by the enzyme of the hydrolysis of chylomicron and very low density lipoprotein triglycerides that are sequestered at the luminal surface of the endothelial cells of the blood capillaries. Furthermore, changes in the activity of the enzyme that occur in particular tissues with changes in physiological status are believed to be responsible for corresponding changes in the uptake of the plasma TGFA by these tissues. Thus, the enzyme probably also performs a directive function in determining the pattern of TGFA removal from the bloodstream. In view of this proposed secondary role of clearing factor lipase, it is clearly important to elucidate the factors which control, and the mechanisms which underlie, the changes in its activity. These questions are considered here in relation to the enzyme in adipose tissue. The activity in this tissue is known to fall markedly on starvation and to rise again on refeeding, and these changes can be directly correlated with corresponding changes in the ability of the tissue to take up TGFA from the bloodstream.

Some information on the factors which may control these changes in adipose tissue enzyme activity has become available as a result of the development of incubation systems in which the low clearing factor lipase activity, characteristic of intact epididymal

71

adipose tissue from fasted animals, increases progressively in
vitro over a period of several hours at 37° to reach a plateau level
not far below that found in the tissue in the fed animal (2, 3).   Such
activity increase is dependent on glucose and insulin and is inhibited
by adrenaline, noradrenaline and adrenocorticotrophic hormone.
Glucagon and thyroid-stimulating hormone have been shown to have
similar inhibitory effects (4).

It is significant that all the hormones which inhibit the rise in
clearing factor lipase activity described above have also been
shown in independent studies to <u>enhance</u> the activity of the so-called
mobilizing lipase in adipose tissue, which is responsible for break-
ing down triglycerides that are stored in the tissue and, therefore,
for mobilizing fatty acids from it (5).   Moreover, insulin is able
to prevent such activation.   This has suggested the possibility of
a single control mechanism affecting differentially the two lipases
concerned respectively with triglyceride deposition in (clearing
factor lipase) and mobilization from (mobilizing lipase) adipose
tissue.   There is already considerable evidence that the activating
effects of hormones on the latter enzyme are mediated through a
rise in the cyclic AMP concentration in the tissue (5).   It is of
interest, therefore, that the rise in adipose tissue clearing factor
lipase activity which occurs under appropriate incubation conditions
in vitro is inhibited in the presence of the dibutyryl derivative of
cyclic AMP (6).   This clearly suggests that tissue cyclic AMP
could be the common mediator of the hormonal actions, a change
in its concentration altering the activity of the two lipases in opposite directions.

Any effect of cyclic AMP on clearing factor lipase activity
could be either direct or indirect.   Thus, a rise in the cyclic
AMP concentration in adipose tissue usually brings about a rise
in the FFA concentration in the tissue because of activation of the
mobilizing lipase (7); and, at least under certain conditions in
vitro, this in turn causes a fall in the tissue ATP concentration
(8, 9, 10).   Either of these two secondary changes could clearly be
the immediate factor influencing the clearing factor lipase activity.
However, correlations between FFA concentration and clearing
factor lipase activity in adipose tissue in a variety of situations in
vivo and in vitro are not always close and changes in ATP concentration in the tissue have not yet been shown to occur in vivo under
conditions when the activity of the enzyme alters.   Thus, the
question of whether any cyclic AMP effect on the enzyme is direct
or indirect remains unsettled at the present time.

The plateau level of enzyme activity that is eventually reached when intact epididymal adipose tissue from fasted rats is incubated for several hours at 37° represents a balance that is achieved at that time between activity increase and activity decrease in the incubation system (3).   The decrease in activity is thought to be accounted for, at least in part, by a pronounced instability of the enzyme at this temperature, and since the enzyme is known to be more stable at 25° than it is at 37°, incubations have also been carried out at 25° (11).   The net increase in activity that is observed at the lower temperature is considerably greater than at the higher.   Moreover, whereas at 37° marked increases in enzyme activity require the presence of heparin in the incubation medium, this is not so at 25°.   The requirement for heparin at 37° is attributable to its ability to extract enzyme from tissues that contain it.   In fact, most of the increase in the enzyme activity at 37° in the presence of heparin is due to enzyme that appears in the incubation medium, the tissue enzyme activity showing little rise.   At 25° and in the absence of heparin, on the other hand, the increase in activity is wholly accounted for by a rise in the activity of enzyme in the tissue.   The observation that a marked rise in activity is only obtained at 37° when heparin is present to extract enzyme from the tissue into the medium, raises the possibility that some factor may normally act within the tissue of the fasted animal at 37° to increase the rate of loss of enzyme activity. Whether such a factor operates in vivo is not known, though there is evidence to show that the high activity of adipose tissue in the fed animal also represents a balance between activity increase and activity decrease in the tissue (12).

Although the physiological action of clearing factor lipase with respect to triglyceride hydrolysis is probably exerted at or close to the endothelial cell surface, the enzyme is also present in association with the fat cells of adipose tissue (13,14).   In the fasting rat, in fact, most of the total activity of the tissue is accounted for by enzyme that is present in the fat cells.   However, in this nutritional state, both the activity of the enzyme and uptake of TGFA by the tissue in vivo are low.   In the fed animal, on the other hand, when both these parameters are high, only a small proportion of the total tissue enzyme is accounted for by that in the fat cells.   Indeed, the fat cell activity remains low and relatively constant whatever the nutritional status of the animal.   This suggests the possibility that this enzyme may be the precursor of the functional enzyme, the activity of which varies so markedly

with changes in nutritional status and which is presumed to be
located at the endothelial cell surface.   Evidence in support of
this view is provided by the finding that the increase in activity
observed when intact epididymal adipose tissue from fasted rats
is incubated in vitro can be reproduced, both with respect to its
pattern and its extent, with fat cells isolated from the tissue (11).
This similarity exists, moreover, whether the comparison is
made at 25° or at 37°.

One important difference between the response of the intact
tissue and of the fat cells isolated from it has been observed (11).
Thus, with the intact tissue the increase in enzyme activity that
occurs at 25° in the absence of heparin takes place wholly within
the tissue, as noted above.   With fat cells, however, the increase
always takes place in the incubation medium, the cell enzyme
activity showing no marked change.   This raises the further possibility, therefore, that a receptor site for the enzyme, which of
course may also be a site for the control of its activity, may exist
in the intact tissue outside the fat cells and perhaps at the endothelial cell surface.

Further work may be expected to show whether control of the
changes in adipose tissue clearing factor lipase activity occurs in
or outside the fat cell and which of the hormonal effects observed
in vitro actually operate in vivo.   However, it is also important
to establish the nature of the changes in activity of the enzyme,
particularly as to whether they involve changes in enzyme amount
or are best accounted for by the conversion of one form of the
enzyme into another of different specific activity.

The increase in clearing factor lipase activity that occurs
when intact adipose tissue is incubated at 37° in vitro is prevented
in the presence of inhibitors of protein synthesis such as puromycin
and cycloheximide (3,15).   Moreover, recent studies with fat cell
systems in a variety of situations in vitro have shown that, there
too, there is a close parallelism between inhibition by cycloheximide
of the clearing factor lipase response and of amino acid incorporation into cell protein (9).   These studies suggest, therefore, that
the increases in enzyme activity in adipose tissue involve stimulation of enzyme synthesis and an increase in the total amount of
enzyme protein present.

The evidence for cyclic AMP involvement, on the other hand,

raises the possibility that the changes in enzyme activity involve conversion of one form of the enzyme into another. Thus, it is well established that this nucleotide plays an important role in the interconversion of different forms of the enzymes concerned in glycogen synthesis and breakdown, and more recent work has shown that its action on the activity of the mobilizing lipase is probably also achieved through the interconversion of different forms of this enzyme (16,17).

Though there is as yet no direct evidence for two forms of clearing factor lipase in adipose tissue, evidence that the enzyme may exist in either a stable or an unstable state in the tissue is already available. Thus, when epididymal adipose tissue from a fed rat is incubated in the presence of puromycin or cycloheximide in vitro at 37°, or when fed rats are injected with puromycin or cycloheximide (3,12), the high clearing factor lipase activity of the tissue declines with a half-life of one to two hours. On the other hand, the low level of enzyme activity characteristic of the tissue in the fasted animal is stable in the presence of cycloheximide or puromycin at 37° (3,15). The possibility exists, therefore, that stable and unstable states of the enzyme characterize the tissue in the fasting and the fed state respectively and may bear a precursor product relationship to each other.

These lines of evidence suggesting, on the one hand, that increases in the activity of clearing factor lipase involve increases in the amount of enzyme protein and, on the other, that the enzyme exists in more than one state, one of which is the precursor of the other, can, of course, be reconciled fairly readily. For example, conversion of the stable state of the enzyme, associated with the fat cells, into an unstable state which is turning over rapidly at the functional site of action of the enzyme at the endothelial cell surface, could induce the synthesis of more of the precursor. However, no evidence for such conversion has yet been obtained, and it is evident that, before such a concept can be advanced with any degree of confidence, much more supporting evidence is required.

The preceding is a shortened form of a paper given at the Fourth International Symposium on Drugs Affecting Lipid Metabolism. A fuller description of the work described is given by Robinson and Wing (11). It was supported by the Medical Research Council, and one of the authors (D. R. W.) is an employee of the Medical Research Council.

REFERENCES

1. Robinson, D.S.   In: Comprehensive Biochemistry.   (Eds.)
   M. Elorkin and E. J. Stotz, Amer. Elsevier (1970) p. 51.
2. Salaman, M. R. and D. S. Robinson.   Biochem. J. 99:640
   (1966).
3. Wing, D. R., M. R. Salaman, and D. S. Robinson. Biochem.
   J. 99:648 (1966).
4. Nestel, P. J. and W. Austin.   Life Sci. 8:157 (1969).
5. Scow, R. O. and S. S. Chernick.   In: Comprehensive Biochemistry.   (Eds.) M. Elorkin and E. J. Stotz, Amer.
   Elsevier (1970) p. 20.
6. Wing, D. R. and D. S. Robinson.   Biochem. J. 109:841 (1968).
7. Nikkila, E. A. and O. Pykalisto.   Biochim. Biophys. Acta
   152:421 (1968).
8. Hepp, D., D. R. Challoner, and R. M. Williams.   J. Biol.
   Chem. 243:4020 (1968).
9. Patten, R. L.   J. Biol. Chem. 245:5577 (1970).
10. Jeanrenaud, B., M. Touabi, S. W. Cushman, and J. J.
    Heindel.   Biochem. J. 122:1P (1971).
11. Robinson, D. S. and D. R. Wing.   Biochem. Soc. Symposium
    33:123 (1972).
12. Wing, D. R., C. J. Fielding, and D. S. Robinson.   Biochem.
    J. 104:45C (1967).
13. Rodbell, M.   J. Biol. Chem. 239:753 (1964).
14. Cunningham, V. J. and D. S. Robinson.   Biochem. J. 112:
    203 (1969).
15. Wing, D. R. and D. S. Robinson.   Biochem. J. 106:667 (1968).
16. Corbin, J. D., E. M. Reimann, D. A. Walsh, and E. G.
    Krebs.   J. Biol. Chem. 245:4849 (1970).
17. Huttunen, J. K., D. Steinberg, and S. E. Mayer.   Proc. Nat.
    Acad. Sci. USA 67:290 (1970).

HORMONAL CONTROL OF LIPOLYSIS IN ADIPOSE TISSUE

Daniel Steinberg, M.D., Ph.D.

Department of Medicine, University of California

San Diego, La Jolla, California

PHYSIOLOGICAL AND CLINICAL IMPLICATIONS OF ALTERATIONS IN RATES OF FREE FATTY ACID MOBILIZATION

It is now generally accepted that the mobilization of free fatty acids from adipose tissue stores is a key metabolic process. Stored triglycerides can only be mobilized as free fatty acids. Thus, mobilization of free fatty acids is a process as important as, or even more important than, mobilization of liver glycogen as glucose. The primary purpose of FFA mobilization is in the provision of caloric substrate to peripheral tissues but there are numerous additional metabolic consequences of FFA mobilization highly relevant to the context of this meeting. Some of these metabolic consequences for which good experimental evidence is available are the following:

1. Increased rate of fat deposition in the liver, which may under appropriate circumstances tend to produce fatty liver;

2. Increased rate of production of ketone bodies, which may be relevant to the genesis of ketosis under some circumstances;

3. Increased rate of production of very low density lipoproteins by the liver, which may be a factor in certain types of hyperlipoproteinemia;

4. Interference with the uptake and utilization of glucose by muscle, which may be a factor in the complex metabolic interrelationships in the diabetic state;

   5.   Effects on the coagulation system, tending to favor intravascular thrombosis.

   Incompletely documented consequences include:

   6.   A tendency to increase overall body metabolism;

   7.   Effects on myocardial contractility;

   8.   An increase in number and firing rate of ectopic foci after
myocardial infarction.

   In view of these many physiologic and pathophysiologic implications of excessively rapid FFA mobilization it is obviously important to understand as well as we can the mechanisms that regulate
the process. The basic elements involved in regulation of FFA mobilization have been extensively reviewed elsewhere and no attempt
will be made here to review the subject comprehensively. Instead,
we would like to present in the time available a brief report on some
recent advances made in our laboratory on the mechanism of action of
lipolytic hormones in adipose tissue. These advances were made possible in the first instance by a successful partial purification of
hormone-sensitive lipase by Huttunen et al. (1,2). In brief, we have
shown that the activation of the enzyme is mediated, probably directly, by cyclic AMP-dependent protein kinase and that the activation
process is correlated with phosphorylation of the enzyme by transfer
of phosphate from the gamma position of ATP (3,4). We will also present some recent findings on monoglyceride lipase activity associated with the purified hormone-sensitive lipase. The monoglyceride
lipase activity is different from the triglyceride lipase activity
in a number of respects, most important of which is the fact that
the monoglyceride lipase activity does not appear to be activated by
protein kinase.

HORMONE-SENSITIVE LIPASE IN ADIPOSE TISSUE

   Although a great deal of work has been published on "hormone-
sensitive lipase" in adipose tissue, it is important to be aware
that all of these studies have concerned themselves with enzyme activity in relatively crude preparations. On the basis of differential properties and partial resolution of enzyme activities it is
fair to say that adipose tissue contains at least 3 different lipase
activities--hormone-sensitive (triglyceride) lipase, monoglyceride
lipase and lipoprotein lipase (5,6). None of these has yet been prepared in pure form from adipose tissue and it is not possible to say
how many different enzymes may be involved in the activities that
have been studied. It is obvious, then, that there are serious potential pitfalls in studies of relatively crude preparations that
contain an uncertain number of lipolytic enzymes. This is particular-

ly true since crude fractions of adipose tissue have been shown to contain lipase-inactivating systems. We shall return to this question of lipase inactivation (or deactivation) toward the end of this paper.

The purification scheme developed by Huttunen et al. for preparation of hormone-sensitive lipase from rat adipose tissue is summarized in Table I and the details have been published (1,2). A key step in the purification involves the flotation of the enzyme at density 1.12. Equilibrium centrifugation in a sucrose density gradient showed the peak of enzyme activity at a density of 1.08-1.09. As expected, then, the purified material proved to be rich in lipid, approximately 50% by weight, and most of the lipid was phospholipid. Sedimentation velocity studies, using ultraviolet scanning, showed a single component with an $S_{20,w}$ of 32-34. Sedimentation equilibrium studies also indicated homogeneity but some of the enzyme protein aggregated and sedimented into the oil phase during the run. Electron microscopy, done by Dr. Thomas F. Roth, showed a predominant particle 160 $\pm$ 20 Angstroms in diameter but in some fields there were very large, membrane-like particles as well. Whether these represent aggregates occurring during the handling of the enzyme or whether they reflect contamination with material of membrane origin remains uncertain. At the end of this discussion we will return to the question of the form in which hormone-sensitive lipase occurs in adipose tissue. The studies on the mechanism of activation reported below were done primarily with enzyme purified through all of the steps shown in Table I.

TABLE I

PURIFICATION OF HORMONE-SENSITIVE LIPASE

Fraction	Yield	Relative specific activity
78,000 x g SUPERNATANT[*]	100%	1.0
pH 5.2 PRECIPITATE	94%	4.5
d < 1.12	42%	11.5
d 1.06 - 1.12	23%	12.1
AGAROSE COLUMN EFFLUENT	19%	27.6
87,000 x g SUPERNATANT[**]	15%	106.0

[*]Total activity, 250 μEqFFA/h; total protein, 435mg
[**]Total activity, 38 μEqFFA/h/ total protein, 0.6mg

MOLECULAR MECHANISM OF ACTIVATION OF HORMONE-SENSITIVE LIPASE

As reviewed elsewhere (7) it has been fairly clear for a number of years that cyclic AMP was somehow involved in lipase activation but the role of cyclic AMP remained to be determined. In 1968 Krebs and coworkers provided the first evidence for a molecular mechanism of cyclic AMP action in muscle phosphorylase activation (8). Their studies showed that cyclic AMP enhanced the activity of protein kinase. Protein kinase in turn converts phosphorylase b kinase to its active form by phosphorylating it; the active form of phosphorylase b kinase in turn converts phosphorylase to its active form, again by a protein-enzyme phosphorylation reaction.

With a partially purified lipase in hand we were able to ask whether a similar mechanism was operative in adipose tissue. In collaboration with Dr. Steven E. Mayer and Dr. Jussi K. Huttunen we carried out preliminary studies utilizing protein kinase partially purified from rabbit muscle. Activation was readily demonstrated in a system containing protein kinase, ATP-magnesium, cyclic AMP and hormone-sensitive lipase. With the complete system, activation ranged from 40-100% whereas little or no activation was observed if any one of the components of the system was omitted. If high concentrations of protein kinase are used the activation is essentially instantaneous. In order to do kinetic studies, the concentration of kinase was sharply reduced. These kinetic studies showed that the reaction was highly specific for cyclic AMP (7,9). Adenosine-5'-monophosphate was without activity at any concentrations tested, up to 10^{-4} M. Cyclic IMP could substitute but required concentrations 10-fold higher. The reaction was also highly specific for ATP, other nucleoside triphosphates being without activity even at concentrations of 10^{-4} M. The apparent K_m values were, for cyclic AMP, 1.1×10^{-7} M, and for ATP, 6×10^{-6} M.

The next question to be explored was that of whether, as in the phosphorylase b kinase activation, there was a transfer of ATP phosphate during activation. When the activation was carried out in the presence of ATP labelled in the terminal phosphate significant radioactivity was transferred to the hormone-sensitive lipase preparation, from 2 to 4 moles P per 10^6 grams of protein. In the absence of kinase, labelling was reduced to less than 15% of that with the complete system. All of the radioactivity was associated with protein, none being present in the lipid extract of the enzyme. Because of the notorious tendency of ATP to adsorb nonspecifically to proteins, control studies were done using ATP labelled in the alpha phosphate and adsorption was in this way corrected for.

In order to test whether the phosphorylation and the activation were indeed causally related, a careful time-course study was carried out. As shown in Fig. 1., there was excellent correlation between the progressive activation of the purified lipase and its progressive

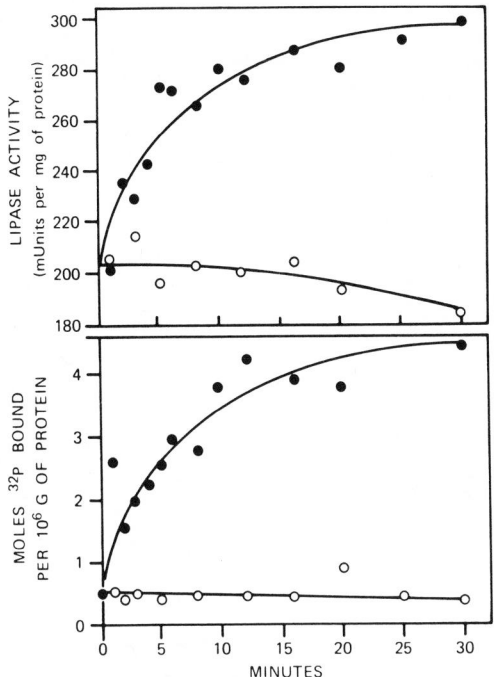

Fig. 1.   Parallel time course of activation (above) and phosphorylation (below) of purified lipase.   Solid symbols with and open symbols without addition of protein kinase.

phosphorylation.   The apparent K_m for phosphorylation and activation were, within experimental error, the same.   While the possibility that parallel but independent phosphorylation and activation
are proceeding cannot be ruled out, the data strongly support the
hypothesis that activation is indeed effected by phosphorylation.

It was necessary to ask whether the activation process demonstrated with the purified enzyme could be related to the hormone-
stimulated activation in intact cells.   Two sets of epididymal fat
pads were incubated prior to homogenization, one in control medium
and one in the presence of epinephrine.   At the end of the pre-incu-
bation period both sets were homogenized and carried through the
fractionation shown in Table I in an absolutely parallel fashion.
At each stage in the purification the degree of protein kinase-depend-
ent activation was determined and the results are shown in Fig. 2
The fractions prepared from control tissues showed activation at each
step, ranging from 60% to 100%.   In contrast, the same fractions derived from hormone-treated tissue showed little or no activation at
any stage in the purification.   These results imply that enzyme prepared from hormone-treated tissue is already fully activated and that
the process of hormone activation in the intact tissue is the same

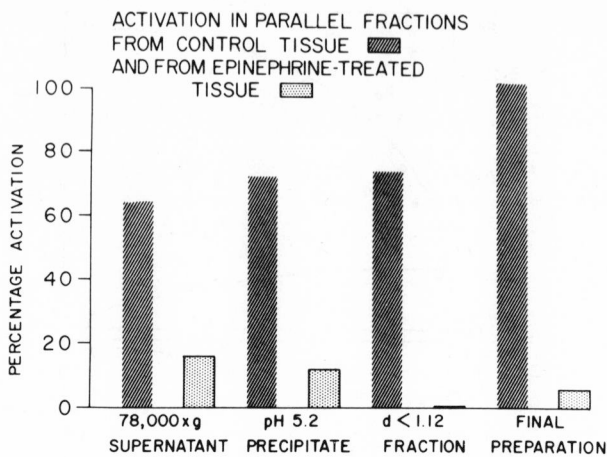

Fig. 2

as that effected by cyclic AMP-dependent protein kinase in the purified system.

These results, then, allow us to expand the "lipolytic cascade" as shown in Fig. 3. The initial reaction of hormone is with an as yet unidentified receptor, probably <u>not</u> identical with adenyl cyclase itself (10). This interaction leads to activation of adenyl cyclase

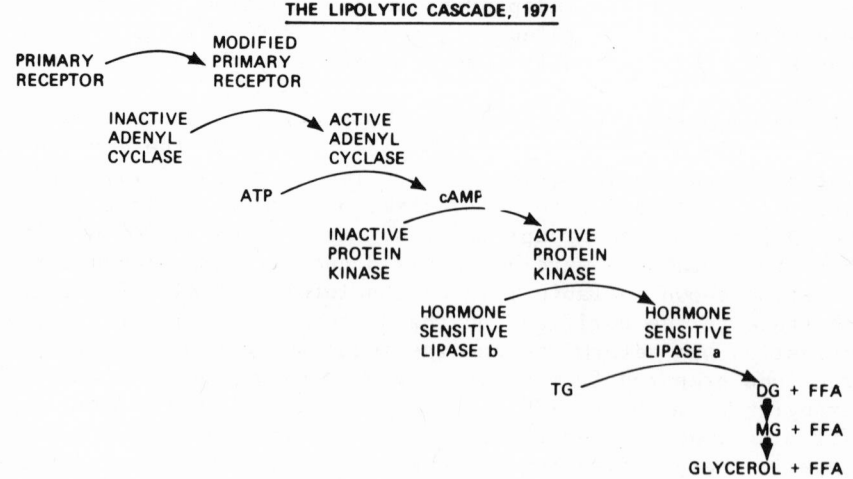

Fig. 3

and an increased rate of formation of cyclic AMP from ATP.   The cyclic AMP in turn activates protein kinase, probably by the mechanism
first proposed by Gill and Garren (11) and by Tao, Salas and Lipmann
(12), namely, combination with a receptor protein moiety leading to
dissociation of the active catalytic unit of protein kinase.   The
latter, in its active form, then phosphorylates the lipase protein
in an ATP-dependent, cyclic AMP-<u>independent</u> reaction.   The question
of whether another step (or steps) intervene between protein kinase
and the activation of lipase—analogous to the activation of phosphorylase b kinase in the muscle phosphorylase system (8)— has been
considered but there is thus far no evidence for such intervening
steps.   Our more recent finding that a second, lower molecular
weight form of hormone-sensitive lipase is also activated directly
by protein kinase makes such a possibility less likely.   Furthermore,
if there were such an intermediate step involved one would anticipate
activation at <u>some</u> rate and under <u>some</u> conditions independent of
cyclic AMP.   Thus far we have not seen that kind of activation with
the purified system.

ACTIVATION IN CRUDER FRACTIONS

     As discussed above, activation of the 100-fold purified enzyme
was completely dependent upon addition of exogenous protein kinase.
However, as shown in Fig. 4., activation in the crude supernatant
fraction could be as effective in the absence of added protein kinase, i.e., only addition of cyclic AMP and of ATP- magnesium was
necessary (7,9). Presumably this activation depends upon endogenous
adipose tissue protein kinase, an enzyme first shown to be present
in adipose tissue by Corbin and Krebs (13).   This is consonant with

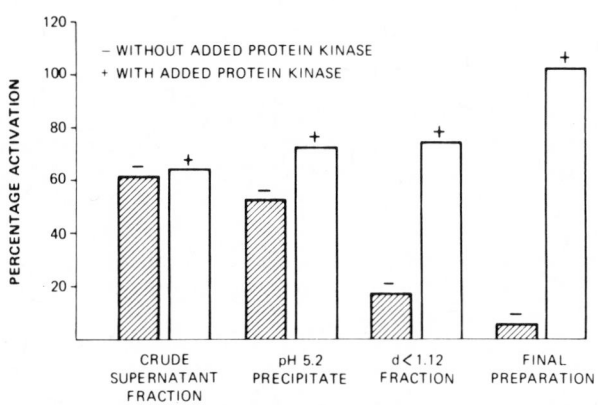

PROTEIN KINASE–DEPENDENCE OF LIPASE ACTIVATION
AT SUCCESSIVE STAGES OF PURIFICATION

Fig. 4

the earlier results of Rizack (14,15) and of Tsai, Belfrage and
Vaughan (16). The latter authors observed activation in crude fractions with cyclic AMP and ATP but were not able to observe any enhancement of activation by the addition of exogenous protein kinase.
Recently Corbin and coworkers (17) utilized the device of adding a
specific protein inhibitor of protein kinase to crude preparations
of adipose tissue to inhibit this endogenous kinase activity. Then
it was possible to show that activation was dependent on addition
of exogenous (rabbit muscle) protein kinase. The earlier results
of Rizack differ in a number of substantive ways from the more recent
experiments and these differences have been discussed elsewhere (7).
The differences may in part stem from participation of the hormone-
sensitive lipase inactivating system discussed below.

It is self-evident that a finely regulated, rapidly responsive
system must include a mechanism for rapid deactivation of lipase.
FFA release can return very rapidly to basal levels following brief
hormonal stimulation and the presence of a lipase inactivating system in crude homogenates has been demonstrated (18). Recently
Manganiello, Murad and Vaughan (19), using isolated adipocytes, have
provided striking evidence of how very rapidly the activated enzyme
can return to its basal state. Their data suggest that within a
minute or less after the addition of a hormone antagonist (propanol
or insulin) epinephrine-stimulated lipolytic activity returns to the
basal value. Little is known at present about this process of enzyme
deactivation but it is clear that it might play an important role in
regulation. On the basis of the studies summarized here, we would
predict that the deactivation of hormone-sensitive lipase can be
effected by a "lipase phosphatase" in analogy with phosphorylase.
Preliminary studies in our laboratory have demonstrated the presence
in crude adipose tissue fractions of an activity that will remove the
labelled phosphate from enzyme previously activated in the presence
of gamma-^{32}P-ATP. Further studies of this activity are in progress.

A SECOND FORM OF HORMONE-SENSITIVE LIPASE IN RAT ADIPOSE TISSUE

Recent studies by Mr. Ray C. Pittman and Mr. Eric Golanty in
our laboratory demonstrate the presence in crude supernatant fractions of epididymal fat of a lower molecular weight lipase that is
also activated by cyclic AMP-dependent protein kinase (20). Only a
fraction of the hormone-sensitive lipase in the 78,000 x g supernatant fraction is recovered in the fraction floating at density 1.12.
That material, as expected, was recovered in or near the void volume
on agarose gel chromatography (Table II). In contrast, the lipolytic activity sedimenting at density 1.12 was mainly in the retained
peak. If the 78,000 x g supernatant fraction is directly applied
to a 4% agarose gel column, one fraction of activatable lipase is
recovered in the void volume and a second peak is recovered at approximately twice the void volume (molecular weight approximately 100,000-

TABLE II

DIFFERENTIAL ELUTION FROM 4% AGAROSE COLUMN
OF d > 1.12 and d < 1.12
LIPASE FRACTIONS PREPARED FROM 1.8×10^5 x g SUPERNATANT[*]

Centrifugal fraction	Percentage of lipase activity in void-volume fraction	Percentage of lipase activity in retained fraction
d > 1.12 (Bottom 3/4)	27%	73%
d < 1.12 (Top 1/4)	100%	None detected

[*]The 1.8×10^5 x g crude supernatant fraction was adjusted to d = 1.12 with concentrated sucrose solution, centrifuged 40 h at 110,000 x g in a 40.3 rotor, and the tubes sliced to yield a top 1/4 and a bottom 3/4. The top and bottom fractions were then subjected to gel filtration on 4% agarose.

200,000). The retained lipolytic activity does not float during centrifugation at density 1.12 and presumably has little or no lipid associated with it although this remains to be established. The partition of hormone-activatable lipase between these two fractions varies from preparation to preparation. On the average, 45% ± 18% was recovered in the void volume peak. The degree of activation observed with the void volume fraction tended to be greater than that for the retained fraction (Table III). It will be important to determine whether these represent different forms of a single hormone-sensitive lipase or whether they represent two distinct enzymes involved in fat mobilization.

Monoglyceride lipase activity. Earlier work provided evidence that there was a monoglyceride lipase activity in rat adipose tissue distinct from the hormone-sensitive triglyceride lipase (5,21). Dr. Renu Heller in our laboratory has recently taken up the study of this monoglyceride lipase activity and followed it through the same purification steps used for the preparation of hormone-sensitive lipase. In the crude 78,000 x g supernatant fraction there is much more monoglyceride lipase activity (mono-olein substrate) than triglyceride lipase activity (triolein substrate). During purification the ratio of monoglyceride lipase activity to triglyceride lipase activity decreases from 15 or 20 to 1 to approximately 5 to 1. Comparison of activities against two substrates with such different physical properties as mono-olein and triolein may be questionable in absolute terms; nevertheless, the change in the ratio of activities is probably significant. Thus it appears that there must be at least two separate monoglyceride lipase activities in the tissue and

TABLE III

CYCLIC AMP-DEPENDENT PROTEIN KINASE ACTIVATION
OF GEL FILTRATION FRACTIONS (n = 6)

Fraction[*]	Percentage activation without cAMP	Percentage activation with cAMP
Void-volume lipase	17% $\pm$ 17%	60% $\pm$ 17%
Retained lipase	2% $\pm$ 7%	34% $\pm$ 15%

[*]The indicated pooled fractions were incubated for 10 minutes at 23° C with 2×10^{-5} M ATP; 1×10^{-2} M MgAc$_2$; 1×10^{-3} M theophylline; 0.02 M tris acetate, pH 8.0; 25 μg/ml rabbit muscle protein kinase; 1×10^{-5} M cAMP, in a final volume of 0.20 ml. Substrate (^{14}C-triolein) was added after 10 minutes and incubation continued at 23° for the assay period, generally 90 minutes. Activation is expressed relative to lipase activity with no added cofactors. Controls with all additions except cAMP and protein kinase, when checked, were comparable to the controls with no added cofactors.

preliminary studies using isoelectric focusing actually suggest that there may be more than two.

The monoglyceride lipase activity behaves differently from the hormone-sensitive lipase in a number of respects. Perhaps the most important of these is that the monoglyceride lipase activity is not enhanced by treatment with the cyclic AMP-protein kinase system that activates the triglyceride lipase. The monoglyceride lipase activity of the purified preparation was not enhanced at all under conditions that yielded 50% activation of the triglyceride lipase activity. The monoglyceride lipase activity in cruder fractions likewise showed little or no activation (22).

Another important difference between the two activities is found in their thermal stability. For example, heating at 50° C for 30 minutes caused little or no inactivation of the triglyceride lipase but 60% of the monoglyceride lipase. Significant differences were seen also in terms of degree of inhibition by 1 M sodium chloride, by isopropanol, and taurodeoxycholate. These results, particularly the absence of activation and the differential thermal stability, suggest that the purified high molecular weight, lipid-rich particle may represent a multi-enzyme complex. However, until the components can be physically separated this conclusion must remain tentative.

EFFECTS OF PROSTAGLANDINS, INSULIN AND NICOTINIC ACID
ON ACTIVATION BY PROTEIN KINASE

The availability of a partially purified lipase and a system
for activation in a cell-free system allowed us to ask whether some
of the important anti-lipolytic agents might have an effect, at
least in part, at the final step in the lipolytic cascade. In collaboration with Miss Alegria Aquino we have looked for effects of
prostaglandins, insulin and nicotinic acid on activation both with
the 100-fold purified lipase (dependent on added rabbit muscle protein kinase) and on activation in the 78,000 x g supernatant fraction (independent of added protein kinase). Activation was not
significantly affected by the addition of prostaglandin E_1 (1 µg/ml),
insulin (400 microunits per ml) or nicotinic acid (4.4 x 10^{-4} M).
These studies were carried out using optimal concentrations of ATP
and cyclic AMP. They do not rule out the possibility that under
conditions where the cofactors may be limiting these substances might
have an effect at this level.

SUMMARY

Because free fatty acid mobilization potentially influences a
wide variety of metabolic processes, drugs that alter FFA mobilization may be useful in a number of clinical situations as well as in
research on fat transport and its consequences. The mechanism of
hormone activation of lipolytic activity in adipose tissue has now
been extended to include a direct demonstration of the molecular
mechanism involved. After hormone stimulation of the adenyl cyclase
system, cyclic AMP activates protein kinase which in turn phosphorylates the lipase enzyme, converting it from a less active to a more
active form. Hormone-sensitive lipase in rat adipose tissue is present both in a high molecular weight, lipid-rich particle and also
in a lower molecular weight, lipid-poor form. Whether or not these
two forms of lipase are interrelated remains to be determined. Further studies on the monoglyceride lipase activity in adipose tissue
show it to be heterogeneous. The partially purified hormone-sensitive lipase retains activity against monoglycerides but this is not
activated by protein kinase. A number of additional differences
between hormone-sensitive lipase and monoglyceride lipase in the
purified preparation have been demonstrated. Studies can now be
undertaken to determine whether drugs or other hormones influence
lipase activation in the later steps. Preliminary studies fail to
show an effect of insulin, prostaglandin E_1 or nicotinic acid.

REFERENCES

1. Huttunen, J.K., J. Ellingboe, R.C. Pittman, and D. Steinberg.
    Biochim. Biophys. Acta 218:333 (1970).
2. Huttunen, J.K., A.A. Aquino and, D. Steinberg. Biochim. Biophys.
    Acta 224:295 (1970).
3. Huttunen, J.K., D. Steinberg and, S.E. Mayer. Proc. Nat. Acad.
    Sci. 67:290 (1970).
4. Huttunen, J.K., D. Steinberg, and S.E. Mayer. Biochem. Biophys.
    Res. Comm. 41:1350 (1970).
5. Vaughan, M., J. Berger, and D. Steinberg. J. Biol. Chem. 239:
    401 (1964).
6. Vaughan, M. and D. Steinberg, in Handbook of Physiology, Adipose
    Tissue. (Eds.) A.E. Renold and G.F. Cahill, Jr., American
    Physiological Society, Washington, D.S. (1965) p. 239.
7. Steinberg, D., in Advances in Cyclic Nucleotide Research, Proc.
    of Int. Conference on Physiol. and Pharmac. of Cyclic AMP,
    vol.1. (Eds.) P. Greengard, G.A. Robison and R. Paoletti,
    Raven Press, New York (1971) in press.
8. Walsh, D.A., J.P. Perkins and E.G. Krebs. J. Biol. Chem. 243:
    3763 (1968).
9. Huttunen, J.K. and D. Steinberg. Biochim. Biophys. Acta 239:
    410 (1971).
10. Rodbell, M., in Adipose Tissue, Regulation and Metabolic Func-
    tions. (Eds.) B. Jeaurenaud and D. Hepp, Academic Press, New
    York (1970).
11. Gill, G.N. and L.D. Garren. Biochem. Biophys. Res. Comm. 39:
    335 (1970).
12. Tao, M., M.L. Salas, and F. Lippman. Proc. Nat. Acad. Sci.(USA)
    67:408 (1970).
13. Corbin, J.D. and E.G. Krebs. Biochem. Biophys. Res. Comm. 36:
    328 (1969).
14. Rizack, M.A. J. Biol. Chem. 236:657 (1961).
15. Rizack, M.A. J. Biol. Chem. 239:352 (1964).
16. Tsai, S.-C., P. Belfrage, and M. Vaughan. J. Lipid Res. 11:466
    (1970).
17. Corbin, J.D., E.M. Reimann, D.A. Walsh, and E.G. Krebs. J. Biol.
    Chem. 245:4849 (1970).
18. Vaughan, M., D. Steinberg, F. Lieberman, and S. Stanley. Life
    Sci. 4:1077 (1965).
19. Manganiello, V.C., F. Murad, and M. Vaughan. J. Biol. Chem.
    246:2195 (1971).
20. Pittman, R.C., E. Golanty, and D. Steinberg. Biochim. Biophys.
    Acta, submitted for publication.
21. Strand, O., M. Vaughan, and D. Steinberg. J. Lipid Res. 5:554
    (1964).
22. Heller, R. and D. Steinberg. Fed. Proc. 30:1090 Abs, (1971).

THE ROLE OF CYCLIC 3'5'-AMP AND ITS DERIVATIVES IN LIPID AND CARBOHYDRATE METABOLISM

R. Paoletti

Institute of Pharmacology and Pharmacognosy

University of Milan, Milan, Italy

Cyclic adenosine-3'5'-monophosphate (CAMP) stimulates in vitro the release of free fatty acids from adipose tissue cells by activating the hormone sensitive lipase. Its activity is potentiated by inhibitors of the phosphodiesterases and it is antagonized by guanosin cyclic-3'5'-monophosphate (CGMP).

The interactions of CAMP and several synthetic derivatives with enzymes involved in lipid and carbohydrate mobilization are investigated and the relations between cyclase activity, prostaglandin formation and tissue regulation of CAMP and CGMP levels are underlined.

BIOCHEMICAL CHANGES IN THE ARTERY WALL DURING GENESIS

AND REGRESSION OF ATHEROMATOUS LESIONS

H. B Lofland, Jr., R. W. St. Clair, and T. B. Clarkson

Arteriosclerosis Research Center, Bowman Gray School

of Medicine, Winston-Salem, North Carolina, U.S.A.

It is generally accepted that the formation of atheromatous lesions represents an interaction between plasma lipids (lipoproteins) and the arterial wall. In most species, including man, qualitative or quantitative changes in plasma lipids result in an accelerated rate of development of atherosclerosis. A growing body of evidence, however, also suggests that the arterial wall itself plays more than a passive role in this process.

Studies from a number of laboratories have described changes in specific biochemical pathways or mechanisms which appear to characterize the developing atherosclerotic lesion. Typical of such studies is the work of Adams, et al. (1), Chobanian (2), Dayton and Hashimoto (3), Eisenberg, et al. (4), Hollander, et al. (5), Portman (6), Stein and Stein (7), Whereat (8), Zemplenyi (9), and Zilversmit (10). This list is by no means inclusive, but rather, points out the diversity of research being conducted on the arterial metabolic aspects of atherosclerosis. For the most part, these studies have dealt with the biochemical aspects of either the developing lesion or of the fully-developed plaque. In recent months, however, evidence has been presented by Armstrong, et al. (11) which indicates that atherosclerotic lesions in primates can be caused to regress to some degree. In the discussion to follow, we will present the results of some studies from our laboratories which deal with several aspects of the progression and regression of atherosclerosis in a variety of animal models.

Lipid Synthesis

We have previously described a perfusion system which allows the intimal surface of isolated arteries to be perfused with a

pulsatile flow of oxygenated serum or tissue culture medium (12).
Using aortas from the atherosclerosis-susceptible White Carneau
pigeon (13) which had been fed cholesterol for several months, and
acetate-2-^{14}C as substrate, we were able to demonstrate the synthesis of fatty acids found in phospholipids, triglycerides, and sterol esters in the artery. Typical results are shown in Table 1.

TABLE I

LIPID SYNTHESIS IN ISOLATED PERFUSED AORTAS
FROM WHITE CARNEAU PIGEONS*

Percent of Total Radioactivity Found in:

Type of Preparation	Free Sterol	Cholesteryl Esters	Triglyceride	Phospholipid
Normal	6	8	51	35
artery	8	4	50	38
Intact dis-	5	31	27	37
eased artery	4	35	37	24
Excised	2	44	42	12
plaque	6	36	39	19

*Values represent results of two separate experiments. (Modi-
fied from J. Lipid Res. 65:112-118,1965.)

The most striking feature of these studies is the marked increase in the synthesis of cholesteryl esters in the intact diseased arteries and in the excised plaques. It is apparent that
the newly synthesized fatty acid becomes esterified to cholesterol
which was preexisting in the arterial wall, since synthesis of the
sterol moiety was minimal.

We have similarly observed increased synthesis of lipids in
diseased areas of perfused aortas of squirrel monkeys (Saimiri
sciureus) (14). As in pigeons, increased amounts of newly synthesized fatty acids are found esterified to cholesterol. Typical
results are shown in Table II.

Similar studies have been carried out in Cebus albifrons monkeys, in which synthesis was studied in both aortas and coronary
arteries. Active synthesis could be demonstrated in both arterial
beds. On the other hand, there did not appear to be marked

TABLE II

INCORPORATION OF ACETATE-1-^{14}C INTO LIPIDS OF THE AORTAS OF SQUIRREL MONKEYS

	Control (N = 4)		Cholesterol-fed (N = 13)		Incorporation Relative to Controls§
	Radioactivity* (dpm/m/g/4 hr)	Acetate-1-^{14}C Incorporated† (mμmoles/g/4 hr)	Radioactivity (dpm/min/g/4 hr)	Acetate-1-^{14}C Incorporated (mμmoles/g/4 hr)	
Thoracic Aorta					
phospholipids¶	106,379± 32,729‡	24	146,735±33,412	33	1.4
triglycerides¶	∇478,265±185,331	109	156,577±27,908	36	0.3
cholesteryl esters¶	2,935± 750	0.7	13,529± 3,200	3.1	4.4
Abdominal Aorta					
phospholipids	62,197± 7,757	14	138,806±37,280	31	2.2
triglycerides	184,598± 66,585	42	170,721±37,017	39	0.9
cholesteryl esters	2,720± 537	0.6	16,346± 9,097	3.7	6.2

*Dpm/min/g lipid-free dry weight/4 hr period of perfusion.
†mμmoles/g lipid-free dry weight/4 hr period of perfusion.
§The relative increase was obtained by dividing acetate incorporation in cholesterol-fed group by that of the control group.
¶The phospholipid, triglyceride, and cholesteryl ester fractions accounted for an average of 90% of the total ^{14}C-labeled lipid recovered.
‡Mean values (± SEM).
∇This value is probably not a representative mean as it was influenced by two very large values.
(Modified from J. Athero. Res. 10:193-206,1969.)

enhancement of sterol esterification, probably due to the fact that the arteries were only slightly diseased (15).

A consistent finding in the above-mentioned studies on lipid synthesis has been the minimal synthesis of cholesterol, which has usually been in the order of a few percent of the total lipid radioactivity. Digitonin-precipitable materials are synthesized, but when they are purified via the dibromide crystallization, the bulk

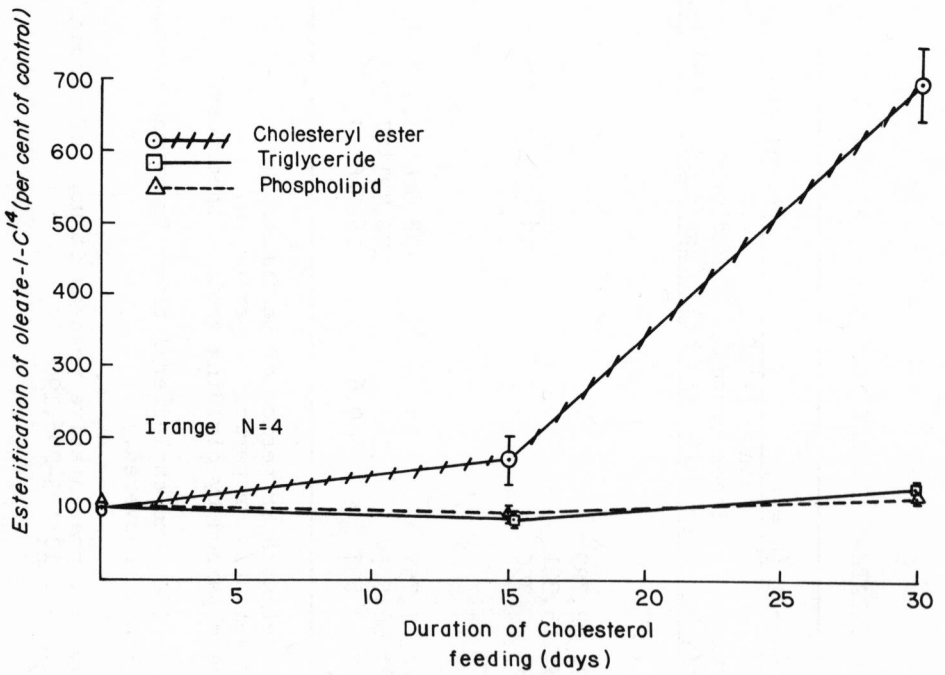

Fig. 1. Influence of short-term cholesterol feeding on incorporation of oleic acid-1-^{14}C into phospholipid, triglyceride, and cholesteryl ester by cell-free preparation of pigeon aorta. Results are the mean and range of 4 determinations. Values are presented as percent of controls, which were birds matched for age and fed a diet containing no added cholesterol. (Reprinted with permission from Circulation Res. 27:213-225,1970.)

of the radioactivity is lost. There is, however, active synthesis
of squalene, a process which appears to be positively correlated
with the severity of atherosclerosis (16).

Sterol Esterification

The studies described above suggested that enhanced sterol esterification is a feature of progressing atherosclerosis. We have
examined this process as a function of the duration of cholesterol
feeding (17) using pigeon aorta. Maximum (>80% of the total) esterifying activity was found to be in the particulate fraction obtained by centrifuging at 105,000XG. As shown in Fig. 1, esterifying activity increased within two weeks after cholesterol feeding
was initiated, and long before atherosclerotic lesions or fatty
streaks were demonstrable. Results indicated that the mechanism of
esterification is probably via the fatty acyl-CoA-cholesterol acyl
transferase, but not via the lecithin-cholesterol-fatty acyl transferase.

Sterol Flux

Almost all studies point to the fact that plasma cholesterol
accounts for almost all of the sterol which accumulates in the artery during atherogenesis. We have studied the dynamics of cholesterol influx and efflux in vivo by the daily oral administration of
cholesterol-1,2-^{3}H to cholesterol-fed pigeons for a period of 30
days, then discontinued. Subgroups of birds were sacrificed short-
ly after isotope feeding was begun, and the aortas were separated
into normal tissue, fatty streaks, and atherosclerotic plaques.
From the ratio of specific activity of cholesterol in the plasma
and that of the tissue, rates of influx were calculated. After the
administration of labeled cholesterol was discontinued, subgroups of
birds were sacrificed at intervals for an additional three months,
and from the slope of the disappearance curve, the rates of cholesterol removal were calculated. Some results are shown in Tables
III and IV.

Results of the experiments indicated that in normal segments of
the artery, the influx of free cholesterol greatly exceeds that of
cholesteryl esters, and the same appears to be true of the rates of
efflux. Normal tissue appears to be in slight negative cholesterol
balance. In contrast, in fatty streaks, influx of cholesteryl esters is increased, and this appears to be even more marked in
plaques, which are seen to be in definite positive cholesterol balance (18). Thus it appears that in areas of the artery where lesions are developing, the arterial wall is actively taking up lipids
from plasma, especially cholesteryl esters.

It has been of interest to examine the mechanism by which cholesterol and its esters are transported from plasma into the

TABLE III

CHANGES IN FREE AND ESTER CHOLESTEROL RADIOACTIVITY IN NORMAL ARTERY,
FATTY STREAKS, AND PLAQUES AT VARIOUS TIME INTERVALS*

Day	Normal Artery Free Cholesterol	Normal Artery Cholesteryl Esters	Fatty Streaks Free Cholesterol	Fatty Streaks Cholesteryl Esters	Plaques Free Cholesterol	Plaques Cholesteryl Esters
18	16,727± 1081	2781± 492	24,970± 2096	11,478± 2787	54,734±11,680	59,100±21,003
24	17,948± 1024	4859±1118	39,310±11,835	31,702±15,361	78,917± 4567	125,628±10,391
31	20,722± 3122	3932±1614	27,526± 5178	8037± 2684	87,075±27,544	111,325±52,636
38	27,546± 2010	5740±1228	36,535± 5719	16,414± 3161	93,201±16,882	134,870±39,021
52	43,603±26,566	3172±1548	37,935± 6043	18,442± 4424	123,891±25,581	178,639±64,723
66	14,204± 569	8826±1750	27,074± 4151	14,808± 3479	86,000±10,132	118,635±50,337
88	8901± 1796	1597± 252	20,274± 5949	8214± 4755	74,858±17,598	89,098±25,869
122	2072± 622	2067±1242	11,572± 5025	4235± 2076	86,660±19,571	103,732±24,445

*Mean values (dpm/g of wet tissue) for 8 birds, at each time interval, followed by the standard errors of the means. (Reprinted with permission from Proc. Soc. Exptl. Biol. Med. 133:1-8, 1970.)

TABLE IV

INFLUX AND EFFLUX OF FREE CHOLESTEROL AND CHOLESTERYL ESTERS
IN NORMAL ARTERY, FATTY STREAKS, AND PLAQUES*

	Free Cholesterol			Cholesteryl Esters		
	Influx	Efflux	Differ-ence	Influx	Efflux	Differ-ence
Normal aorta	71.3	86.4	-15.1	11.9	14.5	- 2.6
Fatty streaks	106.5	75.7	+25.8	49.0	29.6	+19.4
Plaques	198.0	167.0	+31.0	259.0	183.0	+76.0

*Values for influx and efflux represent µg of cholesterol/g of aorta/day. (Reprinted with permission of Proc. Soc. Exptl. Biol. Med. 133:1-8,1970.)

arterial wall. We have developed an organ culture system which allows segments of artery to be maintained in a viable state for up to nine days (19). Using isolated plasma low-density lipoprotein (LDL) labeled with ^{125}I, and ^{3}H-cholesterol, we have conducted preliminary studies on aorta segments from both pigeons and squirrel monkeys. The data, while still in preliminary form, suggest that cholesteryl esters may be transported into the artery as an LDL complex. Free cholesterol appears to enter at a greater rate than does LDL, suggesting that the free form may be transported inward by a mechanism which is different from that of cholesteryl esters.

Lesion Regression

The extent to which atherosclerotic lesions can be caused to regress is a question of importance in regard to human atherosclerosis. We have attempted to study this process, using White Carneau pigeons which have been fed cholesterol for one year, then restored to a pellet diet. Subgroups of birds were sacrificed at the beginning, and after two, four, and eight months of regression. The concentrations of free and ester cholesterol, phospholipids, triglyceride, and collagen were determined in normal artery, fatty streaks, and plaques. The results are shown in Table V. During the regression period, all lipid classes appear to decrease in concentration to some extent. The decrease does not appear to be progressive, however, especially in the concentrations of free and

TABLE V

MEAN VALUES FOR LIPID FRACTIONS IN VARIOUS SEGMENTS
OF PIGEON AORTA BEFORE AND DURING REGRESSION*

Duration of Regression	Type of Tissue	Free Cholesterol[†]	Cholesteryl Esters[†]	Triglycerides[†]	Phospholipids[†]	Collagen[†]
Months		mg/g	mg/g	mg/g	mg/g	% LFDW[§]
0	Normal	2.23±0.19	1.45±0.31	7.01±1.30	5.18±0.37	20.29±0.60
	Fatty streak	5.83±0.88	3.99±0.59	9.77±1.96	5.84±0.25	20.14±0.83
	Plaque	27.05±2.95	26.18±2.86	16.62±1.91	12.52±1.00	21.71±0.83
2	Normal	1.97±0.16	0.77±0.17	4.04±1.13	3.76±0.39	22.99±0.81
	Fatty streak	5.40±0.80	3.40±0.52	6.27±1.47	4.56±0.53	21.90±0.82
	Plaque	19.62±1.75	15.07±2.32	17.40±3.47	10.05±0.81	21.04±1.30
4	Normal	1.67±0.09	0.38±0.05	1.86±0.28	2.16±0.18	25.43±1.05
	Fatty streak	4.00±0.62	1.14±0.18	2.65±0.54	2.73±0.24	25.60±0.93
	Plaque	17.51±2.31	9.71±1.42	5.87±0.78	4.16±0.55	32.65±1.72
8	Normal	1.77±0.13	0.53±0.09	2.15±0.27	6.85±0.28	27.56±1.26
	Fatty streak	4.55±0.92	1.28±0.19	3.60±0.71	7.22±0.26	30.81±2.21
	Plaque	16.86±1.96	11.87±1.97	8.36±1.37	-	38.76±2.75

*Adapted from Clarkson, et al., Circulation abstracts, 1971, in press.
†Each mean value (± SEM) was derived from 7-24 samples of the tissue studied.
§LFDW = Lipid-free dry weight.

esterified cholesterol in plaques. After two months, there appears to be little further change in the concentration of these substances, suggesting that there may be one metabolic pool of cholesterol which is somewhat labile, and another which is more firmly bound within the artery. This finding is consistent with our observations of cholesterol clefts in plaques after eight months of regression. With regression, the plaques became less yellow in appearance, were depressed centrally, and had thicker fibrous caps. It was of interest that the collagen content of plaques, expressed as percent of the lipid-free dry weight, continued to increase during regression. We feel that these studies cast some doubt on the concept of complete regression of advanced lesions of atherosclerosis.

REFERENCES

1. Adams, C. W. M., O. B. Bayliss, and M. Z. M. Ibrahim. J. Path. Bacteriol. 86:421 (1963).
2. Chobanian, A. V. J. Clin. Invest. 47:595 (1968).
3. Dayton, S. and S. Hashimoto. Exptl. Molec. Path. 13:253 (1970).
4. Eisenberg, S., Y. Stein, and O. Stein. Biochim. Biophys. Acta 137:221 (1967).
5. Hollander, W., D. M. Kramsch, M. Farmelant, and I. M. Madoff. J. Clin. Invest. 47:1221 (1968).
6. Portman, O. W. J. Athero. Res. 7:617 (1967).
7. Stein, O. and Y. Stein. Lab. Invest. 23:556 (1970).
8. Whereat, A. F. Exptl. Molec. Path. 7:233 (1967).
9. Zemplenyi, T. J. Athero. Res. 7:725 (1967).
10. Zilversmit, D. B. Ann. N. Y. Acad. Sci. 149:710 (1968).
11. Armstrong, M. L., E. D. Warner, and W. E. Connor. Circulation Res. 27:59 (1970).
12. Lofland, H. B, Jr., D. M. Moury, C. W. Hoffman, and T. B. Clarkson. J. Lipid Res. 6:112 (1965).
13. Clarkson, T. B., R. W. Prichard, M. G. Netsky, and H. B Lofland. A.M.A. Arch. Path. 68:143 (1959).
14. St. Clair, R. W., H. B Lofland, and T. B. Clarkson. J. Athero. Res. 10:193 (1969).
15. Lofland, H. B, Jr., R. W. St. Clair, T. B. Clarkson, B. C. Bullock, and N. D. M. Lehner. Exptl. Molec. Path. 9:57 (1968).
16. St. Clair, R. W., H. B Lofland, Jr., R. W. Prichard, and T. B. Clarkson. Exptl. Molec. Path. 8:201 (1968).
17. St. Clair, R. W., H. B Lofland, and T. B. Clarkson. Circulation Res. 27:213 (1970).
18. Lofland, H. B and T. B. Clarkson. Proc. Soc. Exptl. Biol. Med. 133:1 (1970).
19. St. Clair, R. W. and H. B Lofland, Jr. Proc. Soc. Exptl. Biol. Med., in press.

NEWER ASPECTS OF DRUGS
AFFECTING LIPID METABOLISM

EFFECT OF SOME DRUGS ON FREE FATTY ACIDS AND TRIGLY-CERIDES IN PLASMA AND TISSUES

S.Garattini, M.E.Hess, M.T.Tacconi,E.Veneroni
and A.Bizzi
Istituto di Ricerche Farmacologiche 'Mario

Negri', Via Eritrea, 62 - 20157 MILANO,Italy

INTRODUCTION

Previous studies have shown that marked changes in lipid metabolism occur when the lipase activity of adipose tissue is blocked (1,2,3).

Drugs, known to inhibit lipolytic activity in adipose tissue, such as nicotinic acid,5-carboxy-3-methylpyrazole (5C3MP),5-carboxy-3-methylisoxazole,were used to investigate this problem.

The sequence of the events which occurs after the administration of these compounds has been extensively studied and is the subject of recent reviews (4,5,6).

In an effort to understand better the effects of pyrazole derivatives and of nicotinic acid, we investigated the problem of a possible antagonism by other compounds known to elevate plasma free fatty acids(FFA).

Among these compounds some anorectic drugs,namely amphetamine and fenfluramine were considered (7,8).

In this report some unexpected findings observed after administration of fenfluramine or amphetamine will be presented. Later we will discuss some effects observed during the perfusion of isolated hearts from rats in which the availability of FFA was reduced by inhibiting the lipolytic activity of adipose tissue.

MATERIALS AND METHODS

Male Sprague Dawley rats, average body weight 150 g, were used throughout the experiments.

If not otherwise stated, the animals were deprived of food only at the beginning of the experiments.

Routes of administration, dosage schedules are included in the section on results.

Plasma FFA were measured according to Dole (9) with minor modifications; triglycerides according to Van Handel, Zilversmit and Bowmann (10); glycogen according to Van Handel (11).

Heart perfusions were carried out according to a procedure described previously (12).

R E S U L T S

Some effects of anorectic drugs on lipid metabolism

It has been shown that both amphetamine and fenfluramine evoke a rise in plasma FFA within 15 min after the administration (8).

Since the addition of these compounds to the medium used to incubate adipose tissue did not stimulate the release of FFA or glycerol from adipose tissue, it has been suggested that the rise of plasma FFA might occur through sympathetic stimulation (8).

In spite of the rise of plasma FFA, these compounds caused a decrease in the level of plasma triglycerides in fed rats (Table I).

This effect was maximal between the third and the fourth hr after administration of the drug and in fenfluramine treated rats, was still present 8 hr later.

Liver triglycerides were not affected by amphetamine or fenfluramine, but there was some reduction in heart triglycerides 6 hr after the administration of either drugs (Table II).

The discrepancy between the rise in FFA and the reduction in triglycerides in plasma, plus the difference in time in the appearance of these phenomena, sugge-

TABLE I

EFFECT OF AMPHETAMINE AND FENFLURAMINE ON
PLASMA TRIGLYCERIDES

Interval between treatment and determinations (hr)	Plasma Triglycerides mg/100 ml $\pm$ S.E. after		
	saline	amphetamine 5 mg/kg i.p.	fenfluramine 20 mg/kg i.p.
2	60$\pm$10	36$\pm$5 *	33$\pm$4 *
4	60$\pm$10	23$\pm$2 *	26$\pm$1 *
6	41$\pm$1	39$\pm$2 *	26$\pm$2 *
8	44$\pm$2	36$\pm$1 *	26$\pm$1 *
16	55$\pm$5	68$\pm$3 *	40$\pm$1 *

* p < 0.01 versus saline

sted that the decrease in plasma triglycerides might be
related to the formation of some metabolite.

Results obtained with norfenfluramine (Table III),
the principal metabolite of fenfluramine in rats,showed
that this compound produced the same effect on lipid
metabolism as fenfluramine, in fact it increased FFA
and decreased plasma triglycerides (Table III).

There is therefore the possibility that the effect
on plasma triglycerides could be due to the formation
of norfenfluramine.

Additional studies were primarily concerned with
the mechanism of action of fenfluramine. It was
observed that a pretreatment with fenfluramine
neither affected the rate of clearance when a
triglyceride emulsion was injected (Table IV) nor altered
the lipoprotein lipase activity of serum (Table V).
Likewise, in vitro studies showed that pretreatment with
fenfluramine did not affect the release of VLDL (very
low density lipoprotein) triglyceride from liver slices
(13). Moreover,fenfluramine was effective in decreasing
plasma triglycerides in fed,but not in fasted rats

TABLE II

EFFECT OF AMPHETAMINE AND FENFLURAMINE ON TISSUE
TRIGLYCERIDES

Tissue	Interval between treatment and determinations (hr)	Triglycerides mg/100 g $\pm$ S.E. after		
		saline	amphetamine 5 mg/Kg i.p.	fenflura- mine 20 mg/kg i.p.
Liver	2	424+35	465+17	466+26
	4	424+35	426+48	521+80
	8	401+9	473+61	560+72
	16	463+9	438+32	532+41
Heart	2	105+10	138+4	183+35
	4	-	120+8	111+9
	6	132+10	80+5*	71+4*
	8	156+22	153+8	190+1

* P < 0.01 versus controls

TABLE III

EFFECT OF NORFENFLURAMINE ON PLASMA TG AND FFA

Treatment mg/kg i.p.		Interval between treatment and determinations (min)	Plasma	
			FFA μEq/l $\pm$ S.E.	Triglycerides mg/100 ml $\pm$ S.E.
Saline		-	242+34	46+3
Norfenfluramine	5	60	289+26	42+5
"	5	120	519+42*	41+5
"	5	240	385+42	29+2*
"	5	480	298+48	27+3*

* P < 0.01 against controls .

TABLE   IV

EFFECT OF FENFLURAMINE AND AMPHETAMINE ON THE
CLEARANCE OF A CORN-OIL EMULSION GIVEN I.V.

Time after corn-oil injections (min)	Plasma triglycerides mg/100 ml $\pm$ S.E.		
	Saline + Corn-oil	Amphetamine + Corn-oil	Fenfluramine + Corn-oil
0	47$\pm$4	37$\pm$7	30$\pm$3
1	417$\pm$27	448$\pm$29	452$\pm$42
5	329$\pm$41	360$\pm$53	276$\pm$36
15	151$\pm$12	153$\pm$20	148$\pm$25
30	134$\pm$18	152$\pm$60	77$\pm$24
60	69$\pm$5	55$\pm$7	52$\pm$12

Amphetamine 5 mg/kg i.p. or fenfluramine 20 mg/kg i.p.
were injected at the beginning of the experiment.
The duration of the experiment was 240 min. Corn-oil
emulsion (10 %)was injected i.v. at the dose of
2.5 ml/kg.

(Table VI) and it was able to inhibit the rise in
plasma triglycerides induced by an olive oil load
(Fig. 1).

Consequences of a decreased FFA availability on cardiac contraction

It has been previously observed that a diminution
in FFA availability results in a decrease in the concentration of triglycerides and glycogen in several tissues
(liver,kidney,heart,muscle)(1,3).

Since triglycerides and glycogen constitute two
important stores of energy,it seemed probable that
alteration in physiological functions would occur in
tissues in which triglycerides and glycogen were reduced.

Measurement of contractility of isolated hearts

TABLE V

EFFECT OF A PRETREATMENT WITH FENFLURAMINE OR
AMPHETAMINE ON SERUM CLEARING FACTOR IN VITRO

In vivo Treatment mg/kg	In vitro Clearing activity μEq/l	
	0	15'
Saline	475	550
Amphetamine 5 i.p.	400	475
Fenfluramine 20 i.p.	500	575
Heparin 10 i.v.	800	1650

Amphetamine or fenfluramine were given 240',heparin
was given 5' before sacrifice.
1 ml of serum from treated rats was incubated with 0.5ml
of activated corn-oil(corn-oil 0.3%+ rat serum,1:1 at
37°C for 30') for 15'.

TABLE VI

EFFECT OF FENFLURAMINE AND AMPHETAMINE ON PLASMA
TRIGLYCERIDE OF OVERNIGHT FASTED RATS

Treatment mg/kg i.p.	Time between treatment and determinations (min)	Plasma trigly- cerides mg/100 ml ± S.E.
Saline	-	36±2
Amphetamine 5	120	35±3
Amphetamine 5	240	31±3
Fenfluramine 20	120	34±3
Fenfluramine 20	240	40±2

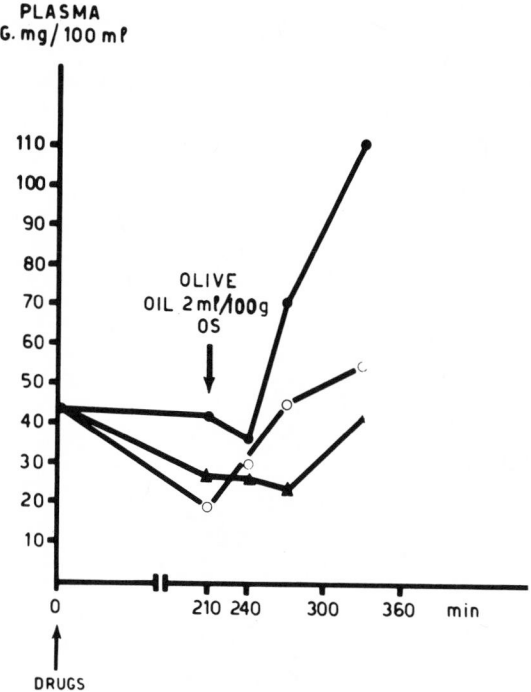

Fig. 1.   Effect of amphetamine and fenfluramine on the absorption of olive oil.
Amphetamine 5 mg/kg i.p. or fenfluramine 20 mg/kg i.p. were
given 120 min before the oral administration of olive oil 20 ml/kg.

● controls   o   amphetamine   ▲ fenfluramine

obtained from normal rats and rats pretreated with
nicotinic acid confirmed this hypothesis.

        Results in Fig. 2 show that both basal and nor-
epinephrine-stimulated force of contraction were lowered
significantly when the concentrations of triglyceride
and glycogen in the heart were decreased (Table VII).
However,the infusion of FFA, glucose or VLDL (12) promptly   restored the contractility of the hearts to normal
levels.

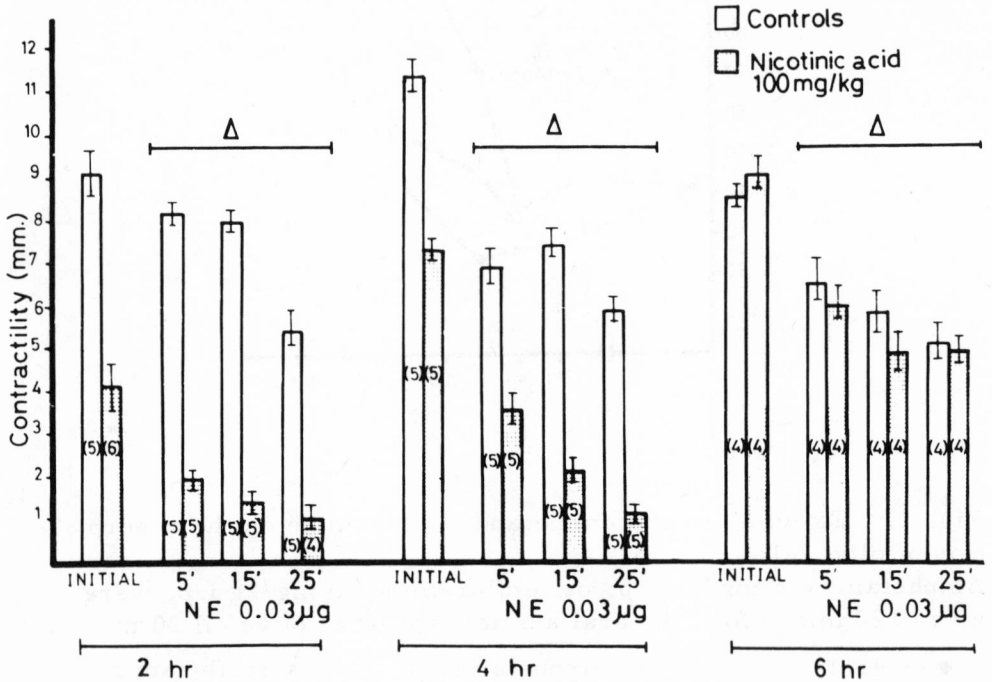

Fig. 2. Effect of nicotinic acid on the force of contraction in isolated rat hearts.

Bars labeled initial indicate force of contractions at start of perfusion. Bars enclosed in △ bracket indicate increase of force of contraction in response to l-norepinephrine infusion.
2, 4, 6 hr means time after in vivo nicotinic acid treatment.

TABLE VII

EFFECT OF NICOTINIC ACID ON HEART TRIGLYCERIDES
AND GLYCOGEN

Time after nicotinic acid treatment (hr)	H e a r t Triglycerides %	Glycogen %
Controls	100	100
2	47 *	12 *
4	65 *	36 *
6	67	170

Nicotinic acid = 100 mg/kg i.p.
* Significantly different from corresponding controls.

DISCUSSION

   It has been observed that amphetamine and fenfluramine, two anorectic drugs which are known to increase
plasma FFA (6, 7),caused a marked reduction in plasma
triglycerides in fed, but not in fasted rats.
This effect was shown to be possibly due to the formation of metabolites,since norfenfluramine,the principal
metabolite of fenfluramine,produced the same effect on
plasma FFA and plasma triglycerides as the parent
compound. The mechanism for this action probably involves changes in lipid absorption,since lowering of plasma
triglycerides occurred only in fed rats and pretreatment of rats with amphetamine reduced markedly the rise
in plasma triglycerides induced by ingestion of olive
oil. The means by which fenfluramine reduces intestinal
absorption are still under investigation. Several
factors may be involved. For example,fenfluramine has
been shown to reduce intestinal motility (A.Bizzi, unpublished data), perhaps by lowering the level of intestinal serotonin, and to decrease the release of pancreatic lipase in vitro (14). If this latter phenomenon
occurs also in vivo the absorption of triglycerides
would be reduced because of the decreased availability
of enzymes necessary to cleave triglycerides in the
intestinal tract. Moreover the reesterification in the
postabsortive intestinal stage may also be affected.

The relative stability of triglycerides concentrations in tissues (hepatic triglycerides were not changed
and cardiac triglycerides were lowered only several
hours after the drug administration) may be related to
the lipolytic effect of these drugs,which results in an
increase in the availability of plasma FFA. The observation that the contractility of the perfused isolated
rat heart was markedly diminished when the concentration
of cardiac triglycerides and glycogen was reduced,
demonstrates that changes in lipid metabolism result
also in alterations of the functional activity.

REFERENCES

1. Carlson, L.A., S.O.Fröberg, and E.R.Nye.Acta Med.
    Scand. 180:571 (1966).
2. Bizzi,A., E.Veneroni, and S.Garattini. J.Pharm.Pharma
    col. 18:611 (1966).
3. Bizzi,A., and S.Garattini. Progr.Biochem.Pharmacol.
    3:320 (1967).
4. Garattini, S., and A.Bizzi. Actualités Pharmacol. 22:
    169 (1969).
5. Kupiecki, F.P. Progr.Biochem.Pharmacol. 6:274(1971).
6. Hasselblatt,A.   Naunyn Schmiedeberg Arch.Pharm. 269:
    331 (1971).
7. Herold, E., F.Kemper, and K.Opitz. Arzneimittelforsch
    15:657 (1965).
8. Bizzi, A., A.Bonaccorsi,S.Jespersen,A.Jori,and S.Ga-
    rattini ,in Amphetamines and Related Compounds .
    (Eds.) E.Costa,and S.Garattini. Raven Press,New York
    (1970) p.577 .
9. Dole, V.P. J.Clin.Invest. 35:150(1956).
10. Handel,E., Van, D.B. Zilversmit, and K.Bowmann .
    J.Lab.Clin.Med. 50:152 (1957).
11. Handel,E.,Van . Anal.Biochem. 11:266 (1965).
12. Hess,M.E.,A.Bizzi,E.Veneroni, and S.Garattini.Amer.
    Heart J., in press (1972).
13. Marsh,J.B., and A.Bizzi . Biochem.Pharmacol.,in
    press (1972).
14. Dannerburg,W.N., and J.W.Ward . Arch.Int.Pharmacodyn.
    191:58 (1971).

EFFECT OF DRUGS ON PLASMA TRIGLYCERIDE METABOLISM

Esko A. Nikkilä

Third Department of Medicine, University of Helsinki

Helsinki, Finland

This paper aims to review the essential information which has accumulated on the mode of action of drugs on the production and utilization of circulating triglycerides. As is natural, main emphasis is paid to the hypolipidemic agents but a brief mention is made also of oral contraceptives as a representative of those drugs which have adverse hyperglyceridemic effects.

Drugs for treatment of hypertriglyceridemia have been actively sought for ten years but very few are available and their therapeutic effect in individual cases is uncertain and often unpredictable. None of these agents has been specifically planned to inhibit the hepatic production of plasma triglycerides or to stimulate the removal of triglycerides from the circulation. This development has been difficult in the past since little has been known of the regulatory steps of plasma triglyceride transport and, particularly, of the mechanisms behind hypertriglyceridemia. Therefore, despite extensive research it has not appeared possible to completely understand the mode of action of any drug currently used for lowering the plasma triglyceride level. It seems at present that many of them have multiple effects on lipid metabolism and no single point of pharmacologic action can be found which alone could account for the decrease of plasma lipid levels. It still might be of interest to deliberately develop drugs which, e.g., increase the activity of lipoprotein lipase or stimulate its synthesis since independently of the primary cause of hyperglyceridemia an increase of the efficiency of utilization of plasma triglycerides certainly lowers their concentration.

The key points of plasma triglyceride metabolism are 1) the liberation of FFA and glycerol from adipose tissue into circulation, 2) hepatic triglyceride synthesis in the secretory pathway, 3) hepatic apolipoprotein synthesis, 4) the secretory process itself (transport from liver cell to plasma) and 5) the lipoprotein-triglyceride lipase activity of peripheral tissues (possibly also of liver). These are also the loci of action of drugs which alter the rates of plasma triglyceride influx or efflux.

CLOFIBRATE AND RELATED DRUGS

Of this group of hypoglyceridemic drugs the clinical experience is limited mostly to chlorophenoxyisobutyrate ethyl ester (clofibrate, CPIB) and a tetralin derivative, methyltetrahydronaphtylphenoxy propionate (TPIA, CIBA Su-13437), which unfortunately has been recently withdrawn from further clinical trials. Even if there is no evidence that these two drugs have a similar mode of action they are treated together below. In fact, very few investigations have been reported on the possible mechanisms by which Su-13437 influences triglyceride metabolism. On the other hand, clofibrate has been extensively studied in both human and rat experiments, in vitro and in vivo, but the manner by which it reduces the plasma triglyceride concentration still remains obscure. Most data have been obtained from rats even though this animal does not show a consistent hypoglyceridemic response to clofibrate (1-3). The vast majority of studies have been made after chronic feeding of the drug and, therefore, the acute effects are poorly explored.

Clofibrate effectively reduces plasma triglyceride level in types III and IV of familial hyperlipoproteinemia and in hyperglyceridemia associated with diabetes. However, the response is variable and often not predictable. Hypertriglyceridemia induced in normal man by a very high sucrose diet is not prevented by the drug (4). On the other hand, in rats clofibrate (or Su-13437) will attenuate the response of plasma triglyceride to dietary carbohydrates (5, 6), to ethanol (7), and to experimental nephrosis (8).

Effect on FFA Metabolism

It has been suggested that clofibrate might decrease plasma triglyceride through a similar antilipolytic action as nitotinic acid (9).   Experimental evidence for this mechanism of action is far from conclusive, however, and the antilipolytic activity, if present at all, is much inferior to that of nicotinic acid and related compounds.   When added to rat adipose tissue incubation medium, clofibrate has been reported to slightly counteract the stimulation of lipolysis by catecholamines (10) but in another study this effect was not observed nor was the lipolytic activity of corticotrophin or growth hormone altered by CPIB (11).   Clofibrate adminis- tered to rats in vivo shows an opposite effect by increasing the glycerol release from incubated fat pads (12).   This finding, again, is difficult to reconcile with a decrease of adenyl cyclase activity of adipose tissue demonstrated recently in clofibrate- treated rats (13).

Several studies on plasma FFA concentration have given some support to the concept on a weak antilipolytic action of clofibrate. The results of early reports on plasma FFA concentration during clofibrate treatment are useless because they did not correct for the interference by drug anion.   More recently, lower fasting plasma FFA levels have been consistently found during CPIB treatment than before it in rats (14,15), dogs (14) and man (16,17). However, in contrast to nicotinic acid the clofibrate is not able to prevent the increase of plasma FFA concentration induced by catecholamines (14,18).

Plasma FFA turnover rate remains substantially unchanged during clofibrate (19, 20) or Su-13437 treatment (21).   Also the uptake of FFA from medium into perfused rat liver is not altered when animals are treated with CPIB (22, 23).

In summary then, it seems possible that clofibrate and re- lated compounds have a slight inhibitory effect on the adipose tissue lipolysis but this hardly plays any significant role in the hypoglyceridemic action of these drugs.   The decrease of plasma FFA level observed during the treatment might be partly second- ary to the lowering of plasma triglyceride level, and the inconsis- tencies of the results obtained with adipose tissue might be due to differences in the feeding pattern of treated and control animals since the drug often decreases the food consumption (13).   Studies on the acute in vivo effects of clofibrate on FFA metabolism, com- parable to those made with nicotinic acid, have not been reported but should be highly desirable.

Effect on Hepatic Synthesis and Release of Triglycerides

Clofibrate administered in high dosage to animals exerts
striking effects on hepatic morphology.   The liver is enlarged
due to increase of the size of hepatocytes (24, 25).   The ultrastructure undergoes characteristic changes, which are apparent
even within a few hours and include increased formation of micro-
bodies, morphological alterations of mitochondria, and proliferation of smooth endoplasmic reticulum (26-28).   These are accompanied by an increase of liver protein (26, 28-31) and phospholipid
(1, 29, 32) whereas the amount of DNA and RNA does not increase
with liver size (28, 33).   The hepatic enlargement by clofibrate
is not accounted for by accumulation of water, fat, or glycogen
(30, 33).   The compound Su-13437 similarly produces hepatomegaly
in rats but at a lower dosage level than clofibrate (34).

It is not known whether similar morphological changes are
produced in the human liver when these drugs are used in the conventional clinical dosage, which on weight basis is only one-tenth
of the amounts given to animals in the experiments referred to
above.   Another unsolved problem is the relationship of structural
alterations of the liver and the lowering of plasma lipid levels
produced by clofibrate.   Anyway, it is difficult to reconcile the
proliferation of hepatic endoplasmic reticulum and decreased triglyceride synthesis.   Stimulation of this subcellular element by
phenobarbital increases acylation of diglyceride but does not alter
hepatic or plasma triglyceride concentration (35).

Under basal conditions the hepatic triglyceride content is not
decreased by clofibrate (25, 36) and it may even be slightly increased (33).   On the other hand, accumulation of fat into the
liver induced by ethanol administration is prevented by CPIB (7,
37).   Some reduction of hepatic triglyceride content has been
shown to occur on treatment of rats with the compound Su-13437
(34).   Contrary to what is expected, clofibrate treatment has been
found to increase the synthesis of liver triglycerides from various
labeled precursors.   Thus, in intact rats clofibrate increases the
incorporation of tritiated water and of radioactive glycerol and
acetate into hepatic triglycerides (32, 33, 38).   Similarly, in perfused liver taken from clofibrate-treated rats the labeling of tissue
triglyceride from palmitate-^{14}C is higher than in the livers of
control animals (23).   Even though the apparently increased incorporation of precursors does not necessarily indicate an accelerated

synthesis but may also be accounted for by retarded removal, these observations support the view that clofibrate does not reduce plasma triglyceride level by inhibiting the overall synthesis of liver triglyceride. The possibility remains, however, that the synthesis of only that part of liver triglyceride which is being secreted directly into the plasma is suppressed, but this change is not detected without separation of storage and secretory triglyceride fractions.

A new possible pathway for the intrahepatic action of drugs of the clofibrate group has been suggested recently by the work of Maragoudakis (39-43). Using purified acetyl coenzyme A carboxyoase of chicken, rat,or monkey liver, he has demonstrated that these compounds act as rather specific inhibitors of this enzyme but do not influence the activity of fatty acid synthetase. In agreement with this enzyme inhibition these drugs have been found to reduce the synthesis of triglyceride fatty acids in cultured mammary cells (44). Whatever the role of this effect may be in the hypoglyceridemic action of these drugs, it is difficult to combine these in vitro findings with the increased incorporation of acetate into liver triglycerides observed in vivo during clofibrate treatment of rats (32, 38).

Studies on the action of clofibrate and its analogues on the release of triglycerides and lipoproteins from rat liver have uniformly demonstrated a definite inhibition at some stage of the secretory process. In isolated perfused rat liver the output of triglycerides into the medium is substantially lowered by administration of CPIB (1, 22, 23), and the incorporation of radioactivity from labeled palmitic acid and glucose into medium triglyceride is markedly reduced (36). Parallel results have been obtained in in vivo experiments on rats, where the plasma triglyceride and apolipoprotein radioactivity after injection of labeled precursors are less in animals given clofibrate than in controls (32, 33, 45). However, these findings cannot be taken as evidence of decreased production without making the unproved assumption that the removal remains uninfluenced by the drug. The observation that plasma triglyceride radioactivity was less in clofibrated-treated rats than in controls also after blocking the elimination with Triton speaks in favor of a real decrease of secretion of triglycerides (45). It is also important to note that the inhibition of triglyceride secretion can be observed within a few hours after a single dose of clofibrate (36, 45).

On the basis of all present evidence cited above it seems
probable that clofibrate blocks some step in the pathway of production and secretion of plasma very low density lipoproteins
(VLDL) (and LDL?) triglycerides in the liver and this forms the
main point of its hypoglyceridemic action, at least in experimental
animals.   The more exact mechanism of this inhibitory effect is
little explored.   Interestingly, Pereira and Holland (36) have
recently shown that clofibrate acutely depresses the α-glycerophosphate levels in the liver possibly through increasing the activity
of glycerophosphate dehydrogenase (26, 46).   As it is known that
increase of hepatic α-glycerophosphate levels (47-49) is accompanied by hyperglyceridemia this observation might provide one
clue to the mechanism of action of clofibrate.   A number of
clofibrate-induced alterations in hepatic enzyme activities have
been reported (26, 28, 50-52) but none of these has been reasonably
linked to the hypoglyceridemic action of the drug.   Again, there
is not the least evidence that these findings and views also apply to
man.

Effect on the Clearance of Plasma
Triglycerides and on Lipoprotein Lipase Activity

The   removal of triglycerides from the plasma occurs by first
order kinetics and the half-life (fractional rate) is partly dependent
on the concentration.   Therefore, it has been difficult to define
the action of any factor in the removal process.   If measurement
shows that under treatment a decrease of concentration is associated with increase of fractional removal rate there remains the
problem of which effect comes first and represents the primary
event.   This dilemma may explain the scarcity of data reporting
on the drug effects on plasma triglyceride efflux.   In one rat study
no influence of clofibrate treatment could be observed either on
plasma triglyceride level or on the removal rate of injected Triton-
hyperlipemic serum triglyceride (3).

There is also a considerable lack of agreement on the possible
influence of clofibrate on lipoprotein lipase activity of adipose
tissue.   In two reports no difference was found in this enzyme
between treated and control rats (7, 12) whereas a third investigation revealed a definite increase of lipoprotein lipase in adipose
tissue homogenate of rats given CPIB and chow diet (53).   In the
latter study there also appeared to be a temporal relationship
between reduction of serum triblyceride and stimulation of lipoprotein lipase.   The uptake of chylomicron fatty acids by adipose

tissue in vitro is probably increased by clofibrate treatment (12).
Postheparin plasma lipolytic activity has been reported to increase
by clofibrate administration (20) but not by Su-13437 (21).

Effect on Plasma Triglyceride Transport in Man

Contrary to the suggestions from animal experiments, the
results of previous turnover studies of plasma triglyceride in man
have generally supported the view that clofibrate and Su-13437 act
mainly by enhancing the removal of plasma tirglycerides. Unfortunately, the published data on this subject are few and incomplete.
Using incorporation of infused palmitic acid-^{14}C into plasma triglyceride as a measure of triglyceride production, Ryan and
Schwartz (19, 54) postulated that reduction of plasma triglyceride
concentration with CPIB in hyperlipemic subjects was not associated with any decrease of production rate but could be accounted
for by increased peripheral clearance of triglycerides. Spritz
(55) came to a similar conclusion by demonstrating that the half-
life of glycerol-labeled endogenous plasma triglycerides was
shortened by clofibrate treatment before any change of concentration had occurred. The fractional removal of intravenous fat
emulsion (Intralipid) is increased after lowering of plasma triglyceride with Su-13437 (21). On the other hand, by chemical measurement of hepatic triglyceride production, Boberg et al. (21)
demonstrated a marked decrease of triglyceride turnover rate
during administration of Su-13437. Recently Sodhi and associates
(56) have studied the metabolism of endogenous triglycerides by
the glycerol-^{3}H labeling technique before and after lowering of
plasma triglycerides with CPIB. The fractional turnover rate
was significantly decreased in six of nine subjects during the treatment but there was no correlation between the changes of fractional rate constant and triglyceride concentration. This result
was believed to indicate that fractional turnover rate is independent
of concentration and is the primary variable influenced by the drug.
However, this apparent lack of correlation could also be interpreted to show that the drug reduced tirglyceride concentration
independently of changes of fractional turnover rate, i.e., by decreasing the influx.

Some time ago we carried out a turnover study (57) which,
incidentally, was very similar to that of Sodhi et al. (56), but instead of clofibrate we used Su-13437 in nine subjects with endogenous hypertriglyceridemia (type IV). The results are shown in

TABLE I

EFFECT OF THE HYPOLIPIDEMIC DRUG Su-13437
ON PLASMA TRIGLYCERIDE TRANSPORT IN NINE
PATIENTS WITH ENDOGENOUS HYPERGLYCERIDEMIA

	Concentration Before During mg/100 ml		Fractional rate Before During h^{-1}		Turnover rate Before During mg/h/kg	
Mean	386	186	0.138	0.178	20.6	13.2
S.D.	195	74	0.053	0.091	4.4	4.3
Change	-52%		+29%		-36%	
p	<0.01		>0.05		<0.001	

Table I and Fig. 1.   In contrast to the observations of Sodhi et al.
(56) it was found that the drug decreased the total plasma triglyceride turnover (production) rate in all cases, whereas a marked
increase of fractional turnover rate was recorded in only three
instances, and the average change of this parameter during the
treatment was not significant.   From these results one must conclude that Su-13437 acts mainly by reducing the production of
plasma triglycerides, but it is possible that the triglyceride removal efficiency may also be improved in some cases.   By using
a nonisotope heparin-infusion method for estimation of triglyceride
transport, Bierman et al. (20) have recently reported very similar
results on the mechanism of action of clofibrate.   In our study,
as in that of Sodhi et al. (56), no significant linear correlation was
apparent between plasma triglyceride concentration and fractional
rate constant.   In fact, the relationship of these two parameters
is not linear but is best described by a hyperbolic curve, which
more or less clearly emerges from the data of both studies (Fig. 2).
This means that at a high triglyceride concentration range, wide
variations of concentration are produced by small changes of production or removal rates (often unmeasurable), whereas at the
lower end of the concentration scale relatively large changes of
flux are needed to produce marked alterations of concentration.
Comparison of the plots in Fig. 2 suggests that actually there is
not very much difference between the two series of drug experiments.   With both the points seem to move downwards along the

hyperbolic curve. From our data a linear transform of the relationship concentration/fractional turnover was made separately
for pretreatment and on-treatment values, and these functions
were statistically compared. This analysis revealed that at a
given triglyceride concentration the fractional rate was less during treatment than before it. This result suggests that the drug
did not influence triglyceride level by increasing the fractional
removal.

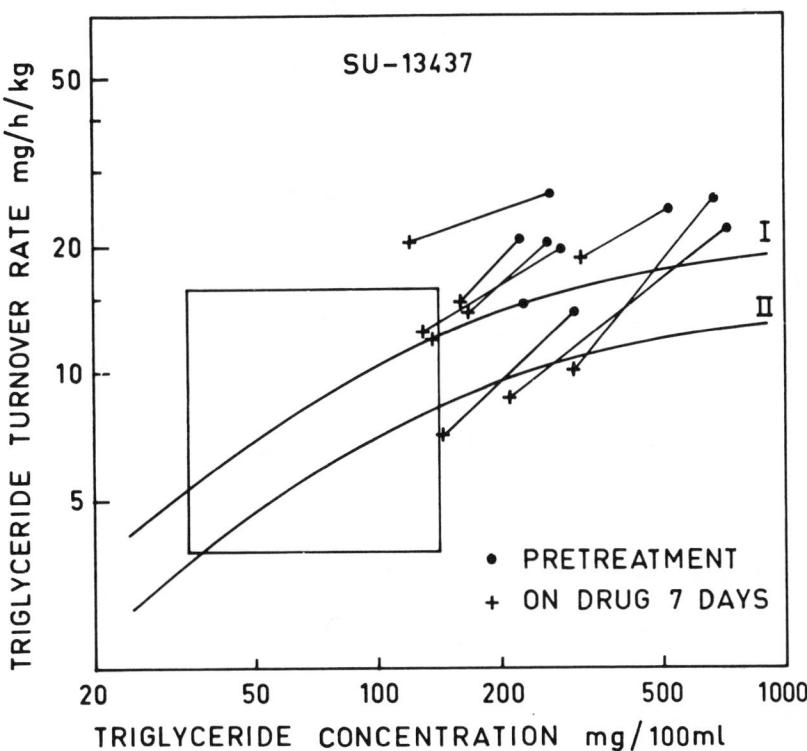

Fig. 1. Changes of plasma triglyceride concentration and turnover
rate in nine hyperglyceridemic patients during treatment with hypolipidemic agent Su-13437. The square delineates the area of normal values, the curves designated I and II describe the correlation
of the two parameters in normal population, which contains two
different kinetic subgroups. Note that every case shows a decrease of turnover and concentration even though there is no definite correlation between the individual values. Black dot = before
treatment, cross = during treatment.

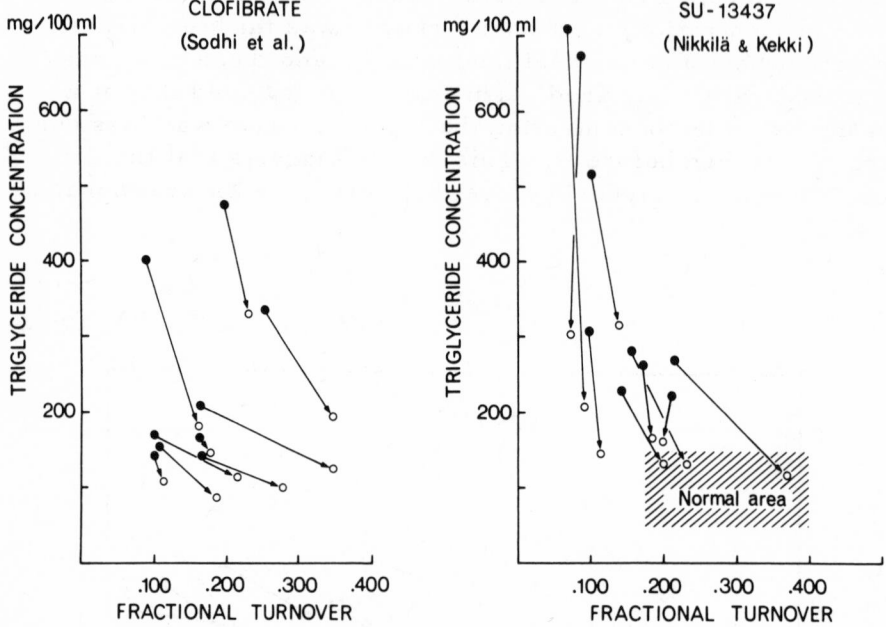

Fig. 2. Correlation of plasma triglyceride concentration and fractional rate constant (fraction per hour) before and during treatment with either clofibrate or its analogue Su-13437.   The black
dots indicate values before treatment, open circles during treatment.   It is seen that with both drugs the values are moving along
a hyperbolic curve.   The essential difference is that in the clofibrate series most patients have starting triglyceride levels below
200 mg/100 ml while in the Su-13437 experiment the patients have
hyperglyceridemia of more severe degree.

Conclusions

The probably sites of action of clofibrate and its analogues on
plasma triglyceride metabolism are presented in Table II.   It is
apparent that some key points have been insufficiently examined
so far.   Particularly the processes of apo-peptide synthesis, its
association with the lipid, and the release of the particle from
hepatic cell are poorly understood and still represent one likely
locus of action of the hypoglyceridemic drugs.

TABLE II

POSSIBLE METABOLIC ACTIONS OF CPIB AND
ANALOGUES IN THE PATHWAYS OF PLASMA
TRIGLYCERIDE PRODUCTION AND UTILIZATION

1.	Release of FFA from adipose tissue	Decreased
2.	Concentration of plasma FFA	Decreased
3.	Hepatic uptake of circulating FFA	No effect
4.	Hepatic α-glycerophosphate content	Decreased
5.	Activity of liver triglyceride "synthesis"	?
6.	Hepatic triglyceride synthesis	Increased?
7.	Hepatic lipogenesis	Decreased
8.	Apolipoprotein synthesis	?
9.	Release of VLDL-triglyceride from the liver	Decreased
10.	Activity of lipoprotein lipase in adipose tissue	Increased?
11.	Uptake of circulating triglycerides at periphery	Increased?

NICOTINIC ACID AND OTHER ANTILIPOLYTIC AGENTS

The different metabolic effects of nicotinic acid have been
thoroughly reviewed in a recent symposium (58) and it is therefore
unnecessary to repeat the details here.   The most marked primary action of this group of drugs is the inhibition of breakdown
of adipose tissue triglycerides.   This effect is probably based on
a decrease of cyclic AMP in fat cells, and the site of action is
adenyl cyclase rather than phosphodiesterase.

The question may be raised as to whether the lowering of
plasma triglyceride concentration by acute or chronic administration of nicotinic acid is completely accounted for by the decreased
transport of FFA and glycerol or is it necessary to assume that
these drugs also have other primary sites of action on triglyceride
metabolism.   With different derivatives of nicotinic acid there
seems to be a good correlation between the antilipolytic activity
in vitro and the lipid lowering effect in vivo (59).   On the other
hand, the average daily plasma FFA concentration is not decreased
during nicotinic acid treatment and may be even higher than in a
comparable placebo group (60, 61).   The acute inhibition of lipolysis with nicotinic acid is followed by a strong rebound elevation of
plasma FFA and fat cell cyclic AMP levels (62-64), and the sum

effect may be an increased rather than reduced plasma FFA concentration and turnover.

Two additional points of action of nicotinic acid have been discussed previously (65, 66). These are the possible depression of hepatic triglyceride synthesis and release, and secondly, activation of lipoprotein lipase.

From a study with isolated perfused rat liver, Mishkel and Webb (23) concluded that chronic treatment of animals with nicotinic acid did not influence hepatic uptake of FFA, their incorporation into tissue triglycerides, or conversion to medium triglycerides. In a similar study but administering nicotinic acid one hour before sacrifice we found that transfer of labeled FFA into medium triglycerides was less in livers of treated animals than in those of controls (65). Also, in in vivo experiments with rats, nicotinic acid decreases the incorporation of injected palmitic acid into plasma triglycerides (65, 67). An example of these studies is shown in Fig. 3. The incorporation of radioactivity from labeled acetate and glucose into liver and plasma triglyceride is also diminished after a single dose of nicotinic acid (65). These results may indicate that nicotinic acid has a direct depressing effect on the synthesis of liver and plasma triglycerides but they can be equally well explained on the basis of inhibition of adipose tissue lipolysis: The decrease of plasma-free glycerol is accompanied by a decline of cytoplasmatic α-glycerophosphate concentration in the liver, and this inhibits synthesis of secretory triglycerides.

The observation that nicotinic acid rapidly increases the lipoprotein lipase activity of adipose tissue (68-70) in fed and fasted rats has been confirmed by several investigators (71-73), even if there is still some uncertainty about the mechanism of this action (66, 71, 73). On the other hand, the postheparin plasma lipolytic activity is not increased by acute or chronic administration of nicotinic acid (66, 74).

As to the influence of nicotinic acid on the removal efficiency of plasma triglycerides it is well possible that this forms one of the main sites of the hypoglyceridemic effect of this drug. Several studies have shown that nicotinic acid accelerates the removal of chylomicron triglycerides and of intravenous fat emulsion from the circulation in rats and man (66, 74-76). The half-life of

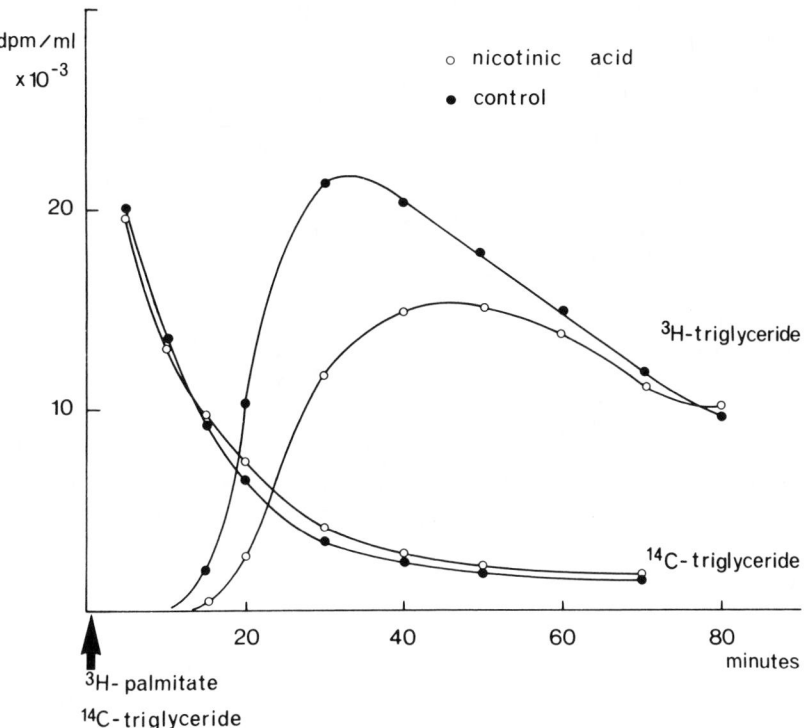

Fig. 3.   Influence of nicotinic acid infusion (iv. 0.5 mg/min) on the rate of disappearance of labeled endogenous plasma triglyceride (^{14}C)-fatty acid and on the appearance of injected ^{3}H-palmitic acid into plasma triglyceride fraction in anesthetized rat.

endogenous plasma triglycerides of rat is also shortened after a single dose of nicotinic acid (66).

Only one study has been reported on the effect of nicotinic acid on plasma triglyceride turnover in man.   Sailer and Bolzano (77) found that the rate of conversion of plasma FFA to plasma triglycerides was markedly decreased on infusion of pyridylcarbinol (Ronicol ^{R}).   This observation is in good agreement with corresponding data obtained in rats (see Table III) and supports the view that the lowering effect of nicotinic acid on plasma triglyceride is at least partly accounted for by reduced production in the liver. We have attempted to study the effect of nicotinic acid on the plasma

TABLE III

PROPOSED SITES FOR THE HYPOGLYCERIDEMIC ACTION OF NICOTINIC ACID AND ITS DERIVATIVES

1.	Release of FFA from adipose tissue	Decreased→ Increased
2.	Concentration of plasma FFA and glycerol	Decreased→ Increased
3.	Hepatic uptake of circulating FFA	Decreased
4.	Hepatic glycerophosphate content	Decreased?
5.	Activity of liver "triglyceride synthetase"	?
6.	Hepatic triglyceride synthesis	Decreased
7.	Hepatic lipogenesis	?
8.	Apolipoprotein synthesis	Decreased?
9.	Release of VLDL-triglyceride from the liver	Decreased
10.	Activity of lipoprotein lipase in adipose tissue	Increased
11.	Peripheral uptake of circulating triglycerides	Increased?

triglyceride kinetics in man by applying the radioglycerol technique but so far with little success since it has been impossible to achieve steady state conditions.

The known effects of nicotinic acid on the pathway of plasma triglyceride synthesis and degradation are summarized in Table III. Even though the mechanism of action of this group of drugs is much better clarified than that of clofibrate, it is not possible to conclude which of the effects is of major importance.

ANABOLIC STEROIDS

Various steroid derivatives with androgenic and/or anabolic activity have been tested for treatment of hypertriglyceridemia on a purely empirical basis. Some of them have effectively reduced plasma triglyceride levels but have not gained general clinical acceptance. Also their mode of action has remained largely obscure. A new approach in this field has been made by Glueck and associates who demonstrated that a progestational steroid, norethindrone, is a potent hypoglyceridemic agent in different types of familial hyperglyceridemia and that the decrease of triglycerides is associated with an increase of postheparin plasma lipolytic activity (78). Recently they have reported similar find-ings with an anabolic synthetic steroid, oxandrolone, which also stimulated the activity of postheparin plasma lipases concurrent with decrease of circulating triglyceride in patients with type III, IV and V hyperlipoproteinemia (79). It remains to be determined whether these two effects are in causal relationship and whether the increase of postheparin plasma lipases reflects an elevated concentration of tissue lipoprotein lipase activities.

ORAL CONTRACEPTIVE STEROIDS

This group of drugs is known to increase plasma triglyceride levels (80, 81) and even to cause gross hyperlipemia (82). The mechanism of this adverse effect has not been clarified even though the finding that postheparin lipolytic activity is decreased by oral contraceptives (81, 83) has suggested that the increase of triglyceride level might be attributed to an impaired elimination of endogenous triglycerides from the circulation. However, this possibility has been recently challenged and no defect in the re-moval of exogenous fat has been detected (84).

To get more information on the mechanism of the hyperglyc-eridemic action of oral contraceptive steroids we determined the parameters of triglyceride transport, shown in Fig. 4, in thirteen women using these drugs and compared the results with those of a group of healthy fertile-aged women who had never used these agents (85). The technique was, again, the radioglycerol proce-dure (57). The results show that oral contraceptives caused a very unusual and definite pattern of changes in plasma triglyceride kinetics. The increase of concentration (average 1.5-fold) was associated with a marked increase of plasma triglyceride produc-tion (total transport, average 1.9-fold), but this was partially compensated for by a simultaneous acceleration of triglyceride removal. The latter effect is revealed by an increase of frac-tional rate constant (in spite of increasing concentration) and a decrease of the K_m removal. Thus, in contrast to earlier views it seems that oral contraceptive steroid combination does not im-pair the removal of circulating triglycerides, but conversely, in-creases the efficiency of efflux. This effect is hardly accounted for by the estrogen component of the pill since the experiments carried out in our laboratory by Dr. Pykälistö show that a single injection of estrogen to male or female rats significantly decreases the lipoprotein lipase activity of adipose tissue (Table IV). On the

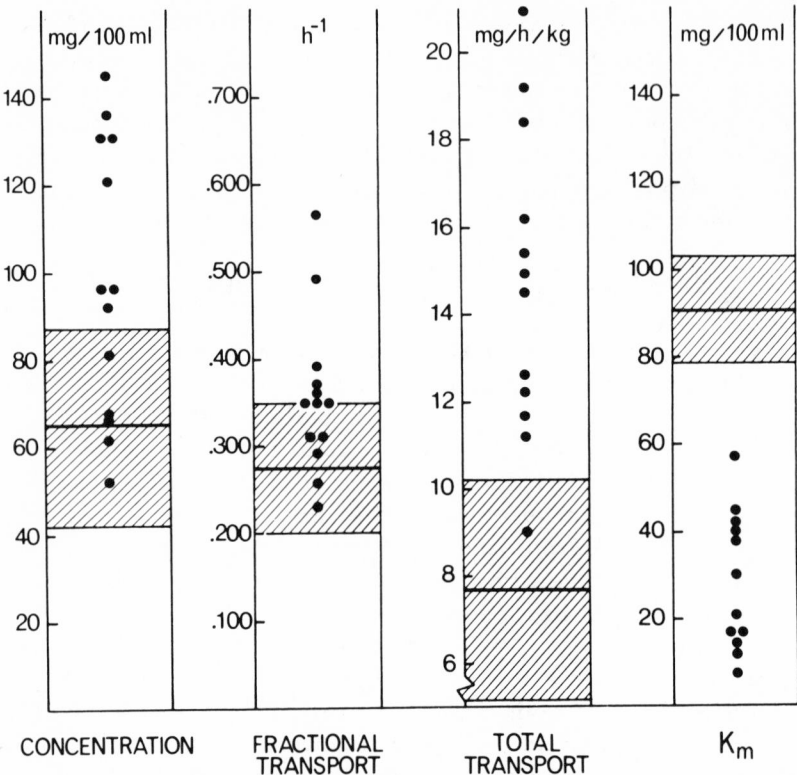

Fig. 4. Parameters of plasma triglyceride metabolism in 13 fertile-aged women taking oral contraceptive drugs (black dots). The hatched area indicates the mean ± one s.d. of healthy young females who never had used contraceptive pills. The Michaelis constant K_m gives the turnover (removal) rate at half-maximal triglyceride concentration and it is inversely correlated to the efficiency of removal.

other hand, the possibility that the progestagen component of the drug might be responsible for the favorable effect on triglyceride removal is compatible with the results of Glueck et al. (78) mentioned above. It is thus evident that like many other adverse side effects of the pill the development of hyperglyceridemia is caused by the estrogen, which increases the production of plasma triglycerides in the liver and possibly also impairs their removal, but the latter effect is counteracted by the progestagen.

TABLE IV

EFFECT OF ESTROGEN ADMINISTRATION (ETHINYL-
ESTRADIOL 3 DAYS) ON PLASMA TRIGLYCERIDE
AND LIPOPROTEIN LIPASE ACTIVITY OF
ADIPOSE TISSUE OF FEMALE RATS (86)

	Control	Estrogen	p
Plasma triglyceride mg/100 ml	107 ± 22	146 ± 36	< 0.05
Postheparin plasma lipase*	1.73 ± 0.21	1.04 ± 0.25	<0.001
Adipose tissue:			
Release of FFA µmoles/g/hr	0.99 ± 0.31	1.70 ± 0.54	<0.05
Lipoprotein lipase µmoles/g/hr	2.95 ± 1.09	1.31 ± 0.60	<0.01

*Samples taken 10 min after injection of heparin, activity meas-
ured with labeled rat plasma triglyceride as substrate, and results expressed as µmoles of FFA liberated per ml per min.

ACKNOWLEDGMENTS

This work has been aided by grants from the Sigrid Jusélius
Foundation, Helsinki, and The Finnish State Medical Research
Council.

REFERENCES

1. Azarnoff, D.L., D.R. Tucker, and G.A. Barr, Metabolism
   14: 959 (1965).
2. Kokatnur, M.G., G.T. Malcom, and R.D. Martinez,
   Metabolism 18: 73 (1969).
3. Byers, S.O. and M. Friedman, Atherosclerosis 11:373
   (1970).
4. Zakim, D. and R.H. Herman, J. Atheroscler. Res. 10: 91
   (1969).
5. Kokatnur, M.G. and G.T. Malcom, Atherosclerosis 12: 193
   (1970).
6. Hess, R. and W.L. Bencze, Experientia 24: 418 (1968).
7. Brown, D.F., Metabolism 15: 868 (1966).
8. Hoak, J.C., W.E. Connor, M.L. Armstrong,and E.D.
   Warner, Lab. Invest. 19: 370 (1968).

9. Thorp, J.M., J. Atheroscler. Res. 3: 351 (1963).

10. Speake, R.N., Progr. biochem. Pharmacol. 2: 372 (1967).

11. Barrett, A.M., Brit. J. Pharmacol. Chemother. 26: 363 (1966).

12. Nestel, P.J. and W. Austin, J. Atheroscler. Res. 8: 827 (1968).

13. Greene, H.L., R.H. Herman,and D. Zakim, Proc. Soc.exp. Biol. Med. 134: 1035 (1970).

14. Barrett, A.M. and J.M. Thorp, Brit. J. Pharmacol. Chemother. 32: 381 (1968).

15. Cenedella, R.J., J.J. Jarrell, and L.H. Saxe, J. Atheroscler. Res. 8: 903 (1968).

16. MacMillan, D.C., M.F. Oliver, J.D. Simpson, and P. Tothill, Lancet 2: 924 (1965).

17. Rifkind, B.M., Metabolism 15: 673 (1966).

18. Duncan, C.H., M.M. Best, and G.L. Robertson, Lancet 1: 191 (1965).

19. Ryan, W.G. and T.B. Schwartz, J. Lab. Clin. Med. 64: 1001 (1964).

20. Bierman, E.L., D. Porte, Jr., and J.D. Brunzell, Clin. Res. 18: 537 (1970).

21. Boberg, J., L.A. Carlson, S.O. Fröberg, and L. Orö, Atherosclerosis 11: 353 (1970).

22. Duncan, C.H., M.M. Best, and A. Despopoulos, Circulation 29: III-7 (1964).

23. Mishkel, M.A. and W.F. Webb, Biochem. Pharmacol. 16: 897 (1967).

24. Paget, G.E., J. Atheroscler. Res. 3: 729 (1963).

25. Best, M.M. and C.H. Duncan, J. Lab. Clin. Med. 64: 634 (1964).

26. Hess, R., W. Stäubli, and W. Riess, Nature 208: 856 (1965).

27. Svoboda, D.J. and D.L. Azarnoff, J. Cell Biol. 30: 442 (1966).

28. Kaneko, A., S. Sakamoto, M. Morita, and T. Onoé, Tohoku J. exp. Med. 99: 81 (1969).

29. Thorp, J.M. and W.S. Waring, Nature 194: 948 (1962).

30. Platt, D.S. and J.M. Thorp, Biochem. Pharmacol. 15: 915 (1966).

31. Kurup, C.K.R., H.N. Aithal, and T. Ramasarma, Biochem. J. 116: 773 (1970).

32. Gould, R.G., E.A. Swyryd, D. Avoy, and B. Coan, Progr. biochem. Pharmacol. 2: 345 (1967).

33. Gould, R.G., E.A. Swyryd, B.J. Coan, and D.R. Avoy, J. Atheroscler. Res. 6: 555 (1966).

34. Best, M.M. and C.H. Duncan, Atherosclerosis 12: 185 (1970).
35. Young, D.L., G. Powell, and W.O. McMillan, J. Lipid Res. 12: 1 (1971).
36. Pereira, J.N. and G.F. Holland, in Atherosclerosis. Proceedings of the Second International Symposium. (Ed.) R.J. Jones, Springer-Verlag, New York (1970) p. 549.
37. Spritz, N. and C.S. Lieber, Proc. Soc. exp. Biol. Med. 121: 147 (1966).
38. Duncan, C.H. and M.M. Best, Circulation 39: III-6 (1969).
39. Maragoudakis, M.E., J. Biol. Chem. 244: 5005 (1969).
40. Maragoudakis, M.E., Biochemistry 9: 413 (1970).
41. Maragoudakis, M.E., J. Biol. Chem. 245: 4136 (1970).
42. Maragoudakis, M.E., in Atherosclerosis. Proceedings of the Second International Symposium. (Ed.) R.J. Jones, Springer-Verlag, New York (1970) p. 554.
43. Maragoudakis, M.E. and H. Hankin, J. Biol. Chem. 246: 348 (1971).
44. Maragoudakis, M.E., J. Biol. Chem. 246: 4046 (1971).
45. Segal, P., P.S. Roheim, and H.A. Eder, Circulation 39: III-182 (1969).
46. Westerfeld, W.W., D.A. Richert, and W.R. Ruegamer, Biochem. Pharmacol. 17: 100 (1968).
47. Nikkilä, E.A. and K. Ojala, Proc. Soc. exp. Biol. Med. 113: 814 (1963).
48. Nikkilä, E.A. and K. Ojala, Life Sci. 3: 1021 (1964).
49. Nikkilä, E.A. and K. Ojala, Life Sci. 4: 937 (1965).
50. Platt, D.S. and B.L. Cockrill, Biochem. Pharmacol. 15: 927 (1966).
51. Schacht, U. and E Granzer, Biochem. Pharmacol. 19: 2963 (1970).
52. Zakim, D., R.S. Paradini, and R.H. Herman, Biochem. Pharmacol. 19: 305 (1970).
53. Tolman, E.L., H.M. Tepperman, and J. Tepperman, Amer. J. Physiol. 218: 1313 (1970).
54. Ryan, W.G. and T.B. Schwartz, Metabolism 14: 1243 (1965).
55. Spritz, N., Circulation 32: II-201 (1965).
56. Sodhi, H.S., B.J. Kudchodkar, and L. Horlick, Metabolism 20: 309 (1971).
57. Nikkilä, E.A. and M. Kekki, Acta Med. Scand. 190: 1971 (in press).
58. Gey, K.F. and L.A. Carlson (Eds.), Nicotinic Acid. Symposium in Flims, Switzerland (1971).

59. Dalton, C., J.B. Quinn, H.J. Crowley, and O.N. Miller, in Nicotinic Acid. Symposium in Flims. (Eds.) K. Gey and L.A. Carlson, Switzerland 1971 (in press).

60. Carlström, S. and S. Laurell, Acta Med. Scand. 184: 121 (1968).

61. Fröberg, S.O., J. Boberg, L.A. Carlson, and M. Eriksson, in Nicotinic Acid. Symposium in Flims. (Eds.) K. Gey and L.A. Carlson, Switzerland 1971 (in press).

62. Carlson, L.A. and L. Orö, Acta Med. Scand. 172: 641 (1962).

63. Pereira, J.N., J. Lipid Res. 8: 239 (1967).

64. Burkard, W.P., H. Lengsfeld, and K.F. Gey, in Nicotinic Acid. Symposium in Flims. (Eds.) K. Gey and L.A. Carlson, Switzerland 1971 (in press).

65. Nikkilä, E.A., in Nicotinic Acid. Symposium in Flims. (Eds.) K. Gey and L.A. Carlson, Switzerland (1971) p. 137.

66. Nikkilä, E.A., in Nicotinic Acid. Symposium in Flims. (Eds.) K. Gey and L.A. Carlson, Switzerland (1971) p. 147.

67. Sólyom, A. and L. Puglisi, Progr. biochem. Pharmacol. 3: 409 (1967).

68. Nikkilä, E.A. and O. Pykälistö, Biochem. Biophys. Acta 152: 421 (1968).

69. Nikkilä, E.A. and O. Pykälistö, Life Sci. 7: 1303 (1968).

70. Nikkilä, E.A. and O. Pykälistö, in Drugs Affecting Lipid Metabolism. (Eds.) W.L. Holmes, L.A. Carlson, and R. Paoletti, Plenum Press, New York (1969) p. 239.

71. Otway, S., D.S. Robinson, M.P. Rogers, and D.R. Wing, in Nicotinic Acid. Symposium in Flims. (Eds.) K. Gey and L. A. Carlson, Switzerland 1971 (in press).

72. Shafrir, E. and Y. Biale, in Nicotinic Acid. Symposium in Flims. (Eds.) K. Gey and L.A. Carlson, Switzerland 1971 (in press).

73. Pykälistö, O., Regulation of the Adipose Tissue Lipoprotein Lipase by Free Fatty Acids. Dissertation, Helsinki, 1970.

74. Boberg, J., L.A. Carlson, S. Fröberg, A. Olsson, L. Orö, and S. Rössner, in Nicotinic Acid. Symposium in Flims. (Eds.) K. Gey and L.A. Carlson, Switzerland 1971 (in press).

75. Jacobs, R.S., M.S. Grebner, and D.L. Cook, Proc. Soc. exp. Biol. Med. 119: 1117 (1965).

76. Barboriak, J.J., R.C. Meade, J. Owenby, R.A. Stiglitz, Arch. Int. Pharmacodyn. 176: 249 (1968).

77. Sailer, S. and K. Bolzano, in Nicotinic Acid. Symposium in Flims. (Eds.) K. Gey and L.A. Carlson, Switzerland 1971 (in press).

78. Glueck, C.J., W.V. Brown, R.I. Levy, H. Greten, and D. S. Fredrickson, Lancet 1: 1290 (1969).
79. Glueck, C.J., Metabolism 20: 691 (1971).
80. Wynn, V., J.W.H. Doar, and G.L. Mills, Lancet 2: 720 (1966).
81. Hazzard, W.R., M.I. Spiger, J.D. Bagdade, and E.L. Bierman, New Engl. J. Med. 280: 471 (1969).
82. Zorrilla, E., M. Hulse, A. Hernandez, and H. Gershberg, J. Clin. Endocrin. Metab. 28: 1793 (1968).
83. Ham, J.M. and R. Rose, Amer. J. Obstet. Gynec. 105: 628 (1969).
84. Hazzard, W.R., M.J. Spiger, and E.L. Bierman, in Metabolic Effects of Gonadal Hormone and Contraceptive Steroids. (Eds.) H.A. Salhanick, D.M. Kipnis, and R.L. Vande Wiele, Plenum Press, New York (1969) p. 232.
85. Nikkilä, E.A. and M. Kekki, Metabolism 20: 1971 (in press).
86. Pykälistö, O. and E.A. Nikkilä, 1971, to be published.

THE ECONOMY OF CHOLESTEROL IN MAN: DRUG EFFECTS

E. H. Ahrens, Jr.

The Rockefeller University, New York, New York

A partial list of the factors controlling the movement and storage of cholesterol in man must include: intake; absorption; lipoprotein synthesis and transport capacity; tissue equilibria with plasma cholesterol; endogenous synthesis; conversion to bile acids; pool sizes; excretion rates and pathways. All of these can now be defined with directness and exactitude except for measurement of pool sizes and of tissue-plasma equilibria, utilizing sterol balance and isotope kinetic techniques. Although pool sizes can be estimated by isotope kinetics, as yet we have no independent means by which to verify these estimates.

Examples will be given of the effects on cholesterol metabolism of various drug and diet interventions. From the evidence accumulated since 1960 the conclusion is inescapable that changes in plasma cholesterol concentration are only weakly indicative of changes in total body economy of cholesterol. Indeed, in terms of the chain of events leading to atherosclerosis, it may be more important to know the degree of saturation of tissue stores with cholesterol than to know the "head of pressure" of plasma lipoprotein cholesterol.

EFFECTS OF DRUGS ON THE METABOLISM OF BILE ACIDS

N. B. Myant

Medical Research Council Lipid Metabolism Unit

Hammersmith Hospital, London, W12 OHS

Bile acids are the main end products of the breakdown of cholesterol and their metabolism is intimately linked with that of cholesterol. Hence, the study of the effects of drugs on bile acid metabolism, apart from its intrinsic interest, is relevant to the problem of hypercholesterolaemia. Drugs that modify bile acid metabolism may also be used to produce experimental situations that provide information as to how sterol metabolism is regulated. In this review I shall describe briefly those steps in the synthesis and subsequent fate of bile acids that are likely to be susceptible to the actions of drugs and I shall then discuss the effects of various agents, including hormones and certain dietary factors, that are known to influence bile acid metabolism.

NORMAL PHYSIOLOGY OF BILE ACIDS

Synthesis

In rats and human beings the principal bile acids synthesized in the liver are cholic and chenodeoxycholic acids. The first step in the formation of cholic acid is the 7α-hydroxylation of cholesterol (1). This is followed by further modifications to the nucleus, including the introduction of a 12α-OH group. After completion of these changes in the nucleus, three carbon atoms are removed from the side chain by oxidative cleavage (Fig. 1). The main pathway for the formation of chenodeoxycholic acid is probably analogous to that for cholic acid, but some chenodeoxycholic acid may be formed by another pathway in which oxidation of the side chain precedes the changes in the nucleus (2). Before leaving the liver, the bile acids are conjugated with glycine or taurine by the formation of peptide bonds.

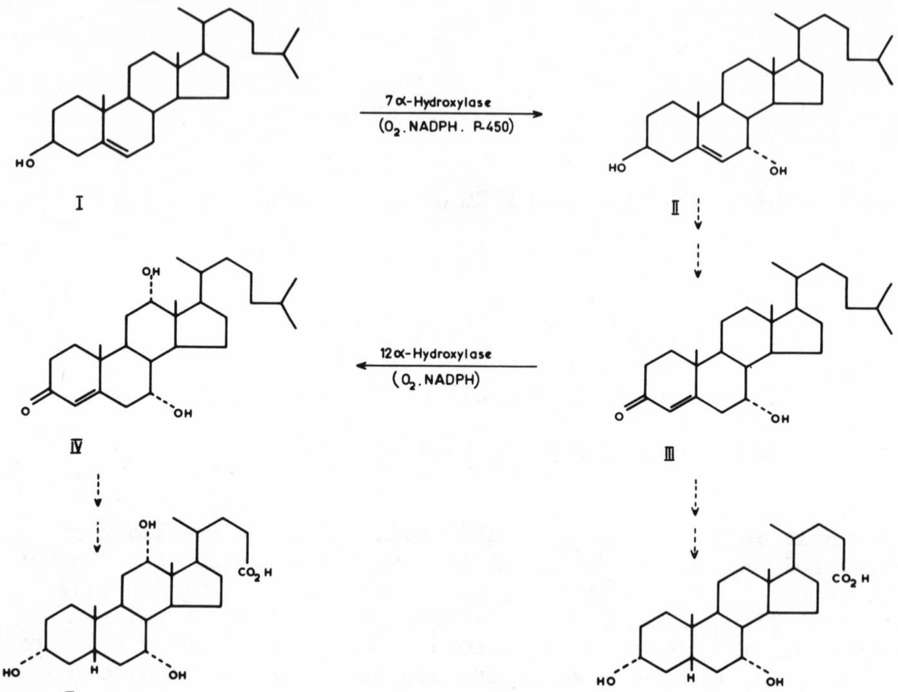

Fig. 1.   Some intermediates in the formation of bile acids from
cholesterol.   I, Cholesterol;   II, 7α-hydroxycholesterol;
III, 7α-hydroxycholest-4-en-3-one;   IV, 7α,12α-dihydroxycholest-4-
en-3-one;   V, cholic acid;   VI, chenodeoxycholic acid.

The formation of 7α-hydroxycholesterol in the liver is
catalyzed by a microsomal enzyme system (3).   The overall reaction
is highly complex but consists essentially in the introduction of
one atom of molecular oxygen into the cholesterol nucleus, the
other oxygen atom being reduced to water by NADPH in the presence
of cytochrome P-450 and NADPH-cytochrome c reductase:

$$\text{Cholesterol} + O_2 + \text{NADPH} + H^+ \xrightarrow[\substack{(\text{NADPH-c} \\ \text{reductase})}]{(\text{P-450})} \begin{array}{l} \text{7α-Hydroxycholesterol} + \\ \text{NADP}^+ + H_2O \end{array}$$

The term "cholesterol 7α-hydroxylase" is used rather loosely for
the enzyme system that catalyzes the overall reaction.

Indirect evidence suggests that the 7α-hydroxylation of
cholesterol is the rate-limiting step in bile acid formation (4)
and is therefore the step whose modification is most likely to
affect the rate of conversion of cholesterol into bile acids.

The concentration of P-450 in liver microsomes appears to be rate-limiting for the hydroxylation of some drugs, such as phenobarbital (5), suggesting that P-450 may be rate-limiting for the 7α-hydroxylation of cholesterol. If this were so, it might provide a foot-hold for attempts to modify this important reaction, since the P-450 of liver microsomes is inducible by drugs. Current evidence on this point is conflicting. Shefer et al. (6) found that liver microsomes from rats treated with phenobarbital, a drug that increases microsomal P-450 concentration, converted more [14C]-cholesterol into [14C] 7α-hydroxycholesterol than normal liver microsomes. Others (7, 8, 9), however, have not found any stimulatory effect of phenobarbital on the 7α-hydroxylation of cholesterol. Moreover, when rats are treated with cholestyramine the 7α-hydroxylation of cholesterol by their liver microsomes is stimulated (6), but there is no increase in microsomal P-450 concentration (Table 1). This result is not consistent with the view that P-450 is rate-limiting for 7α-hydroxylation. It is unlikely, therefore, that the concentration of P-450 in liver microsomes determines the rate of formation of the first intermediate in the synthesis of bile acids from cholesterol. Hence, there is little reason to expect that attempts to increase the catabolism of cholesterol by modifying the concentration of P-450 in the liver would be successful.

TABLE 1

EFFECT OF CHOLESTYRAMINE ON THE FORMATION OF 7α-HYDROXYCHOLESTEROL FROM CHOLESTEROL, THE ACTIVITY OF NADPH-c REDUCTASE AND THE CONCENTRATION OF CYTOCHROME P-450 IN RAT LIVER MICROSOMES

Treatment	Formation of 7α-OH cholesterol (nmoles/mg of protein/hr)	P-450 (nmoles/mg of protein)	NADPH-c reductase (nmoles/mg of protein/min)
Standard diet	3.5	1.44	117
Standard diet + 5% cholestyramine	7.0	1.38	96

Livers pooled from six rats were used for each set of values. The preparation and incubation of the microsomal suspension (6) and assay methods for 7α-hydroxycholesterol (10), P-450 and NADPH-c reductase (11, 12) are described elsewhere. (K.A. Mitropoulos and S. Balasubramaniam, unpublished observations.)

The introduction of the 12α-OH group into the steroid nucleus (Fig. 1) is catalyzed by a microsomal enzyme system that requires molecular O_2 and NADPH but not P-450 (13). This reaction is important because it occurs at the branch point in the main pathway for the formation of cholic and chenodeoxycholic acids. It is thus possible that changes in 12α-hydroxylase activity may influence the relative rates of formation of these two acids. The specificity of the 12α-hydroxylase in rat liver is such that it cannot catalyze the introduction of the 12α-OH group unless the side chain of the substrate is intact. Hence 26-hydroxy-cholesterol can be converted into chenodeoxycholic but not into cholic acid in vivo (14). As we shall see, the influence of thyroid hormone on bile acid metabolism is probably due partly to an effect on 12α-hydroxylation.

Enterohepatic Circulation

The bile acids undergo an enterohepatic circulation in which about 95% of the bile acid entering the duodenum is reabsorbed via the portal vein, the small quantity that escapes reabsorption being excreted in the faeces. Bile acids returning to the liver are extracted from the plasma and re-excreted in the bile. In the steady state, the loss of bile acids in the faeces is balanced by synthesis from cholesterol at an equal rate. During their passage down the intestine the bile acids are modified by the actions of bacteria present in the lower ileum, caecum and colon. In man, the main bacterial modifications are deconjugation to give free bile acids, and 7α-dehydroxylation, giving rise to the secondary bile acids, deoxycholic and lithocholic acids. In the absence of bacteria in the intestine, as in animals treated with antibiotics, these transformations do not occur and so the pattern of bile acids excreted in the faeces is identical with that in the bile. Free bile acids, including some of the secondary bile acids with modified ring-systems, are absorbed from the intestine, reconjugated in the liver and excreted in the bile.

Intestinal Absorption

The bile acids are absorbed from the intestine by active transport in the ileum and by passive diffusion which, under appropriate conditions, may occur throughout most of the intestinal tract (15). Active transport is most rapid for the more polar bile acids and the K_m value for active transport (the intraluminal concentration at which half the maximal rate is achieved) is considerably greater for free than for conjugated bile acids. Bile acids are absorbed by passive diffusion mainly when they are in nonionized form. Conjugated bile acids, being relatively strong acids, are almost completely ionized at the pH of the intestinal lumen. Hence, they are not available for absorption by passive nonionic diffusion, but are absorbed by active transport in the ileum. Free bile acids, on the other hand, are to a considerable extent nnionized in the intestinal lumen. Under normal conditions, deconjugating bacteria are not present in the jejunum. However, free bile acids are formed in the ileum and their absorption by passive nonionic diffusion at this level of the intestine may well contribute substantially to the overall absorption of bile acids. The manner in which chemo-therapeutic agents may affect this process is considered below.

Regulation

Bile acid synthesis is regulated by negative feedback, the bile acids returning to the liver via the portal vein inhibiting their own synthesis, probably by repression of cholesterol 7α-hydroxylase. Thus, when the enterohepatic circulation is inter-rupted by a bile fistula, bile acid synthesis is stimulated and 7α-hydroxylase activity increases (16). Interference with the return of bile acids to the liver also leads to an increase in hepatic synthesis of cholesterol, either by a direct effect on cholesterol synthesis or indirectly by diminishing the absorption of cholesterol.

EFFECTS OF DRUGS

Cholestyramine and Other Unabsorbable Drugs

Cholestyramine is an anionic exchange resin that binds bile acids in the intestinal lumen when given by mouth in the chloride form. It therefore interferes with the return of bile acids to the liver and so releases bile acid synthesis from feedback inhibition of 7α-hydroxylase (Table 2). As we have seen, diminished reabsorption of bile acids also leads to increased hepatic synthesis of cholesterol. However, in many species, including man, the increase in cholesterol synthesis is not sufficient to compensate for the increase in cholesterol catabo-lism and the net result is therefore a fall in plasma cholesterol concentration. In rats (17) and pigs (18) cholestyramine does not lower the plasma cholesterol level, despite a marked effect on faecal excretion of bile acids.

When given to human subjects at a dose level of 20 g/day cholestyramine causes a five- to tenfold increase in the faecal output of bile acids, but usually has little effect on fat absorption. Presumably, the increase in bile acid synthesis in the liver is sufficient to maintain a concentration of bile acids in the jejunum that is adequate for the formation of mixed micelles in the presence of cholestyramine. Cholestyramine at this dose level may increase the faecal excretion of neutral

sterols by interfering with their absorption.   When larger doses
of cholestyramine are given the increased excretion of neutral fat
may be sufficient to cause steatorrhea (19).

        In most patients with primary hyperbetalipoproteinaemia,
cholestyramine lowers the plasma cholesterol level and may cause
the disappearance of skin xanthomata if these are present.   Since
it is essentially nontoxic, it is therefore the treatment of
choice for this disease, either alone or in combination with other
measures.   However, in the rare homozygous form of familial
hyperbetalipoproteinaemia (FH) cholestyramine generally has little
or no effect on the plasma cholesterol level or on the skin
lesions.   This is probably because in these patients the increase
in cholesterol synthesis balances the increase in cholesterol
catabolism, so that there is no net decrease in the amount of
exchangeable cholesterol in the whole body (20).   Fig. 2 shows
the effect of cholestyramine on the metabolism of bile acids and
cholesterol in a boy with FH in the homozygous form.   Before
the investigation was begun, a liver biopsy was taken for measurement of cholesterol synthesis from acetate.   His plasma
cholesterol was then labelled with intravenous $[4-^{14}C]$ cholesterol
and measurements were made at weekly intervals on the specific
activity of his plasma cholesterol and on the faecal output of
bile acids and neutral sterols.   After a control period of seven
weeks he was given cholestyramine (16 g/day for three weeks,
followed by 30 g/day) and a second liver biopsy was taken for
measurement of cholesterol synthesis.   Treatment with cholestyramine increased the faecal output of bile acids from 195 $\pm$ 28 to
1222 $\pm$ 100 mg/day, but had only a slight effect on neutral sterol
excretion.   There was a slight fall in plasma cholesterol level
but no change in the appearance of the skin xanthomata.   Within
a few days of the first dose of cholestyramine the rate of fall of
specific activity of the plasma cholesterol increased, suggesting
that the treatment had increased the rate of synthesis of
cholesterol from endogenous, and therefore nonradioactive,
precursors.   In agreement with this, cholestyramine caused a
four- to fivefold stimulation of hepatic synthesis of cholesterol
in vitro.

        Although cholestyramine alone is usually ineffective in the
treatment of homozygous FH, we have had some success in the treatment of this condition by combining cholestyramine with nicotinic
acid (21), a drug that appears to inhibit hepatic synthesis of
cholesterol and may thus counteract the stimulatory effect of
cholestyramine on cholesterol synthesis.

        The failure of cholestyramine alone to produce a worthwhile
effect on the plasma cholesterol level in these patients raises
two questions.   First, is their capacity to increase bile acid
synthesis in response to interruption of the enterohepatic circulation less than that of normal subjects?   Second, are the doses

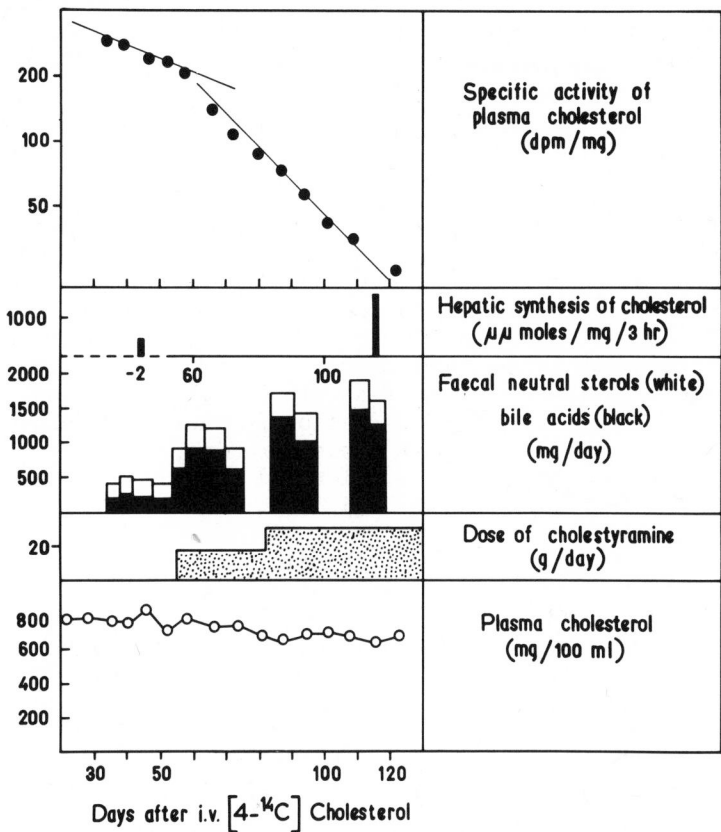

Fig. 2.   Effect of cholestyramine on plasma cholesterol concentration, faecal steroid excretion and hepatic synthesis of cholesterol in a 10-year-old boy suffering from familial hyperbetalipoproteinaemia in the homozygous form. The methods used were those described elsewhere (20, 23).   (C.D. Moutafis, P.W. Adams, N.B. Myant and V. Wynn, unpublished observations.)

of cholestyramine given to these patients sufficient to elicit a maximal stimulation of cholesterol catabolism?   The answer to the first question is that patients with homozygous FH have, if anything, a greater capacity for increasing bile acid output than heterozygous patients (22).   This makes it unlikely that the hypercholesterolaemia of FH is due to an intrinsic inability to synthesize bile acids at the normal rate, or to defective regulation of bile acid synthesis, although Miettinen (24) has reported

a smaller increase in faecal bile acid excretion in response to
cholestyramine in hypercholesterolaemic than in normal subjects.
The second question is more difficult to answer.   In four of the
hypercholesterolaemic patients studied by Moutafis and Myant (22),
bile acid output in the presence of 30 g of cholestyramine/day
was only slightly above that in the presence of 20 g/day, suggesting that the degree of interruption of the enterohepatic circulation brought about by 30 g/day is almost sufficient to induce
maximal synthesis of bile acids.   If this is so, any attempt to
increase the degree of interruption by increasing the dose of
cholestyramine, or by combining cholestyramine with other measures
designed to interfere with the reabsorption of bile acids, would
not be advantageous.   However, the output of bile acids in
patients treated with large doses of cholestyramine seldom exceeds
2 g/day, whereas in the presence of a bile fistula, when the
interruption is total, bile acid excretion in adults may exceed
3 g/day (25).   This suggests that cholestyramine, even when given
in the largest doses that could be tolerated for long-term treatment, does not induce maximal synthesis of bile acids.

     Neomycin, an unabsorbable antibiotic, lowers the plasma
cholesterol level in man (26) and in cholesterol-fed chicks (27).
When given to hypercholesterolaemic patients it increases the
faecal excretion of neutral sterols and bile acids (28, 29).
The effect on plasma cholesterol concentration is perhaps due to
a combination of decreased absorption of cholesterol and increased
catabolism brought about by partial interruption of the enterohepatic circulation of bile acids.   N-Methyl neomycin, an
analogue of neomycin that retains its basic properties but is not
an antibiotic, also lowers the plasma cholesterol level and
increases bile acid excretion in chicks (30).   This suggests that
the effect of neomycin on bile acid and sterol excretion is due to
its polybasic character (it has six amino groups per molecule),
rather than to its antibiotic properties.   De Somer et al. (27)
have shown that neomycin precipitates bile salts from aqueous
solutions in vitro and have suggested that it precipitates bile
salts in the intestinal lumen and thus prevents the formation of
mixed micelles in vivo.   However, it would be unwise to ignore
the possibility that part of the effect of neomycin on the plasma
cholesterol in man is due to its antibiotic action, since Samuel
et al. (27a) have shown that the effect of several oral antibiotics
(including neomycin) on the plasma cholesterol level is related
directly to their ability to suppress 7α-dehydroxylation of bile
acids by faecal bacteria.

     Several other unabsorbable substances have been found to
lower the plasma cholesterol concentration in man and in experimental animals by promoting the faecal excretion of neutral or
acidic steroids.   Some of these substances (31, 32) may act in
a nonspecific way by increasing intestinal motility, or perhaps
by modifying the microbial flora of the intestine.   Others,

however, such as DEAE-Sephadex (a modified dextran) and DEAE-
cellulose, increase bile acid excretion by acting as anion
exchangers (33).   DEAE-Sephadex has been reported to lower the
plasma cholesterol concentration and to increase faecal excretion
of bile acids in hypercholesterolaemic patients (34).   The effect
of unabsorbable dietary constituents on bile acid metabolism is
discussed in more detail below.

Hormones

The plasma cholesterol concentration is lower in women
during the reproductive period than in men of comparable age.
Attempts to explain this difference in terms of effects of sex
hormones on bile acid formation have led to conflicting results.
Isolated liver mitochondria from female rats and from castrated
or estrogen-treated male rats oxidize the side chain of cholesterol more rapidly than those from normal male rats (35).   These
findings suggest that estrogens stimulate bile acid formation from
cholesterol.   However, Boyd (36) found that the rate of conversion
of cholesterol to bile acids in vivo was not affected in female
rats by castration or in male rats by treatment with estrogen.

Thyroid hormone lowers the plasma cholesterol concentration
not only in myxedematous patients but also in hypercholesterolaemic subjects with normal thyroid function.   This had led to the
use of thyroid hormones and their analogues in the treatment of
primary hypercholesterolaemia and, hence, to intensive interest
in the mode of action of these hormones on cholesterol metabolism.
Thyroxine stimulates endogenous synthesis of cholesterol in human
subjects (37) and in rats (38).   However, it also stimulates the
mechanisms responsible for the removal of exchangeable cholesterol
from the body, this effect presumably outweighing the effect on
cholesterol synthesis (39).   Part of the effect on removal is due
to increased excretion of sterols, but in intact rats thyroid
hormone also increases the output of total bile acid (40).
Table 2 shows the influence of triiodothyronine and of an anti-
thyroid drug on the daily production of cholic and chenodeoxycholic acids in groups of rats in which the enterohepatic circulation of bile acids was intact.   In these experiments, triiodothyronine had two distinct effects on bile acid production.   It
stimulated the output of total bile acids to 60% above the control
value and it changed the ratio of chenodeoxycholic to cholic acid
production from the normal value of 0.25 to a value of 0.74.
Propylthiouracil had no significant influence on total bile acid
production or on the chenodeoxycholic/cholic acid ratio.

Observations on the metabolism of cholesterol by cell-free
fractions of liver from rats treated with thyroid hormones have
gone some way towards explaining these effects.   Liver mitochondria from rats treated with thyroxine or triiodothyronine have
an enhanced capacity for oxidative cleavage of the side-chain of

TABLE 2

EFFECT OF L-TRIIODOTHYRONINE AND PROPYLTHIOURACIL
ON THE PRODUCTION OF BILE ACIDS IN INTACT RATS

| Treatment | Bile acid production (mg/day) | | | Chenodeoxycholic Cholic |
	Cholic	Chenodeoxy-cholic	Total	
None	4.0	1.0	5.0	0.25
Triiodothyronine	4.6	3.4	8.0	0.74
Propylthiouracil	3.6	1.0	4.6	0.28

Bile acid output was estimated from the pool size and half-life of each bile acid.   Modified from Strand (40).

cholesterol (41) and of 3α,7α,12α-trihydroxycholestane (42), the last intermediate in the biosynthesis of cholic acid before the cleavage of the side chain.   Since a 12α-OH group cannot be introduced into the steroid nucleus once the side chain has been oxidized, increased oxidation of the side chain before modification to the ring system would tend to increase the formation of chenodeoxycholic acid (the primary bile acid lacking a 12α-OH group) at the expense of that of cholic acid.   This explanation of the increased chenodeoxycholic/cholic acid ratio in thyrotoxic rats would only be valid if sterol molecules in the intact liver cell can reach the side-chain-cleaving enzymes in the mitochondria before they have been 12α-hydroxylated.   That this may, in fact, occur is suggested by the finding that about 30% of the $[^{14}C]$-cholesterol taken up by the livers of rats injected intravenously with $[^{14}C]$cholesterol is present in the mitochondrial fraction 10 minutes after the injection (43).   Moreover, the fraction of the injected dose that is taken up by liver mitochondria is increased by treating the rats with thyroxine (43).   Mitropoulos and Myant (2) have shown that isolated liver mitochondria are capable of cleaving the side chain of cholesterol before any modification to the ring system has occurred, as shown by the formation of 3β-hydroxychol-5-enoic acid from cholesterol (Fig. 3).   It is possible, therefore, that the increased production of chenodeoxycholic acid in thyrotoxic rats is due, at least in part, to stimulation of the mitochondrial cleavage of the side chain at a stage preceding 12α-hydroxylation.   Mitropoulos et al. (44) have also shown that 12α-hydroxylase activity of rat liver microsomes is depressed by treating the animals with thyroxine and is stimulated by thyroidectomy. These changes are accompanied by parallel alterations in the concentration of cytochrome P-450 (Table 3).

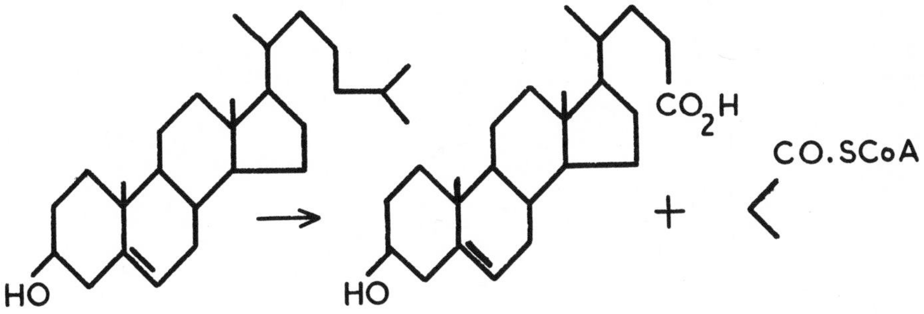

Fig. 3. The mitochondrial conversion of cholesterol (I) into 3β-hydroxychol-5-enoic acid (II) and propionyl-CoA (III) by oxidative cleavage of the side chain before modification to the ring system.

TABLE 3

EFFECT OF THYROXINE TREATMENT AND THYROIDECTOMY ON 12α-HYDROXYLASE ACTIVITY AND CYTOCHROME P-450 CONCENTRATION IN RAT-LIVER MICROSOMES

Rats	12α-Hydroxylase	P-450
Control	100	100
Thyroxine-treated (100 µg/day for 7 days)	49	51
Thyroidectomized (17 days)	153	123

Modified from Mitropoulos et al. (44).

A combination of increased side chain cleavage at an early
stage in bile acid formation and depression of 12α-hydroxylase
activity provides a satisfactory explanation of the relative and
absolute increase in chenodeoxycholic acid production in thyrotoxic rats, but leaves open the question as to why there is an
increase in total bile acid production.

In man, the influence of the thyroid on bile acid metabolism appears to be less marked than in rats. In myxedema the
daily production of cholic acid, estimated from the pool size and
half-life of [^{14}C]cholic acid, is subnormal and is increased by
treatment with thyroid hormone (45). On the other hand, treatment with thyroxine does not significantly increase the faecal
excretion of total bile acids in hypothyroid subjects (34).
Hellström and Lindstedt (45) found that the chenodeoxycholic/
cholic acid ratio in the bile was higher in a group of thyrotoxic
patients than in normal subjects, but the difference was not
statistically significant.

Vitamins

Nicotinic acid, if given in doses of at least 1 g/day,
lowers the plasma cholesterol concentration in normal and hypercholesterolaemic human subjects. This effect is accompanied by
inhibition of endogenous synthesis of cholesterol (46, 21).
Nicotinic acid given to rats increases the capacity of their liver
mitochondria for oxidizing the side chain of cholesterol in vitro
(47), raising the possibility that nicotinic acid also stimulates
bile acid formation in vivo. However, Miettinen (46) found no
significant stimulation of the faecal excretion of total bile
acids in hypercholesterolaemic patients treated with nicotinic
acid in doses sufficient to bring about a substantial fall in the
plasma cholesterol concentration.

In pyridoxine-deficient rats, the production of bile acids
is increased to twice the normal level and there is an increase in
the chenodeoxycholic/cholic acid ratio in the bile (48).   There
is also a marked decrease in the ratio of taurine- to glycine-
conjugated bile acids (48), due possibly to a shortage of taurine
in the liver, since the decarboxylation step in the formation of
taurine from cysteic acid requires pyridoxal phosphate.

Diet and Intestinal Micro-organisms

The composition of the food and the nature of the
intestinal micro-organisms have a marked influence on the
metabolism of bile acids. Both these factors are relevant to
the subject of this discussion. In the first place, an understanding of the way in which specific components of the diet

affect the enterohepatic circulation of bile acids could lead to
the development of useful therapeutic agents.   Secondly, modification of the intestinal flora by chemotherapeutic drugs may influence bile acid metabolism.

Portman and Murphy (49) showed that the half-life of cholic
acid is longer, and that the daily output of cholic acid and its
metabolites is less, when rats are fed a purified sucrose diet
than when they are fed Purina Chow.   When the purified diet is
supplemented with 20% cellulose fiber, the half-life of cholic acid
is diminished and the daily output is increased (Table 4), suggesting that the fibrous residue of a normal diet in some way limits
the reabsorption of bile acids and so promotes their excretion in
the faeces.   The addition of a chemotherapeutic drug to the diet

TABLE 4

EFFECT OF DIET AND OF SUCCINYLSULPHATHIAZOLE ON THE HALF-LIFE AND TURNOVER OF CHOLIC ACID IN RATS

	Diet	Half-life (days)	Turnover (mg/kg/day)
1.	Chow	2.0	36.4
2.	Purified sucrose	4.2	7.7
3.	Purified sucrose + 20% fiber	1.4	23.4
4.	Chow + sulpha	6.6	17.2
5.	Purified sucrose + 20% fiber + sulpha	5.4	8.0

Diets 4 and 5 contained 0.5% of succinylsulphathiazole.
Modified from Portman and Murphy (49) and Portman (51).

diminishes the production of cholic acid (50, 51) and
reverses the effect of cellulose fiber on the half-life and daily
production of cholic acid in rats fed a purified diet (Table 4).
The diminished output of bile acids in rats fed residue-free diets
or chemotherapeutic agents is frequently accompanied by a rise in
the plasma cholesterol concentration (51).

These findings have led to the suggestion (51, 1) that the
effect of diet on the turnover and excretion of bile acids is
mediated by effects on the microbial flora of the intestine, the

presence of fiber favouring the growth of bacteria that convert
conjugated primary bile acids into metabolites that are less
readily absorbed.   In keeping with this idea, the half-life of
cholic acid in germ-free rats is three times that in conventional
rats (52).   However, in view of the many factors that determine
bile acid absorption, it is impossible to predict what effect
increased formation of bile acid metabolites would have on the net
reabsorption of bile acids by a normal intestinal tract. V_{max}
for active ileal transport of deoxycholate is less than that for
cholate.   Moreover, since the K_m for active transport of free
bile acids is higher than that for conjugated acids, free bile
acids would compete unfavourably with conjugated acids for active
transport.   To this extent, the presence in the small intestine
of bacteria capable of deconjugating and dehydroxylating bile
acids would be expected to diminish reabsorption by active transport.   On the other hand, free bile acids, having a relatively
high pK_a, would be available for transport by passive nonionic
diffusion in the ileum.   The extent to which changes in the diet
may, in fact, alter bile acid excretion by influencing bacterial
modification of bile salts in the intestine can only be determined
experimentally from observations on the nature of the bile acids
in the ileum and large intestine in animals given different diets,
combined with measurement of the rates of absorption of different
bile acid mixtures at these levels of the intestine.

        Gustafsson et al. (52) found that when germ-free rats were
infected with C. perfringens there was no increase in the faecal
excretion of labelled taurocholate, though significant deconjugation of the taurocholate took place in the infected animals.
More recently, Kellogg et al. (53) have shown that infection of
germ-free rats with a strain of C. perfringens that deconjugates
all tauro-conjugated bile salts in the intestine does not
increase the faecal excretion of total bile acids.   These results
suggest that the difference in bile acid turnover of germ-free and
conventional rats is not due to the presence of deconjugating
micro-organisms in the conventional animals.   However, results
obtained with germ-free animals should be interpreted with
caution, since the intestinal tract of the germ-free rat has an
abnormally large caecum, and its motility is abnormally slow (54).
Possibly, these abnormalities are not reversed by a brief period
of infection with a single strain of micro-organism.

        The effect of chemotherapeutic drugs on the turnover of
cholic acid in conventional rats, and the abnormal bile acid
metabolism in germ-free rats, leave little doubt that the
composition of the intestinal flora has a marked influence on the
enterohepatic circulation of bile salts.   However, the effects
of diet on bile acid metabolism are not necessarily mediated by
changes in the nature and quantity of the micro-organisms in the
intestine.   Differences in the output of bile acids in conventional rats on different diets are not correlated with differences

in the pattern of bile acids in the faeces (55). Moreover, the turnover of cholic acid in germ-free rats fed Chow pellets is six times that in germ-free rats fed a purified diet with no fiber (56), showing that the composition of the diet can affect bile acid metabolism in conditions in which there can be no question of a change in intestinal flora. One possible explanation for this is that normal diets contain substances that bind bile acids in the intestinal lumen.

Gustafsson and Norman (57) have shown that about half the cholic acid and its metabolites present in the caecum of conventional rats is not extractable by phosphate buffer, whether the rats are fed "pellets" or a fiber-free diet. They have also shown that labelled bile acids become nonextractable when added to the contents of a rat's caecum and that adsorption by caecal contents is greater for free than for conjugated acids. Adsorption of bile acids to substances in the caecum could influence their reabsorption from the intestine, in so far as absorption of bile acids can take place from the caecum and colon. The nature of the dietary components that bind bile acids in the intestine is not fully understood. Eastwood and Hamilton (58) have shown that lignin, a nonabsorbable constituent of vegetable matter, binds bile acids, the binding capacity being greater for free than for conjugated bile acids. Binding of bile acids is not due to anionic exchange, but may be due to "hydrophobic bonding" similar to that responsible for the formation of detergent micelles. Lignin in the diet may well be responsible for some of the binding of bile acids by intestinal contents of animals given a nonpurified diet, and its presence in the caecum of rats fed normal diets may explain why the caecal contents of such animals bind free bile acids to a greater extent than conjugated acids. However, lignin cannot be the only substance present in the intestinal lumen capable of binding bile acids, since Gustafsson and Norman (57) observed binding of bile acids in the caecal contents and faeces of conventional rats given a fiber-free diet. Possibly, the micro-organisms present in the intestine of conventional rats bind bile acids in the absence of insoluble food residue, since bile acids are not adsorbed by the caecal contents or faeces of germ-free rats given a diet with no fiber (57). There is no evidence that cellulose binds bile acids, either in vitro or in the intestinal lumen.

In summary, it is clear that diet and the intestinal flora interact to influence the metabolism of bile salts in an extremely complex way and that no simple explanation of all the known facts is yet possible. It seems probable that in rats a normal rate of turnover of bile acids takes place only in the presence of both micro-organisms and insoluble food residue in the intestine. The presence of food residue may act partly by stimulating intestinal motility, partly by adsorbing bile salts and thus diminishing their availability for reabsorption, and partly by

modifying the intestinal flora. The bacteria in the rat intestine
may act by converting bile salts into metabolites that are less
readily absorbed by active transport and are more readily bound by
food residue and other bile-acid adsorbents in the intestinal
lumen; bacteria may also be necessary for normal intestinal
motility and may themselves adsorb bile acids.   In view of the
large number of factors that influence the intestinal phase of
bile acid metabolism, it is hardly surprising that marked
individual variations in the excretion of bile acids by human
beings have often been observed.   Finally, it should be noted that
observations on bile acid metabolism in rats are not necessarily
applicable to man, since several oral antibiotics, including
neomycin, lower the plasma cholesterol in man whereas they increase
it in rats.

REFERENCES

1. Danielsson, H.   Advanc. Lipid Res. 1: 335 (1963).
2. Mitropoulos, K. A. and N. B. Myant.   Biochem. J. 103:472
    (1967).
3. Danielsson, H. and K. Einarsson.   Acta chem. scand. 18:831
    (1964).
4. Myant, N. B., in The Biological Basis of Medicine, Vol. 2.
    (Eds.) E. E. Bittar and N. Bittar, Academic Press, London
    (1968) p. 193.
5. Ernster, L. and S. Orrenius.   Fed. Proc. 24:1190 (1965).
6. Shefer, S., S. Hauser, and E. H. Mosbach.   J. Lipid Res.
    9: 328 (1968).
7. Einarsson, K. and G. Johansson.   Europ. J. Biochem. 6: 293
    (1968).
8. Boyd, G. S., N. A. Scholan, and J. R. Mitton, in Drugs
    Affecting Lipid Metabolism, Proc. III Int. Symp., Milan,
    1968 (Eds.) W. L. Holmes, L. A. Carlson, and R. Paoletti,
    Plenum Press, New York (1969) p. 443.
9. Mitropoulos, K. A. and N. B. Myant.   Unpublished observa-
    tions.
10. Balasubramaniam, S. and K. A. Mitropoulos.   Biochem. J.,
    in press.
11. Omura, T. and R. Sato.   J. biol. Chem. 239:2370 (1964).
12. Phillips, A. H. and R. G. Langdon.   J. biol. Chem. 237:2652
    (1962).
13. Suzuki, M., K. A. Mitropoulos, and N. B. Myant.   Biochem.
    Biophys. Res. Commun. 30:516 (1968).
14. Danielsson, H.   Arkiv Kemi 17:373 (1961).
15. Dietschy, J. M.   J. Lipid Res. 9:297 (1968).
16. Danielsson, H., K. Einarsson, and G. Johansson.   Europ J.
    Biochem. 2:44 (1967).
17. Huff, J. W., J. L. Gilfillan, and V. M. Hunt.   Proc. Soc.
    exp. Biol. (N.Y.) 114:352 (1963).

18. Schneider, D. L., D. G. Gallo, and H. P. Sarett. Proc. Soc. exp. Biol. (N.Y.) 121:1244 (1966).
19. Hashim, S. A., S. S. Bergen, Jr., and T. B. Van Itallie. Proc. Soc. exp. Biol. (N.Y.) 106:173 (1961).
20. Moutafis, C. D. and N. B. Myant. Clin. Sci. 37:443 (1969).
21. Moutafis, C. D. and N. B. Myant, in Metabolic Effects of Nicotinic Acid and Its Derivatives. (Eds.) K. F. Gey and L. A. Carlson, Hans Huber, Berne (1971) p. 659.
22. Moutafis, C. D. and N. B. Myant. Unpublished observations presented at IV Int. Symp. Drugs Affecting Lipid Metabolism, Philadelphia, 1971.
23. Moutafis, C. D. and N. B. Myant. Clin. Sci. 34:541 (1968).
24. Miettinen, T. A., in Atherosclerosis, Proc. II Int. Symp. (Ed.) R. J. Jones, Springer-Verlag, New York (1970) p. 558.
25. Carey, J. B., Jr. and G. Williams. Gastroenterology 56:1249 (1969).
26. Samuel, P. and A. Steiner. Proc. Soc. exp. Biol. (N.Y.) 100:193 (1959).
27. De Somer, P., H. Vanderhaeghe, and H. Eyssen. Nature, Lond. 204:1306 (1964).
27a. Samuel, P., E. Meilman, and I. Sekowski. J. clin. Invest 48:73a (1969).
28. Goldsmith, G. A., J. G. Hamilton, and O. N. Miller. Arch. int. Med. 105:512 (1960).
29. Powell, R. C., W. T. Nunes, R. S. Harding, and J. B. Vacca. Amer. J. clin. Nutr. 11:156 (1962).
30. Eyssen, H., E. Evrard, and H. Vanderhaeghe. J. Lab. clin. Med. 68:753 (1966).
31. Lin, T. M., K. S. Kim, E. Karvinen, and A. C. Ivy. Amer. J. Physiol. 188:66 (1957).
32. Forman, D. T., J. E. Garvin, J. E. Forestner, and C. B. Taylor. Proc. Soc. exp. Biol. (N.Y.) 127:1060 (1968).
33. Parkinson, T. M. J. Lipid Res. 8:24 (1967).
34. Miettinen, T. A., in Atherosclerosis, Proc. II Int. Symp. (Ed. R. J. Jones), Springer-Verlag, New York (1970) p. 508.
35. Kritchevsky, D., E. Staple, J. L. Rabinowitz, and M. J. Whitehouse. Amer. J. Physiol. 200:519 (1961).
36. Boyd, G. S., in The Control of Lipid Metabolism, Biochem. Soc. Symp. No. 24 (Ed.) J. K. Grant, Academic Press, London (1963) p. 79.
37. Gould, R. G., in Hormones and Atherosclerosis, Proc. Conf. Brighton, Utah, 1958 (Ed.) G. Pincus, Academic Press, New York (1959) p. 75.
38. Fletcher, K. and N. B. Myant. J. Physiol. 144:361 (1958).
39. Myant, N. B., in Lipid Pharmacology. (Ed.) R. Paoletti, Academic Press, New York (1964) p. 299.
40. Strand, O. J. Lipid Res. 4:305 (1963).
41. Mitropoulos, K. A. and N. B. Myant. Biochem. J. 94:594 (1965).
42. Berséus, O. Acta chem. scand. 19:2131 (1965).
43. Suzuki, M., K. A. Mitropoulos, and N. B. Myant. Biochim.

biophys. Acta 184:455 (1969).

44. Mitropoulos, K. A., M. Suzuki, N. B. Myant, and H. Danielsson.
     FEBS Letters 1:13 (1968).
45. Hellström, K. and S. Lindstedt.   J. Lab. clin. Med. 63:666
     (1964).
46. Miettinen, T. A.   Clin. chim. Acta 20:43 (1968).
47. Kritchevsky, D., M. W. Whitehouse, and E. Staple.
     J. Lipid Res. 1:154 (1960).
48. Avery, M., Thèse de Grade de Docteur es Sciences, Université
     Laval, Québec (1970).
49. Portman, O. W. and P. Murphy.   Arch. Biochem. Biophys.
     76:367 (1958).
50. Lindstedt, S. and A. Norman.   Acta physiol. scand. 38:129
     (1956).
51. Portman, O. W.   Amer. J. clin. Nutr. 8:462 (1960).
52. Gustafsson, B. E., S. Bergström, S. Lindstedt, and A. Norman.
     Proc. Soc. exp. Biol. (N.Y.) 94:467 (1957).
53. Kellogg, T. F., P. L. Knight, and B. S. Wostmann.
     J. Lipid Res. 11:362 (1970).
54. Abrams, G. D. and J. E. Bishop.   Proc. Soc. exp. Biol. (N.Y.)
     126:301 (1963).
55. Gustafsson, B. E. and A. Norman.   Biochem. J. 23:627 (1969).
56. Gustafsson, B. E. and A. Norman.   Brit. J. Nutr. 23:429
     (1969).
57. Gustafsson, B. E. and A. Norman.   Scand. J. Gastroenterol.
     3:625 (1968).
58. Eastwood, M. A. and D. Hamilton.   Biochim. biophys. Acta
     152:165 (1968).

HYPOLIPIDEMIC DRUGS AND LIPOPROTEIN METABOLISM

Robert I. Levy and Terry Langer

Section on Lipoproteins, Molecular Disease Branch

National Heart & Lung Institute, Bethesda, Md. 20014

Insight into the mechanism of action and efficacy of hypolipidemic drugs has awaited the development of the current concepts of lipid transport (1). Fundamental is the fact that the blood fats-- cholesterol, phospholipid,and triglyceride-- do not circulate free in the plasma. Lipids exist in a soluble form in the blood only because they are bound to protein. These proteins serve as detergents and solubilize the otherwise insoluble lipid. It is as lipid protein complexes or lipoproteins that all fat enters and leaves the blood stream.

A mass of clinical data has been gathered over the last 10 years to indicate that "hypercholesterolemia" and "hypertriglyceridemia" do not define specific disease entities. Hyperlipidemia is a symptom of a heterogeneous group of disorders that differ in clinical manifestations, prognosis and responsiveness to therapy. It has now become clear that hyperlipidemia must be translated into hyperlipoproteinemia for proper diagnosis and management(2).

Clinical interest in the hyperlipoproteinemias in man has stimulated a search for new pharmacologic agents for the treatment of these disorders. Since plasma lipids circulate in the form of lipoproteins, ultimately the changes in plasma lipid levels induced by drugs must reflect changes in lipoprotein concentrations. Though a drug may have a primary effect on the metabolism of cholesterol, triglyceride, or fatty acids,it is the secondary effect on lipoprotein metabolism which is actually expressed as an alteration in plasma lipid concentrations. Some drugs, moreoever, may directly influence the synthesis or catabolism of lipoproteins either by regulating the availability of non-lipid precursors or by directly

155

modulating the synthesis and degradation of the intact lipoproteins
or apoproteins.

It is now clear that to understand completely the mechanism by
which a drug affects plasma lipid concentrations, one must carefully
study the effect the drug has on lipoprotein metabolism in addition
to any direct effect the drug may have on the metabolism of specific
lipids. Today, to stress this point, I would like to describe some
of our observations on the perturbations produced by drugs on the
metabolism of plasma low density lipoproteins (LDL).

Methods

Patients with well-documented familial type II hyperlipoproteinemia (heterozygotes), as well as normal volunteers over age 21
with no personal or family history or physical findings of hyperlipidemia and with normal plasma lipid and lipoprotein levels,
served as subjects. During the entire study period, the subjects
were housed as inpatients on the metabolic wards of the Clinical
Center of the National Institutes of Health. Diet and weight were
held constant. All subjects were fed an isocaloric diet providing
20% of the calories from protein, 40% from fat, and 40% from carbohydrates. The diets contained less than 300 milligrams of choles-
terol/day and were high in polyunsaturated fats (p/s ratio = 2).
The patients were considered to be in a metabolic steady state prior
to any study as judged from their constant body weight, stable
plasma concentrations of total and LDL cholesterol, triglyceride,
and the absence of intercurrent infection or fever. The turnover
of LDL was studied twice in each subject. One study was done with
the subject on diet and placebo or drug for 4 to 6 weeks. The
second study was performed 4 - 6 weeks later after the institution
or drug or placebo therapy to its maximum dosage and the establishment of a new steady state. The order of placebo and drug were
varied randomly. Cholestyramine and cholestyramine placebo were
provided courtesy of Mead Johnson. Cholestyramine or its placebo
was given in 4 divided doses daily: 24 g of the active medication
per day. When nicotinic acid was given no placebo was used; here
diet alone was compared to diet and drug. In the normal subjects
1 g of nicotinic acid TID (3 g/day) was used. In the subjects with
type II hyperlipoproteinemia, 1.5 or 2 g of nicotinic acid (TID)
was the regimen employed (4.5 - 6 g/day). No alteration in hepatic
or hematologic functions was noted during the periods of drug
administration. Saturated solution of potassium iodide, 1 g daily
in divided doses, was administered throughout each study to inhibit
the uptake of radioiodine by the thyroid.

Preparation of labeled LDL (Fig. 1). After an overnight fast
plasma was collected in EDTA using the technique of plasmaphoresis.
The LDL of density 1.019 to 1.063 were isolated and purified by
preparative ultracentrifugation (3). Each isolation involved a

single ultracentrifugation at D1.019, a second centrifugation at
D1.063,followed by at least one wash of the D1.063 supernatant
through saline at the same density. Each preparation of LDL was
examined for the presence of protein contaminants by immunoelectro-
phoresis using antisera specific for albumin and alpha lipoprotein;
none were found. Evidence for denaturation was sought by observing
the distribution of the radioactive label after electrophoresis
and repeated ultracentrifugation. Better than 98% of the label
could always be recovered in the LDL band on electrophoresis; over
97% of the radioactivity was recoverable in the LDL density range
D1.019 to 1.063 upon recentrifugation (4).

On two occasions the labeled LDL was injected into animals and
screened for evidence of biologically denatured material; none was
found. The LDL was radioiodinated with ^{125}I by a modification of
the iodine myochloride method of McFarlane (5), dialyzed to remove
unbound iodine, sterilized by ultrafiltration, and tested for
pyrogens prior to administration. In all cases more than 98% of
the label was bound to the protein moiety of the LDL (4).

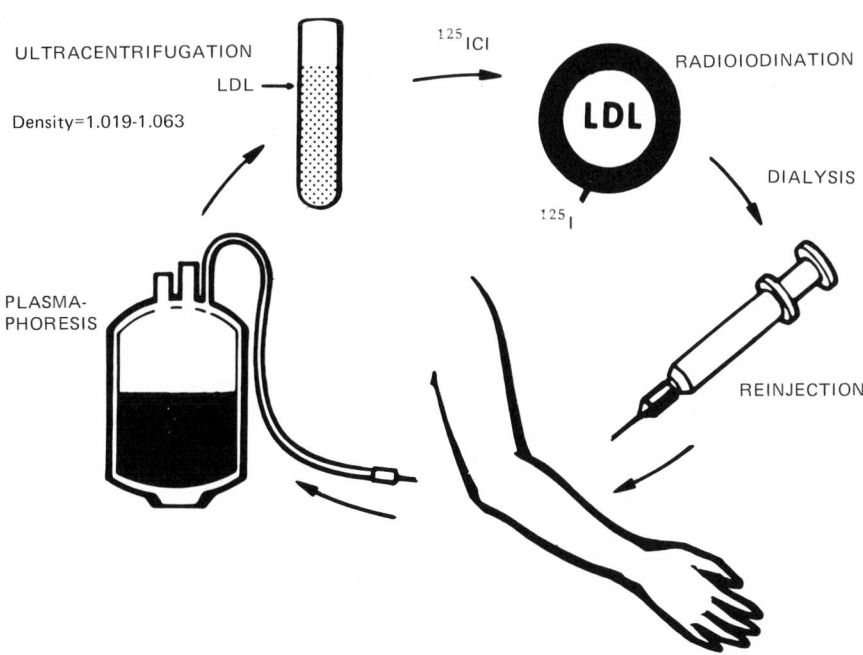

Fig. 1.   Preparation of ^{125}I-LDL.

Turnover studies. Twenty-five to 50 µc of ^{125}I-LDL was injected intravenously into the fasting subject, and serial blood
samples and 24-hour urine collections were obtained for 14 days.
Plasma total cholesterol was determined daily. LDL cholesterol and
triglycerides were measured 5 times during the 14-day study. The
decay of plasma radioactivity was plotted against time on semi-
logarithmic scales, and in all studies the curve could be resolved
into two exponential components. The fractional catabolic rate (FCR)
of LDL (the fraction of the intravascular LDL pool catabolized per
unit time) and the distribution of the LDL between the plasma and
extravascular space were calculated from the slopes and intercepts
of the two exponentials resolved from the plasma decay curve by the
method of Nosslin (6). In addition, an independent estimation of
the FCR was obtained by determining the daily ratio of urinary
radioactivity excretion to the mean plasma radioactivity during the
collection. The synthetic rate of LDL protein was calculated from
the product of the FCR and the plasma pool of LDL protein. The LDL
protein concentration was determined by direct analysis of the protein concentration of density 1.019 to 1.063 LDL.

Observation of LDL metabolism in man demonstrated that the
metabolism of LDL can be described by a simple two-compartmental
model consisting of an intravascular pool containing 65-75% of the
protein and an extravascular compartment. The model is depicted
in Figure 2.

It can be seen that the concentration of LDL in the plasma can
be altered by changes in the synthesis, catabolism, or distribution
of LDL.

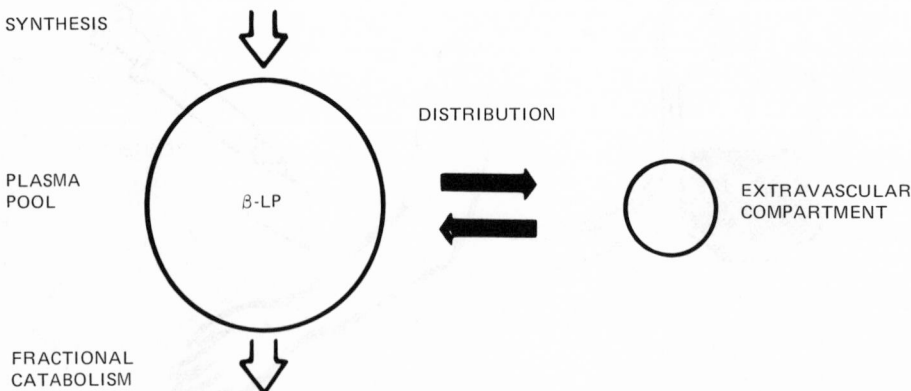

Fig. 2.   Schematic representation of two compartmental model of
βLp LDL turnover.

Results

The administration of cholestyramine in a dosage of 24 g per day to 6 subjects with familial type II hyperlipoproteinemia resulted in a mean reduction of LDL cholesterol concentrations of 32% (Fig. 3). This was associated with an increase in the catabolic rate of LDL from 22.7 ± 1.7% of the IV pool per day to 32.3 ± 3.8% of the IV pool per day. The synthetic rate of the LDL remained unchanged as did its distribution, suggesting that cholestyramine lowered the level of LDL in these patients by accelerating LDL catabolism.

The administration of nicotinic acid, in contrast, another potent hypolipidemic agent, in a dosage of 3 to 6 g/day had a very different effect while producing a similar lowering of cholesterol and LDL in 2 type II and 2 normal subjects. Administration of nicotinic acid resulted in a 20 - 30% fall in cholesterol and 25 - 45% fall in LDL cholesterol concentration. In these studies, however, there was no significant alteration in the biologic T-1/2

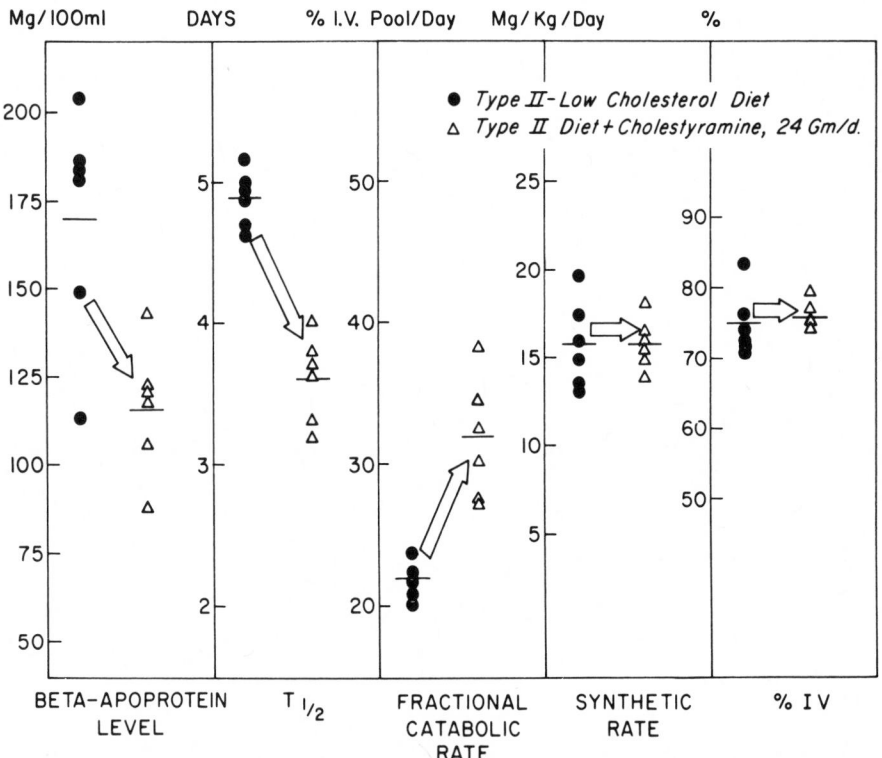

Fig. 3. The effects of cholestyramine on LDL turnover.

(half-life of the slow exponential component), the fractional
catabolic rate,or in the distribution of the LDL (Fig. 4).
Nicotinic acid therapy, rather, was associated with a marked
decrease in the absolute synthetic rate of the LDL protein.

Discussion

The differentiation of the hyperlipoproteinemias in man has
stimulated a new and active approach to the management of these
disorders. It has become abundantly clear that proper selection of
hypolipidemic agents, associated with appropriate dietary manipula-
tion,can allow the normalization of plasma lipid levels in most
affected patients (7). Why these drugs work at all and specifically
in some types of hyperlipoproteinemia and not in others is still
not clear.

In the past there has been a tendency of many to focus attention on hepatic cholesterol metabolism and its control, losing sight
of the fact that it is the <u>availability of circulating lipoproteins</u>
and <u>not the total hepatic cholesterol</u> pool that determines the amount
of cholesterol in plasma at any time. Numerous disease states have
been recognized that did not and could not fit with this view of
relating rates of hepatic cholesterol synthesis to plasma cholesterol levels. It has been clear that one cannot explain, for
example, the increased levels of cholesterol seen in hypothyroidism

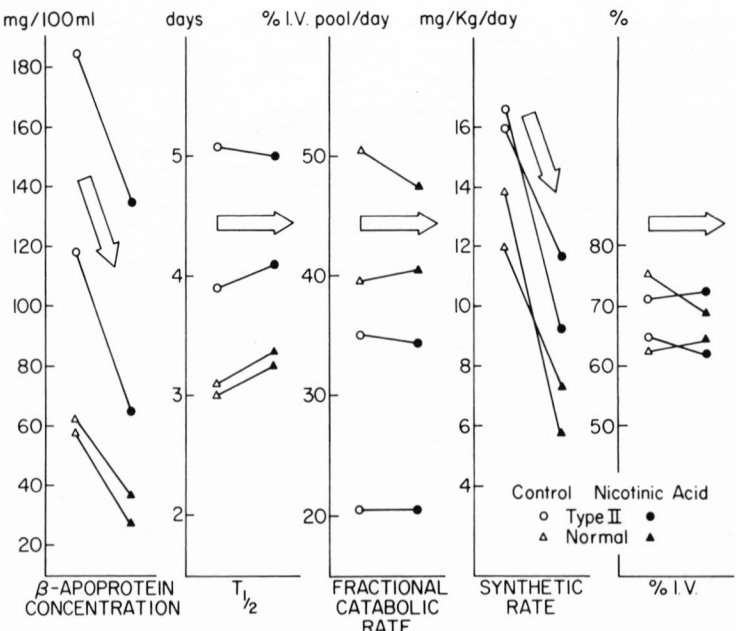

Fig. 4.   The effect of nicotinic acid on LDL turnover.

on the basis of increased cholesterol synthesis, since in hypothyroidism synthesis in the liver is actually decreased. Similarly,
decreased cholesterol biosynthesis does not explain the decreased
levels of plasma cholesterol found in hyperthyroidism.

This conceptual approach that placed emphasis on intermediary
lipid metabolism rather than on lipoprotein metabolism has also
hindered understanding of the mechanism of action of most lipid-
lowering drugs. Cholestyramine, for example, supposedly has a well-
understood mechanism of action. It binds bile acids in the intestine and prevents their reabsorption, thereby leading to increased
turnover of bile acids and, hence, an increased breakdown of cholesterol (8). That cholestyramine therefore lowers cholesterol levels
by increasing cholesterol catabolism at first glance seems clear.
However, a review of cholesterol balance studies reveals that de
novo cholesterol synthesis in the liver increases to balance completely the increased cholesterol degradation induced by cholestyramine (9). Why, then, if cholesterol synthesis affects the
plasma cholesterol levels, should the plasma cholesterol level fall?
Studies on the metabolism of the ^{125}I-labeled LDL, the major
carrier of cholesterol in the plasma, reveal that the levels of
LDL are reduced by cholestyramine, not by any change in intravascular/
extravascular distribution or by a decrease in the rate of synthesis
of lipoprotein. Rather, cholestyramine acts by increasing the fractional catabolic rate of the lipoprotein protein moiety. Why
cholestyramine should act by increased lipoprotein clearance is not
clear. It points out the fact that we really understand very little
about the determinants and even the sites of lipoprotein degradation.
Other drugs that seem to work by increasing the removal of lipoproteins from the plasma would include D-thyroxin (10) and probably
neomycin.

Nicotinic acid does not seem to work this way. Though nicotinic acid clearly is an effective cholesterol-lowering agent in
normal subjects as well as in subjects with hyperlipoproteinemia,
the mechanism by which it lowers plasma cholesterol has not been
totally understood (11). No effect of nicotinic acid has clearly
and reproducibly been demonstrated on cholesterol biosynthesis,
degradation, or bile acid formation. Studies of beta lipoprotein
turnover in normal subjects and patients with hyperlipoproteinemia
reveal that nicotinic acid lowers plasma LDL levels, not by changing
lipoprotein distribution and, in contrast to cholestyramine, not by
changing the rate of clearance of LDL. Nicotinic acid lowers LDL
levels by markedly decreasing the rate of synthesis of LDL. The
mechanisms involved in the suppression of LDL synthesis associated
with the nicotinic acid administration remain conjectural. It is
plausible to explain this effect by extending the observations
made on the effects of nicotinic acid on the release of fatty acids
from adipose tissue (12). VLDL can now be shown to be the precursor
of most, if not all, plasma LDL. Normally de novo synthesis or

increased hepatic influx of triglyceride precursors increases VLDL
production. VLDL or more specifically the apoLDL portion of VLDL
is rapidly catabolized in vivo and converted to LDL. A reduction
in the synthesis of VLDL would result in a measurable decrease in
the amount of LDL produced (13). The observation that the fall in
cholesterol and LDL induced by nicotinic acid lags considerably
behind that of triglycerides and VLDL would fit entirely with the
marked difference in the biologic half-life observed between VLDL
(about 6 hours) and LDL (3 to 5 days).

We thus can now differentiate hypolipidemic drugs into at
lease two, and perhaps three, different groups (Table 1): those
that act by decreasing lipoprotein synthesis, those that promote
lipoprotein degradation, and perhaps eventually those that affect
the intravascular/extravascular distribution of the lipoproteins.
The primary effects of each and every one of these drugs may be on
lipid or protein precursors of the lipoprotein, but their lipid-
lowering effect clearly relates to the effect they have on the circulating lipoproteins.

We can perhaps gain some insight into why certain hypolipidemic
drugs and diets are specifically effective in some types of hyperlipoproteinemias and not in others (2, 7). For example, in familial
type II hyperlipoproteinemia, the large excesses of plasma LDL appear
to result from defective clearance of LDL (14). It is not surprising
that drugs that increase LDL clearance would have a high degree of
efficacy in type II, while drugs that apparently do not affect
lipoprotein clearance like nicotinic acid and clofibrate have lesser
effectiveness in type II. In type III, where there is a defect in the
normal interconversion of VLDL to LDL (15), drugs that effect VLDL
production like nicotinic acid are exquisitely effective.

TABLE I

MECHANISM OF ACTION OF HYPOLIPIDEMIC DRUGS

Decreased Lipoprotein Synthesis	Increased Lipoprotein Catabolism	Alteration in Lipoprotein Distribution
Nicotinic Acid	Cholestyramine	?
Clofibrate (?)	D-thyroxine	
	Neomycin (?)	

We can also, perhaps for the first time, understand the synergism possible through the use of combinations of hypolipidemic drugs. For example, nicotinic acid is usually only effective in high dosages in the treatment of subjects with type II. A combination of nicotinic acid and cholestyramine in type II homozygotes, however, has recently been reported to be extremely effective (2). This synergism can plausibly be explained in that this combination employs drugs that act at the opposite ends of LDL metabolism. Nicotinic acid decreases LDL synthesis while cholestyramine increases its degradation.

One fact is clearly apparent as a result of these studies: we cannot and should not focus only on the intermediary metabolism of cholesterol or other lipids in attempting to study the mechanism of action of lipid-lowering drugs or the pathogenesis of lipid transport disorders. Study of the metabolism of the circulating plasma lipoproteins can provide us with a great insight into lipid transport, its disorders and the action of hypolipidemic drugs.

REFERENCES

1. Fredrickson, D. S., R. I. Levy and R. S. Lees. New Eng. J. Med. 276:34 (1967).
2. Fredrickson, D. S. and R. I. Levy in The Metabolic Basis of Inherited Disease. (Eds.) J. B. Stanbury, J. B. Wyngaarden and D. S. Fredrickson, McGraw-Hill, New York, in press (1972)
3. Havel, R. J., H. A. Eder and J. H. Bragdon. J. Clin. Invest. 34:1345 (1955).
4. Langer, T., W. Strober and R. I. Levy, in preparation.
5. McFarlane, A. S. Nature (London) 182:53 (1958).
6. Nosslin, B. in Metabolism of Human Gamma Globulin. (Ed.) S. B. Anderson, Blackwell Sci. Publ., Oxford (1964) p. 34.
7. Levy, R. I. and D. S. Fredrickson. Postgrad. Med. 47:130 (1970).
8. Hashim, S. A. and T. B. VanItallie. J. A. M. A. 192:289(1965).
9. Goodman, D. S. and R. P. Noble. J. Clin. Invest. 47:231(1968).
10. Walton, K. W., P. J. Scott, P. W. Dykes and J. W. L. Davies. Clin. Sci. 29:217 (1965).
11. Kritchevsky, D. in Proceedings of the Workshop on the Metabolic Effects of Nicotinic Acid, Flims. Switzerland (1970) in press.
12. Carlson, L. A., L. Orö and J. Ostman. J. Ather. Res. 8:667 (1968).
13. Levy, R. I., D. Bilheimer and S. Eisenberg. Biochem. Soc. Symposium. In press (1972).
14. Langer, T., W. Strober and R. I. Levy. J. Clin. Invest. 48:49a (1969).
15. Bilheimer, D. W., S. Eisenberg and R. I. Levy. A.H.A.Abstract Circulation. Vol. 44:II-56, 1971.

SERUM AND TISSUE LIPID METABOLISM AND EFFECT OF NICOTINIC ACID IN DIFFERENT TYPES OF HYPERLIPIDEMIA

Lars A. Carlson and Göran Walldius

Department of Geriatrics, Uppsala University
Uppsala and King Gustaf V:th Research Institute
Stockholm, Sweden

It is necessary with the increasing use of drugs affecting lipid metabolism (DALM) to obtain a much more complete picture of the mode of action of all these drugs. Although it is obvious we would like to stress the fact that if we have two drugs which are equally effective in lowering a given plasma lipoprotein family, this does by no means imply that their effects on lipid metabolism are the same in other tissues, including the arterial wall.

Several laboratories are studying the mechanisms by which drugs lower different plasma lipoproteins as has been reported at this meeting. We have felt that another important area which must be studied is the effect of DALM on lipid pools in other tissues than plasma. Arteries are of course the most important tissue in this regard but knowledge about other tissues is certainly also needed. The developement of technique for fine needle biopsy has now made it possible to take repeat biopsies of different tissues such as adipose (1) and skeletal muscle (2) for analysis of lipid metabolism.

We have started studies along these lines the aim being to evaluate the effect of DALM on tissue lipid metabolism. In this report the effect of nicotinic acid on plasma and tissue lipids and also data on cholesterol content of adipose tissue in different types of hyperlipidemia will be discussed.

MATERIAL AND METHODS

Patients

The effect of nicotinic acid on plasma lipids in different hyperlipidemias and on skeletal muscle composition
was studied in male outpatients at the Lipid Outpatient
Clinic, Department of Medicine, Karolinska Hospital (in
collaboration with Drs S. Fröberg and L. Orö). The patients had been given general advice on dietary habits
comprising avoidance of visible animal fat, changing from
butter to a polyunsaturated margarine and drinking skim
milk. There was no great emphasis or control of this advice, and the patients had been on this regime usually at
least six months before start of the study. The patients
either had asymptomatic hyperlipidemia or clinical signs
of atherosclerosis. No treatment was started until at
least six months had passed from any acute vascular episode. Patients with endocrine or other major diseases are
not included. The mean age was 54 years, range 27-73 and
mean body weight 78 kg, range 63-83. Nicotinic acid ·was
given in the form of plain nicotinic acid, buffered with
sodium bicarbonate (Nicangin^R, Draco, Lund, Sweden). Treatment was started by giving 1/4 of a gram three times daily
after meals. The dose was increased by further 1/4 of a
gram every fourth day until 1 or $1\frac{1}{2}$ g three times daily
was reached. This dose schedule was used to accustom the
patients to the flush which they had been carefully inst-
ructed about.

The composition and cell size of adipose tissue was
studied on in- and outpatients at the Department of Geriatrics, Uppsala. The patients had been referred to us
mainly because of coronary or peripheral atherosclerosis,
"primary" hyperlipidemia, or because of reduced glucose
tolerance (k-value below 1.1 after an intravenous glucose
tolerance test). Blood samples and adipose tissue biopsies
were taken before any therapeutic regimes were started.

Sampling

Blood was taken between 7 and 9 a.m. after fasting
overnight, allowed to clot at room temperature and serum
recovered after centrifugation. For lipid analysis the
sera were either extracted immediately or kept at -15^{0}C
for later analysis. For lipoprotein analysis EDTA was added to a final concentration of 0.01 %. Lipoprotein electrophoresis on paper was carried out on the day of sampling. Separation of lipoprotein families in the preparative

ultracentrifuge was begun on the day of sampling or 1 or
2 days later after storage at $+4^0$C.

Skeletal muscle biopsies were taken from the lateral
femoral muscle (2) in the fasting state in the morning.

Adipose tissue pieces were obtained from subcutaneous
abdominal fat below the umbilicus (5, 22). The biopsy was
taken before blood was drawn for lipid analysis.

In the intravenous glucose tolerance test 0.5 g/kg
body weight was given in the fasting state the same morning biopsy and blood samples were taken. Some patients
were also investigated several weeks preceding the day of
biopsy.

Methods

Determination of serum cholesterol and triglycerides,
lipoprotein electrophoresis and the analysis of lipoprotein families separated in the preparative ultracentrifuge
have been described in detail previously (see 3). Analysis
of skeletal muscle lipids and glycogen has also been described earlier (4). Fat cell size was determined according
to Sjöström et al. (5). Adipose tissue free cholesterol
and triglycerides were determined by extraction with chlo-
roform-methanol, separation of triglycerides and free cholesterol by thinlayer chromatography and determination by
the methods described above. Esterified cholesterol is not
included by this method and is less than 10 % of free cholesterol. This method for cholesterol determination in
adipose tissue shows good agreement when cholesterol was
determined after precipitation with digitonin (6).

Classification of Hyperlipidemia

The classification of hyperlipidemia was done according to the WHO-group report (7). All patients with Type
III hyperlipidemia were characterized by a high ratio
cholesterol/triglycerides in the very low density lipoprotein fraction (<1.006), which fraction also had β-
mobility on paper electrophoresis.

RESULTS

Effect of Nicotinic Acid on Serum Lipids in
Different Types of Hyperlipidemia

The effect of treatment for 1 month with 3 g daily
of nicotinic acid in patients with Types II A, II B, III,
IV and V is summarized in Tables I-III. A significant
lowering of both cholesterol and triglycerides was obtained in all types. The percentage decrease as summarized
in Table III was more pronounced for triglycerides than
for cholesterol. From the percentage figures the hypolipidemic effect of nicotinic acid was most pronounced in patients with Type V and III followed by Type II B hyperlipidemia.

TABLE I

EFFECT OF NICOTINIC ACID ON SERUM CHOLESTEROL
(CHOL) AND TRIGLYCERIDES (TG) IN MEN HAVING
DIFFERENT TYPES OF HYPERLIPIDEMIA

Mean Values before and after and Mean Decrease
($\pm$SEM) in Response to 3 g Daily for 1 Month

Type		II A	II B	IV
	n	17	26	39
CHOL mg/100 ml	Before	337	336	258
	After	299	270	232
	Decrease	38 ± 15	66 ± 10	26 ± 4
	p[1]	< 0.01	<0.001	< 0.001
TG mmol/l	Before	1.63	2.93	2.71
	After	1.20	1.76	1.92
	Decrease	0.43 ± 0.05	1.17 ± 0.15	0.79 ± 0.12
	p[1]	<0.001	<0.001	< 0.001

1) Statistical significance of the decrease

Effect of Nicotinic Acid on Skeletal Muscle Lipids

Treatment with nicotinic acid for 2-4 months lowered
the triglyceride concentration of skeletal muscle by 28 %
(Table IV). The level of phospholipids remained unchanged,

TABLE II

EFFECT OF NICOTINIC ACID ON SERUM CHOLESTEROL
(CHOL) AND TRIGLYCERIDES (TG) IN MEN HAVING
TYPE III AND TYPE V HYPERLIPIDEMIA

Individual Values before and after 3 g Daily
for 1 Month

	Case	PP	AS	KK	RH	EP	AA
	Type	III	III	III	III	V	V
CHOL	Before	375	897	490	536	763	998
mg/100 ml	After	252	339	323	228	205	394
TG	Before	5.90	18.7	6.61	6.68	81.0	90.5
mmol/l	After	2.42	5.32	3.42	3.33	4.82	12.7

TABLE III

PERCENTAGE DECREASE OF SERUM CHOLESTEROL (CHOL)
AND TRIGLYCERIDES (TG) BY NICOTINIC ACID IN DIF-
FERENT TYPES OF HYPERLIPIDEMIA

Mean Values after Treatment with 3 g Daily for
1 Month

Type	II A	II B	III	IV	V
CHOL	11	20	50	10	67
TG	26	40	62	29	91
n	17	26	4	39	2

however. As is evident the patients had quite pronounced
hyperlipidemia with a mean serum triglyceride value of
about 6 mmol/l. There was, however, no relationship between
the type and degree of hyperlipidemia and the concentration
in skeletal muscle of triglycerides or phospholipids.

Fat Cell Size (FCS) in Different Types
of Hyperlipidemia

In a group of patients with normal plasma lipoprotein
pattern the mean fat cell size (89 μ) was lower than fat
cell size in patients with hyperlipidemia Type II A (97 μ),

TABLE IV

EFFECT OF NICOTINIC ACID ON SKELETAL MUSCLE
LIPIDS IN HYPERLIPIDEMIA

Mean Value before and Percentage Decrease in
Response to 3-4.5 g Daily for 2-4 Months in
15 Patients

SERUM		SKELETAL MUSCLE			
TRIGLYCERIDES		TRIGLYCERIDES		PHOSPHOLIPIDS	
Before mmol/l	Decrease %	Before µmol/g	Decrease %	Before mg/g	Decrease %
6.28	62	17.7	28	9.0	1
	p < 0.01		p < 0.01		p > 0.05

Type II B (92 µ) and Type IV (95 µ). None of these differences is, however, statistically significant. Results and
characteristics of the patients are given in Table V. The
highest individual fat cell size (128 µ) was obtained from
a healthy 59-year old woman with a Type IV hyperlipidemia.
The lowest value (56 µ) was found in a man with normal lipoprotein pattern and suffering from intermittent claudication.

Of 15 subjects referred because of asymptomatic glucose intolerance 9 had normal serum lipids and 6 had Type
IV hyperlipidemia. Fat cell size in the 9 patients with
normal lipoproteins (k-value of $0.89 \pm .08$; mean $\pm$ SEM) was
on the average 88 µ. Fat cell size in the 6 patients with
Type IV hyperlipidemia (k-value $0.84 \pm .07$) was on the average 102 µ, a difference which is significant on the one
per cent level.

Cholesterol Concentration in Adipose Tissue
(ATC) in Different Types of Hyperlipidemia

Adipose tissue cholesterol concentration has been
calculated in two ways, either per unit triglyceride or
per cell. When expressed as mg cholesterol per mmol triglycerides (mg/mM TG) the group with normal lipid values had
the highest concentration, 1.13 mg/mM TG. All hyperlipidemic groups had lower values, 1.01, 1.05 and 0.99 mg/mM TG

TABLE V

FAT CELL SIZE (FCS), CHOLESTEROL CONCENTRATION IN ADIPOSE TISSUE (ATC), SERUM CHOLESTEROL (SC) AND TRIGLYCERIDE (STG) CONCENTRATIONS IN DIFFE-RENT TYPES OF HYPERLIPIDEMIA

	N[1]	II A	II B	IV
n	33	8	11	30
FCS (μ)	89.4±2.3	97.1±4.2	91.8±3.0	94.8±2.4
ATC (mg/mM TG)	1.13±.05	1.01±.12	1.05±.17	0.99±.03*
ATC (ng/cell)	0.51±.04	0.56±.08	0.49±.08	0.54±.05
SC (mg/100 ml)	239.5±5.9	325.0±13.5	349.6±11.8	256.0±6.1
STG (mmol/l)	1.67±.05	1.76±.16	3.36±.39	3.60±.44
Age (year)	54±1.8 (39-76)[3]	58.3±2.9 (50-70)	57.2±2.8 (44-68)	56.9±1.9 (33-79)
Weight (kg)	73.5±2.0 (56-105)	67.5±3.2 (56-79)	76.0±3.0 (63-94)	76.4±2.1 (61-103)
Body index $\left(\frac{W}{H-100}\right)$[2]	0.99±.03 (0.65-1.32)	1.04±.06 (0.85-1.39)	1.09±.04 (0.89-1.36)	1.07±.03 (0.86-1.57)

1/ N = normal serum lipoprotein pattern; 2/ W = weight, H = height in cm; 3/ Range

* $p < .05$

for Type II A, II B and Type IV respectively (Table V).
There was a statistically significant difference (p < .05)
between the concentrations in the normal group and the
concentrations found in patients with Type IV pattern.
There was no significant difference in the serum cholesterol (SC) concentration in these two groups. When expressed
as nanogram cholesterol per cell in adipose tissue (ng/
cell) no statistically significant difference was obtained between the groups. Concentrations per cell were
0.51; 0.56; 0.49; 0.54 in normal, Type II A, Type II B
and Type IV patients.

There was a highly significant correlation (Table VI)
between cholesterol concentration per cell and fat cell
size in patients with normal lipoprotein pattern and Type
IV lipoprotein pattern, with r-values .72 and .90 respectively (Table VI). These high correlations were not obtained in the smaller groups of patients with Type II A
or Type II B pattern, their r-values being .53 and .25
respectively (not significant).

TABLE VI

CORRELATION COEFFICIENTS FOR SERUM LIPIDS, FAT
CELL SIZE AND CONCENTRATION OF CHOLESTEROL IN
ADIPOSE TISSUE IN DIFFERENT TYPES OF HYPERLI-
PIDEMIA

	$N^{1/}$	II A	II B	IV
n	33	8	11	30
FCS (μ)- ATC (ng/cell)	.72***	.53	.25	.90***
FCS (μ)- ATC (mg/mM TG)	-.26	-.23	-.11	.09
SC (mg/100 ml)- ATC (mg/mM TG)	.14	.16	.19	.33
SC (mg/100 ml)- ATC (ng/cell)	.20	.16	-.09	-.01
STG (mM/1)- ATC (mg/mM TG)	-.21	-.40	.27	.09
STG (mM/1)- ATC (ng/cell)	-.05	-.06	-.09	-.11
SC (mg/100 ml)- FCS (μ)	.11	.07	-.43	-.15
STG (mM/1)- FCS (μ)	.13	.46	-.39	-.23

1/ N = normal serum lipoprotein pattern
*** p < .001

There was no correlation between adipose tissue cholesterol (mg/mM TG) and fat cell size.

Neither serum cholesterol concentration nor serum
triglyceride (STG) concentration did correlate with adipose tissue cholesterol concentration (Table VI).

No correlation was seen between serum cholesterol or
serum triglyceride concentration and fat cell size (Table
VI).

The 9 patients with glucose intolerance but normal
plasma lipoprotein pattern had an adipose tissue cholesterol concentration of $0.41 \pm .04$ ng/cell and the corresponding group of 6 patients with intolerance but Type IV lipoprotein pattern and greater fat cell size had a significantly higher mean value for adipose tissue cholesterol
concentration of $0.61 \pm .07$ ng/cell (p < .025)

DISCUSSION

Effect of Nicotinic Acid on Serum Lipids

The finding of Altschul et al. (8) that nicotinic
acid lowers serum cholesterol levels has been repeatedly
confirmed and extended to include also serum triglycerides (for review see 9). In fact the results presented here
indicate that nicotinic acid excerts a more pronounced
effect on triglyceride levels than on cholesterol at least
from the percentage point of view. The more detailed information on the effects of nicotinic acid obtained here
after classifying the hyperlipidemia into so called types (7) has revealed quite different response between these types. The more major lipid transport abnormalities,
as encountered in Types III and V, had the most dramatic
lowering of their serum lipid levels. As it is likely that
a major mechanism responsible for hypertriglyceridemia is
a reduction in removal from plasma (10, 11, 12) which
should be more pronounced the more intense the hyperlipoproteinemia is, the dramatic reduction of plasma triglyceride levels suggests that the treatment with nicotinic
acid had considerably improved triglyceride clearance from
blood. In accordance with this we have previously reported increase in the intravenous fat tolerance (13) and reduced alimentary lipemia (14) in man after treatment with
nicotinic acid. Similar observations have been made by
Nikkilä (15). These data strongly suggest that nicotinic
acid improves the removal of triglycerides from blood. In
this connection it is of considerable interest that the

activity of lipoprotein lipase - an enzyme system believed
to play an important role in removal of both endogenous
and exogenous triglycerides from blood - is increased in
rat adipose tissue by nicotinic acid (see 15). In man,
however, postheparin lipoprotein lipase activity is not
increased by treatment with nicotinic acid (13, 15).

Decreased secretion of lipoproteins into plasma as a
direct effect of the antilipolytic action of nicotinic
acid has also been suggested as mechanism for the hypolipidemic effect of this compound (16). Support of this view
has been obtained by Langer and Levy (17), who demonstrated that nicotinic acid treatment reduced the synthetic
rate of low density lipoproteins in patients with Type
II A hyperlipidemia. It is of interest that both reduced
synthesis as well as increased removal of triglyceride
rich lipoproteins may be referred to a single mode of action. Nicotinic acid is known to lower the levels of cyclic AMP in adipose tissue (18, see also 9). Low levels of
cyclic AMP may cause reduced fat mobilizing lipolysis (18)
and increased lipoprotein lipase activity (19), the former effect leading to reduced hepatic secretion of lipoproteins because of reduced inflow of precursor fatty acids
and the latter possibly causing increased removal of triglycerides from blood. Both these mechanisms, possibly
induced by a lowering of cyclic AMP in adipose tissue,
would tend to lower serum lipoprotein levels. It is not
unlikely that the importance of these two mechanisms may
vary between different types of hyperlipidemia.

Effect of Nicotinic Acid on Skeletal Muscle Lipids

Within a couple of hours after giving rats nicotinic
acid skeletal muscle triglyceride concentration is reduced (20). This effect is most likely explained by the inhibition of fat mobilizing lipolysis by nicotinic acid
causing reduced FFA flux to muscle tissue. It is not possible from this study to say if the lowering observed during chronic treatment with nicotinic acid was due to reduced FFA availability as this was not measured. Previous
studies have suggested, however, that the FFA availability
might be increased during the 24 hour period during nicotinic acid treatment (14, 21, see 9) because of the over-
shoot phenomenon (16). An alternative explanation for the
reduction in muscle triglycerides would be that there
exists an equilibrium between triglycerides in plasma and
tissues. However, this does not seem to fit with the fact
that there was no good correlation between the degree of
hyperlipidemia and muscle triglyceride concentration.

There was no weight decrease of the patients during the
treatment. The phospholipid concentration of the muscle
remained unchanged. This fits with the concept that while
the triglycerides are a metabolically active pool, the
phospholipids are mainly structural.

Adipose Tissue Characteristics in Hyperlipidemia

The new findings are that the concentration of free
cholesterol per cell in adipose tissue is related to fat
cell size in patients with normal and Type IV lipoprotein
pattern. Free cholesterol in adipose tissue expressed as
mg/mM TG was higher in patients with normal lipid pattern
than in those with Type IV pattern. In small cells the
per cent membrane material relative to triglycerides is
probably higher than in large expanded cells. Our findings might suggest that the main part of cholesterol in
fat cells is located in the cell membrane systems. In
patients with Type II A and II B lipoprotein patterns these relationships were not obtained. There were no significant differences in the concentration of free cholesterol expressed as mg/mM TG or ng/cell as compared to normal
or Type IV patients. There are several possible explanations for this lack of correlation, for example few patients, mixed clinical disorders, other cell types than
fat cells or numbers of fat cells, or possibly altered
cholesterol metabolism or storage.

The plasma or triglyceride concentration did not correlate with adipose tissue cholesterol concentration. This
does not exclude plasma triglyceride concentration as an
important determinant of adipose tissue cholesterol content. Prolonged positive caloric balance results in an
accumulation of TG in a normal or increased number of fat
cells in adipose tissue as discussed by Björntorp-Sjöström
(22).

In these studies we have also found that the combination of glucose intolerance, small fat cells and low cholesterol content (ng/cell) in adipose tissue is not related to hypertriglyceridemia, whereas large fat cells, high
concentration of free cholesterol in adipose tissue in
connection with pathological intravenous glucose tolerance
test is related to hypertriglyceridemia. There was no significantly different concentration of cholesterol when
expressed as mg/mM TG between these two groups. There was
no difference in plasma cholesterol concentration. These
patients with Type IV hyperlipidemia and pathological k-
value were quite different in body composition (BI = 1.20)

when compared with normals showing low k-values. The body
index was far above 1.0 which is considered as a normal
index when total body fat is not in excess.

These findings suggest that total body fat contains
a large free cholesterol pool. Since the concentration in
adipose tissue is in the range of 1 g per kg body fat
and total body fat can vary between 20 and 100 kg, the
total pool of free cholesterol in this tissue may range
from 20 to 100 grams.

There are other pools of cholesterol in the body of
similar magnitude. We find that skeletal muscle concentration of cholesterol is about 1 mg/g which gives us a
body pool of about 30 g. The liver content of cholesterol
is about 10 g.

What happens with these cholesterol pools during
treatment with diet and/or DALM is currently under investigation.

SUMMARY

The effect of treatment with 3 g daily of nicotinic
acid for one month on serum triglycerides and cholesterol
was studied in patients having hyperlipidemia of Type II
A, II B, III, IV and V. Significant reductions were obtained of both serum lipids in all types. The percentage
decrease of triglycerides was greater than that of cholesterol. The most dramatic reductions of serum lipids
(between 50 and 90 %) were obtained in patients with Type
III and V hyperlipidemia.

After two to four months treatment with nicotinic
acid the concentration of skeletal muscle triglycerides
but not phospholipids had decreased.

Fat cell size did not differ between various types
of hyperlipidemia. Adipose tissue free cholesterol concentration was slightly less in the group of patients with
Type IV hyperlipidemia when expressed per unit triglyceride. Fat cell cholesterol content, however, did not vary
between the different types. In the groups of patients
with normal lipids and with Type IV pattern there was a
strong correlation between fat cell content of cholesterol
and fat cell size. There was no correlation between the
serum lipids and either fat cell size or adipose tissue
cholesterol.

A group of subjects with asymptomatic glucose intolerance could be subdivided into two groups, one having
small fat cells, low adipose tissue cholesterol concentration and normal serum triglycerides, and the other having
large fat cells, high adipose tissue cholesterol concentration and hypertriglyceridemia.

Supported by grants from the Swedish Medical Research Council (19x-204-08), Konung Gustaf V:s 80-årsfond
and Loo och Hans Ostermans fond för medicinsk forskning.

REFERENCES

1. Hirsch, J., J.W. Farquhar, E.H. Ahrens, M.L. Peter-
    son, and W. Stoffel. Am. J. Clin. Nutr. 8:499 (1960).
2. Bergström, J. Scand. J. Clin. Lab. Invest. Suppl.
    68:23 (1962).
3. Carlson, L.A. and B. Kolmodin-Hedman. Acta Med.
    Scand., in press (1971).
4. Carlson, L.A., L.G. Ekelund, and S. Fröberg. Europ.
    J. Clin. Invest. 1:248 (1971).
5. Sjöström, L., P. Björntorp, and J. Vrana. J. Lipid
    Res. 12:521 (1971).
6. Walldius, G., to be published.
7. Beaumont, L., L.A. Carlson, G.R. Cooper, Z. Fejfar,
    D.S. Fredrickson, and T. Strasser. Bull. Wld. Hlth.
    Org. 43:891 (1970).
8. Altschul, R., A. Hoffer, and J.D. Stephen. Arch.
    Biochem. 54:558 (1955).
9. Gey, K.F. and L.A. Carlson (Eds.). Metabolic Effects
    of Nicotinic Acid and Its Derivatives. Hans Huber
    Publisher, Bern (1971).
10. Boberg, J., L.A. Carlson, and D. Hallberg. J. Athe-
    roscler. Res. 9:159 (1969).
11. Havel, R.J., in Atherosclerosis: Proceedings of the
    Second International Symposium. (Ed.) R.J. Jones,
    Springer-Verlag, Berlin-Heidelberg-New York (1970)
    p. 210.
12. Boberg, J., L.A. Carlson, U. Freyschuss, B.W. Las-
    sers, and M. Wahlqvist. Europ. J. Clin. Invest.,
    in press (1972).
13. Boberg, J., L.A. Carlson, S. Fröberg, A. Olsson,
    L. Orö and S. Rössner, in Metabolic Effects of Nico-
    tinic Acid and Its Derivatives. (Eds.) K.F. Gey and
    L.A. Carlson, Hans Huber Publisher, Bern (1971) p.
    465.

14. Fröberg, S., J. Boberg, L.A. Carlson, and M. Erics-
     son, in Metabolic Effects of Nicotinic Acid and Its
     Derivatives. (Eds.) K.F. Gey and L.A. Carlson, Hans
     Huber Publisher, Bern (1971) p. 167.
15. Nikkilä, E., in Metabolic Effects of Nicotinic Acid
     and Its Derivatives. (Eds.) K.F. Gey and L.A. Carl-
     son, Hans Huber Publisher, Bern (1971) p. 487.
16. Carlson, L.A. and L. Orö. Acta Med. Scand. 172:641
     (1962).
17. Langer, T. and R.I. Levy, in Metabolic Effects of
     Nicotinic Acid and Its Derivatives. (Eds.) K.F. Gey
     and L.A. Carlson, Hans Huber Publisher, Bern (1971)
     p. 641.
18. Butcher, R.W., C.E. Baird, and E.W. Sutherland. J.
     Biol. Chem. 243:1705 (1968).
19. Wing, D.R. and D.S. Robinson. Biochem. J. 109:841
     (1968).
20. Carlson, L.A., S. Fröberg, and E.R. Nye. Acta Med.
     Scand. 180:571 (1966).
21. Carlström, S. and S. Laurell. Acta Med. Scand. 184:
     121 (1968).
22. Björntorp, P. and L. Sjöström. Metabolism 20:703
     (1971).

THE COMBINED USE OF CLOFIBRATE AND ANION EXCHANGE

IN THE TREATMENT OF HYPERCHOLESTEROLEMIA

A. N. Howard, D. E. Hyams[*] and R. Courtenay Evans

Dept. of Investigative Medicine, University of Cambridge

and Chesterton Hospital, Cambridge, England

The use of anion exchange resins for the treatment of type II hyperlipoproteinemia is now well established, and one such resin, cholestyramine, has received considerable attention (1, 2). This class of drug acts by preferentially binding bile acids in the intestine and facilitating their increased excretion. Since cholesterol is the precursor of bile acids in the liver, total body cholesterol decreases and there is a subsequent fall in plasma cholesterol. Cholestyramine is found to be only moderately effective because the liver compensates by synthesizing more cholesterol from acetate (3). Also, the proportion of bile acids sequestered in the intestine is small (about 5-10%) compared with the total available (4). For these reasons, effective treatment is obtained with only large doses (12-35 g/day) of the resin. In type II hypercholesterolemic patients even 32 g/day gives a mean decrease of only 22% (5).

Earlier preparations of cholestyramine, such as Cuemid (Merck), were found to be unpalatable due to the smell, taste and texture of the impure resin. A purified product called Questran (Mead Johnson) is much better tolerated, and the use of additives and flavorings has provided a medication which is not unpleasant. However, some patients are unable to continue therapy because of

[*] Present address: Department of Geriatric Medicine (Guy's Hospital), New Cross Hospital, London, S.E. 14.

gastrointestinal disorders, such as acidity or constipation. For
the above reasons there is a need for the investigation of alternative resins, especially with respect to finding one with increased
activity and fewer side effects.

Parkinson (6) found that the cellulose and dextran anion
exchangers bound bile salts in vitro in the same way as cholestyramine. Of the substances examined, DEAE (diethyl amino ethyl)
Sephadex, a dextran polymer containing quaternary ammonium
groups, was the most active. In addition, DEAE Sephadex
reduced serum cholesterol in normocholesterolemic cockerels
and dogs and cholesterol-fed cockerels. Since this resin is a
tasteless powder, forming a smooth gel with water, it was potentially more acceptable to the patient. Experments were therefore carried out to compare its efficacy and acceptability with
cholestyramine.

Because cholestyramine is only moderately effective, its
combination with other drugs has been examined by other workers
and nicotinic acid has proved especially useful (7). In the present
work, attempts were made to increase the potency of the anion
exchange resin by the use of clofibrate, which has a completely
different mechanism of action.

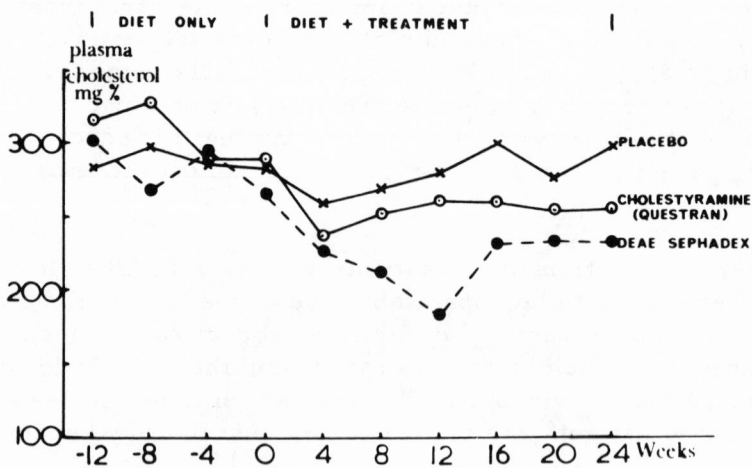

Fig. 1.   Effect of cholestyramine and DEAE Sephadex on plasma
cholesterol (5 patients/group).

COMPARISON OF DEAE SEPHADEX AND CHOLESTYRAMINE

Three groups of hypercholesterolemic patients (5 per group, each containing one type IV and four type II pattern lipoprotein disorders) were given a low cholesterol, low saturated fat diet (8). After a three-month base line period their treatment consisted of either a placebo resin, DEAE Sephadex or cholestyramine (Questran) given in water 12 g/day.

As shown in Fig. 1, both DEAE Sephadex and cholestyramine lowered plasma cholesterol consistently over a six-month period. Although the mean reduction with DEAE Sephadex (15%) was greater than with cholestyramine (12%) the difference was not significant. Plasma triglycerides were unaffected by both resins. Both groups of patients tolerated the resins fairly well, although the incidence of side effects was considerably less with DEAE Sephadex. In our experience the acceptability of DEAE Sephadex is excellent and it would seem a useful alternative to cholestyramine in the patients who complain of unpalatability or gastrointestinal disturbances.

ANION EXCHANGE RESINS AND CLOFIBRATE

Short Term Studies with Separate Dosage

In initial experiments, the dose of clofibrate (Atromid-S, 1.5 g/day) was given one-half hour before meals and the resin (15 g/day) with meals. This was to avoid any interference with the absorption of clofibrate. Six patients with type II lipoprotein pattern and three normals were asked to remain on their normal diet and were then given for two weeks either clofibrate, DEAE Sephadex or both drugs. Each treatment was followed by a period of no treatment for two weeks and was carried out at random. As shown in Table I, the combination of DEAE Sephadex and clofibrate produced a mean lowering of 33% which was greater than the sum of the two drugs separately (7% for clofibrate and 13% for DEAE Sephadex). Thus, the combination acted synergistically. Fig. 2 shows results of 11 patients treated with the combination for two and four weeks. The mean decreases were 34% and 35% respectively.

Treatment with clofibrate and cholestyramine combined was not so effective and only three out of 11 patients showed as good a

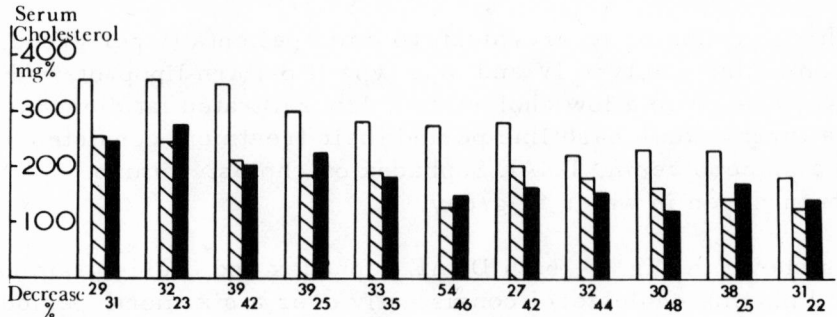

Fig. 2.   Effect of DEAE Sephadex (15 g/day) and clofibrate
(1.5 g/day) on serum cholesterol.

☐ base line   ◩ 2 weeks   ■ 4 weeks

TABLE I

SYNERGISM OF DEAE SEPHADEX (15 g/day)
AND CLOFIBRATE (1.5 g/day)

	CLOFIBRATE			DEAE SEPHADEX			CLOFIBRATE AND DEAE SEPHADEX		
Weeks	0 mg%	2	Change %	0 mg%	2	Change %	0 mg%	2	Change %
Patient									
1	279	267	4	308	253	15	296	182	39
2	208	182	13	200	189	6	279	186	33
3	308	236	23	218	183	16	272	125	54
4	248	183	26	262	274	+5	278	202	27
5	240	218	9	236	196	17	270	180	32
6	261	262	0	215	180	16	248	187	26
7	204	227	+11	233	204	12	230	175	24
8	245	245	0	224	184	18	230	162	30
9	253	253	0	246	186	24	228	142	38
MEAN			7			13			33

response as with DEAE Sephadex.   Nevertheless, a number of
patients showed an improvement with clofibrate and cholestyramine

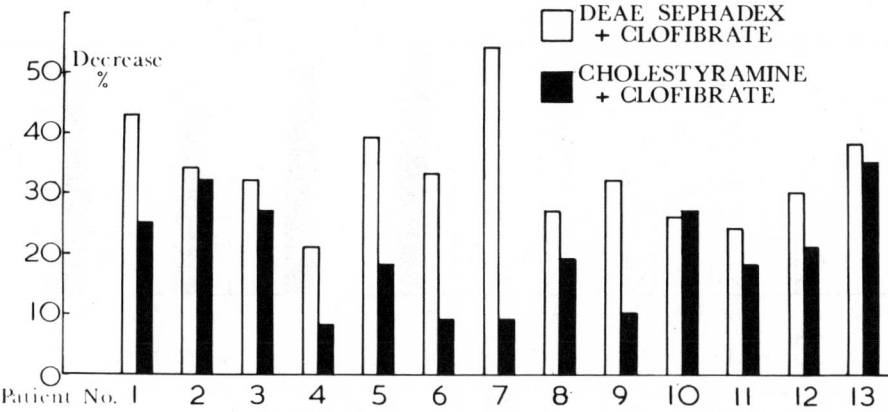

Fig. 3. Comparison of clofibrate (1.5 g/day) with either DEAE Sephadex (15 g/day) or cholestyramine (15 g/day): % decrease in serum cholesterol after two weeks treatment.

than each separately (Fig. 3) and the reason for the difference between the resins could be due to the greater binding power of DEAE Sephadex for bile acids (6).

Simultaneous Dosage of Clofibrate and DEAE Sephadex

Recent work has shown that neither cholestyramine nor DEAE Sephadex interferes appreciably with the absorption of clofibrate (9) and there is no need to give the drugs separately. In subsequent work, both drugs were given with meals and typical results are shown in Fig. 4. Although the combination is most useful in type II lipoprotein abnormality, an improvement in response is also seen in type IV patients. As expected, the decrease is proportional to the quantity of resin administered. Thus, 18 g/day DEAE Sephadex and clofibrate gives a mean lowering of 40% compared with about 20% for 9 g/day of the resin. Increases of clofibrate above 1.5 g/day have not been considered desirable and there is no evidence that an increased dose of clofibrate gives an appreciable improvement. As expected, elevated triglycerides are normalized by the combination with resins as obtained with clofibrate alone.

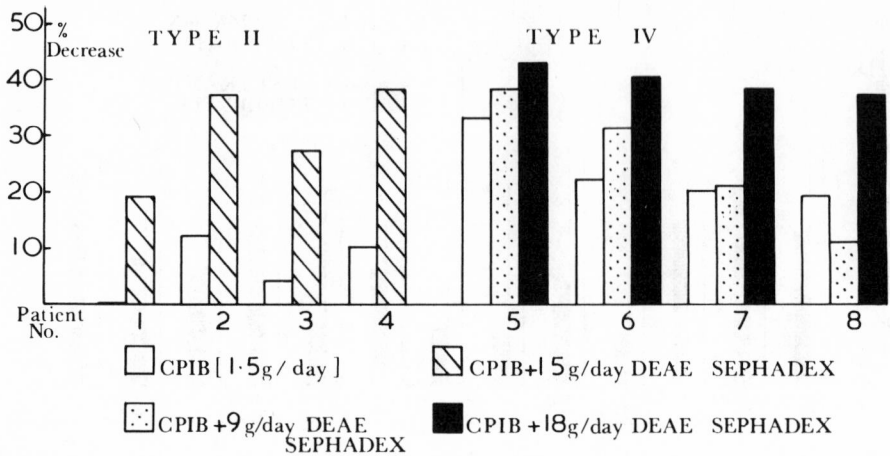

Fig. 4.   Different doses of DEAE Sephadex and clofibrate given
simultaneously in type II and type IV patients: % decrease in
serum cholesterol from base line after treatment for two weeks.

Long Term Studies

Administration of clofibrate and DEAE Sephadex over a
longer period are still in progress.   In six type II heterozygous
patients with type II disease treatment with clofibrate gave only a
small response (Fig. 5).   The addition of DEAE Sephadex (12 g/day)
gave a mean decrease of 35% and the effect was sustained after
20 weeks of treatment.   So far there is no evidence of resistance
developing in such patients.

Synergism of Clofibrate and Anion Exchange Resins

The proposed modes of action of clofibrate are numerous
(10,11).   Beneficial actions have been reported on lipoprotein,
cholesterol and triglyceride metabolism, all of which would assist
the hypocholesterolemic effect of anion exchange resins.   Of
special importance is the effect of clofibrate in increasing the
weight of bile acids secreted into the intestine as seen in the dog
(12) and the rat (13).   If this effect occurred in man, then clofibrate would increase the quantity of bile acids available for
sequestering by the resin.   Although in man clofibrate gives no
increase in the excretion of bile acids, fecal cholesterol is
increased (14).

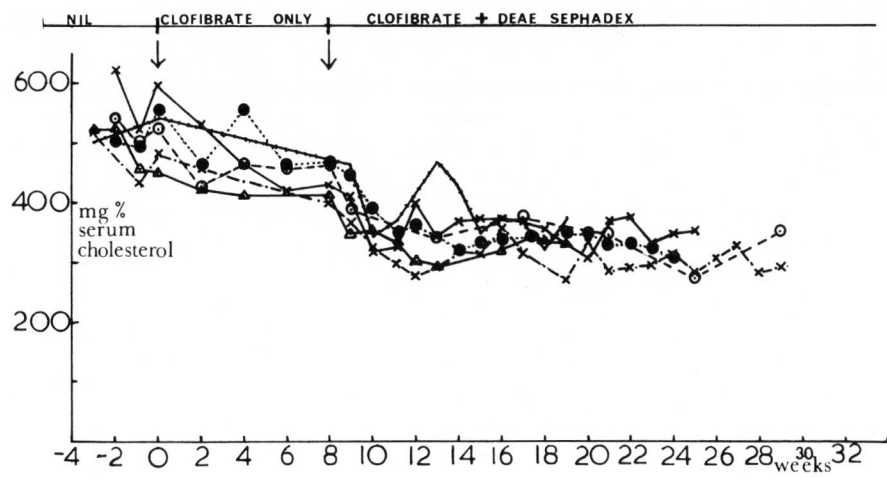

Fig. 5.   Longer term administration of DEAE Sephadex (12 g/day)
and clofibrate (1.5 g/day) after initial treatment with clofibrate
only: effect on serum cholesterol.

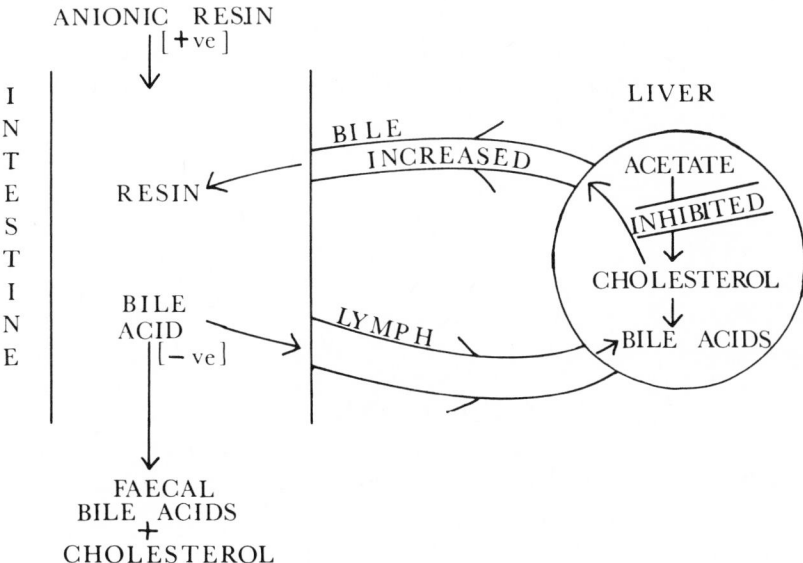

Fig. 6.   The combined action of clofibrate and anion exchange
resins.

When anion exchange resins are given, the liver compensates for the loss of bile acids by synthesizing more cholesterol from acetate.   Clofibrate has an important action in inhibiting cholesterol biosynthesis (15).   Furthermore, Cayen and Dvornik (16) showed that in the rat, clofibrate is able to depress the increased acetate incorporation into cholesterol produced by cholestyramine. Both the choleretic effect of clofibrate and its inhibition of cholesterol biosynthesis, could explain its synergism with anion exchange resins (Fig. 6).

CONCLUSIONS

DEAE Sephadex is a palatable and well-tolerated anion exchange resin which is as effective as cholestyramine when administered alone.   When the anion exchange resins were combined with clofibrate, synergism occurred.   Simultaneous dosage of DEAE Sephadex (15 g/day) and clofibrate (1.5 g/day) was particularly effective in all patients studied and produced a mean fall in plasma cholesterol of 35%.   This therapy is particularly useful in those patients who are resistant to clofibrate alone.

Much attention has been devoted in the past to the production of a single drug which would lower plasma lipids, yet so far no such compound has been evolved which is effective in all cases needing treatment.   The use of two drugs, each with a different mode of action, as illustrated here, would seem to offer a greater chance of success.

ACKNOWLEDGMENTS

This work was supported by a grant from the United Cambridge Hospitals.   Mead Johnson (Evansville, Ind.) and Pharmacia (Uppsala, Sweden) generously donated supplied of Questran and DEAE Sephadex, respectively.

REFERENCES

1. Bergen, S. S., Jr. and T. B. van Itallie.   Ann. Intern. Med. 58:355 (1963).
2. Hashim, S. A. and T. B. van Itallie.   J. Amer. Med. Assn. 192:289 (1965).
3. Goodman, D. S. and R. P. Noble.   J. Clin. Invest. 47:231 (1968).

4. van Itallie, T. B. and S. A. Hashim.   Med. Clin. N. Amer. <u>47</u>:629 (1963).
5. Miettinen, T. A.   In, <u>Atherosclerosis</u>, Proc. 2nd Int. Symp. (Ed.) R. J. Jones, Springer-Verlag, Berlin (1970) p. 508.
6. Parkinson, T. M.   J. Lipid Res. <u>8</u>:24 (1967).
7. Smith, D. H. and E. Gaman.   Fed. Proc. <u>19</u>:236 (1960).
8. Howard, A. N. and D. E. Hyams.   Brit. Med. J. <u>3</u>:25 (1971).
9. Hyams, D. E., A. N. Howard, and R. C. Evans.   (In preparation).
10. Steinberg, D.   In, <u>Atherosclerosis</u>, Proc. 2nd Int. Symp. (Ed.) R. J. Jones, Springer-Verlag, Berlin (1970) p. 500.
11. Pereira, J. N. and G. F. Holland.   In, <u>Atherosclerosis</u>, Proc. 2nd Int. Symp.   (Ed.) R. J. Jones, Springer-Verlag, Berlin (1970) p. 549.
12. Horning, M. and E. Horning (1970).   Unpublished observations.
13. Hess, R. (1970).   Unpublished observations.
14. Grundy, S. M., E. H. Ahrens, Jr., G. Salen, and E. Quintao.   J. Clin. Invest. <u>48</u>:33a (1969).
15. Gould, R. G. and E. A. Swyryd.   Progr. Biochem. Pharm. <u>4</u>: 191 (1968).
16. Cayen, M. N. and D. Dvornik.   Canad. J. Biochem. <u>48</u>:1022 (1970).

CAN HEART DISEASE BE POSTPONED OR PREVENTED?

ATHEROGENIC AND THROMBOGENIC MOSAIC

Irvine H. Page

Research Division, Cleveland Clinic, Cleveland, Ohio

The prevention of coronary heart disease, from the viewpoint of numbers, will certainly be the greatest achievement of modern medicine. Despite the recent foray of politicians into cancer research, simple arithmetic shows the urgency of the heart disease problem. Oddly, many seem to believe prevention of coronary heart disease would help only the aged and infirm, but the young business executive is far from immune. Obviously, prevention would more likely be achieved if we knew the cause of athero-sclerosis.

The question I will pose is whether there is a single cause. I realize how committed my generation is to the single-cause dogma, but now younger generations seem quite as firmly hooked on it. The opposing view of multifaceted or multifactorial etiology is contemptuously considered miasma, woolly thinking, or impure science.

I hesitate to mention this, but many years ago I proposed that the mechanisms of hypertension were many and varied, that they were all involved and integrated to different degrees in determining the final set of arterial blood pressure at levels best adapted to perfusion of the tissues. This mosaic was conceived as an equili-brated system; the regulating system of a genetically determined body. Changing interactions of these mechanisms produced the varied clinical manifestations of arterial hypertension. Such a hypothesis gives a place for such sophisticated mechanisms as

control by feedback and even such chemical control mechanisms
as allostery.   It aims to provide a structure on which to hang all
the mechanisms concerned with maintaining the wholeness of the
body.

I fully realize that this mosaic theory has caused some acute
pain in varied parts of the anatomy.   Others have accepted it but
called it simplistic, which it certainly is.   But its chief function
of maintaining a structure onto which new facts can be added in an
orderly and meaningful fashion should not be lost.

I am sure you have anticipated what I am up to.   I warned you
years ago that atherosclerosis was my next victim for the mosaic
hypothesis.   Now I think we know enough about the multiplicity of
mechanisms of atherogenesis to try and climb out of the miasma
of the one mechanism concept.   We can no longer be "cholesterol
doctors" or "cholesterol is all bosh doctors."   After decades of
research there still is no single cause that can be blamed.   Even
the question, "Do you believe diet is the cause of atherosclerosis,"
is beginning to sound tired.   I think you will agree we are now
moving out in many directions, any one, or all of which, may prove
of vital importance to prevention and even cure.   While fully
recognizing that coronary atherosclerosis is the main substrate on
which myocardial infarction rests, it may by no means be the only
factor involved.   If George Mann is correct, the Masai live well
with extensive atherosclerosis, and suffer little or no myocardial
infarction.

We made a correlative study of patients referred to the Cleveland Clinic for coronary angiography because of suspected coronary
disease, comparing the angiograms with the blood lipid patterns.
Most of the patients could have been correctly diagnosed with either
procedure alone, which shows not only the close correlation of high
lipid values with visible coronary atherosclerosis but the perspi-
cacity of referring physicians because their diagnosis by clinical
means alone was usually correct.

Though I fully accept the close relationship of elevation of
blood lipids with accelerated atherogenesis, I am not persuaded
that there are not several other important factors in the precipitation of thrombosis and myocardial infarction.   Understandably
most of us draw our views from one patient while concurrently
giving lip service to statisticians and double-blind studies, especially
so if that patient is you!

Therefore, without even a preliminary "by your leave," I will use myself as a prototype of the atherogenic and thrombogenic mosaic. Many of our friends have espoused unpopular mechanisms of atherogenesis and some have proved to be probably correct. You will remember the catecholamines, sticky platelets, poor collaterals, hemorrhage into placques, emotional fatigue, decreased thrombolysis, etc. To combine these with the old war horses of elevated blood lipids, femaleness, smoking, genetic factors, lack of exercise, obesity, elevated uric acid, and chronic stress into a meaningful pattern does indeed require a mosaic or something like it.

My own troubles began four years ago. After decades of telling the public and doctors how to prevent heart attacks, I grossly disregarded my own advice and got well repaid for it. I was presiding at the final meeting of the National Diet-Heart Study in Chicago. It was a grueling meeting and I was determined that we submit a unified report, not like the double headed monster on lipoproteins. I am sure you know all of us on the committee well enough to appreciate that individuality is not lost in our democracy. I was exhausted when it was over and "ran" to the airport only to find that all planes were canceled because of a heavy storm. Instead of accepting it, I thought with thousands of other travelers that I could get home somehow. Nine hours later I did. The next day was unconscionably hot and humid but nothing would deter me from playing three sets of tennis "to make me feel better." I should add that I possess a very peculiar thirst center. Instead of being thirsty during, or just after having loss of water, there is a six to eight hour lag. It was just about at the end of that six hours that my heart attack occurred. The rest is all boring detail of how to be a good patient without really being one.

Here are the things that I consider important: (1) my blood cholesterol had averaged around 300 mg with a moderately high pre-beta fraction for many years, (2) my father died at 66 with extensive atherosclerosis and was a heavy whole-milk drinker all his life, (3) I was a week-end athlete, (4) I was enjoying "chronic emotional fatigue," (5) the Chicago episode must have mobilized a large amount of catecholamines and free fatty acids since I had nothing to eat, (6) dehydration with hemoconcentration due to sweating during tennis must have been severe and it was not repaired, (7) my platelets must have stuck together like Scotch tape, (8) I smoked cigarettes more freely that I usually did.

It is just such a conglomeration of potentially atherogenic and thrombogenic mechanisms that spells trouble.   This is not to say there are not many other ways of arriving at the point of having a heart attack.   The mosaic will keep you up to date on other ways in case you are interested.

My last point is the problems with which this panel is charged. "Can we prevent heart attacks?"   If I knew, we would not have a panel.   Being an experimentalist at heart, my policy is to try something if there seems to me to be substantial evidence in its favor, even though not proved.   I would rather take a low cholesterol, high polyunsaturated fat diet "in moderation" and without making a tiresome social fetish of it, on the bet that after another decade it will be shown to have been beneficial.   If I wait for ten years to find out and it turns out to be right, then I am ten years older and ten years closer to meeting my ancestors by way of my defective coronary arteries.   Just so, while I do not know whether saphenous vein bypass as developed by Dr. Favaloro will be a long term success, I would be willing to have the operation if I were in acute pain and a serious obstruction had been shown to be present by the Sones-Shirey angiographic technique.   I would even go so far as to believe that a myocardial infarction had been headed off by such an operation performed at the right time.

Thus, my answer is that prevention consists in the development of a way of life with which you as a person are content to live without making a martyr of yourself.   With few exceptions such as smoking, you will be able to follow the injunction: moderation in all things, but don't miss anything.   Life must still be to live, not to live to prevent!   For most things, life demands a price, usually a small one.   Just be sure the price is not too high and you don't get short-changed.

On a more fundamental level, I suspect that the problem of atherogenesis has some similarity to the one Jules Hirsch had concerning the nature of adipose cells and "liposomes."   In short, if you can tell me how to manipulate the lipophilic quality of atherocytes, I will tell you how to convert a Twiggy into a Jayne Mansfield. The difference between men and most women is that the latter know where to deposit fat and we men do not.

RISK FACTORS IN CORONARY HEART DISEASE: POSSIBILITIES OF PREVENTION IN THE FEDERAL REPUBLIC OF WEST GERMANY

G. Schettler

Medical Clinic, University of Heidelberg Medical

School, Heidelberg, Germany

According to new international statistical data published by WHO, the United States has the highest mortality rate due to coronary disease since 1956. These rates have, in general, remained constant. From 1956 to 1967, however, there has been a continuous increase in mortality rates in all West European countries and in Japan, and it is unlikely that those rates are due to statistical errors. Among the West European countries, Finland has the highest mortality rate. Within these countries there exists regional differences: there are marked differences in mortality rates due to myocardial infarction between East and West Finland, between North and South Italy, between the Baltic region and the Caspian districts of Russia, between North and South Japan. The situation in the Federal Republic of West Germany for the period 1948 to 1970 is as follows: the total number of cardiovascular deaths rose from 2600 in 1948 to 38,000 in 1956, 56,000 in 1960, and 66,000 in 1964; and the rise has continued. The number of deaths in 1968, 1969 and 1970 was 95,000, 104,000 and 125,000, respectively. We do not have exact statistical data representative of the first years after World War II. According to reports from the Institutes of Pathology and large clinics, it is evident that the incidence of myocardial infarctions was extremely low. There were not more than approximately 2000 deaths due to myocardial infarction in 1948. There is no doubt that the striking increase of myocardial infarctions in the Federal Republic since 1948 parallels the normalizing situation in the food markets. In 1971, we expect an even higher death rate. If we count the number of patients who

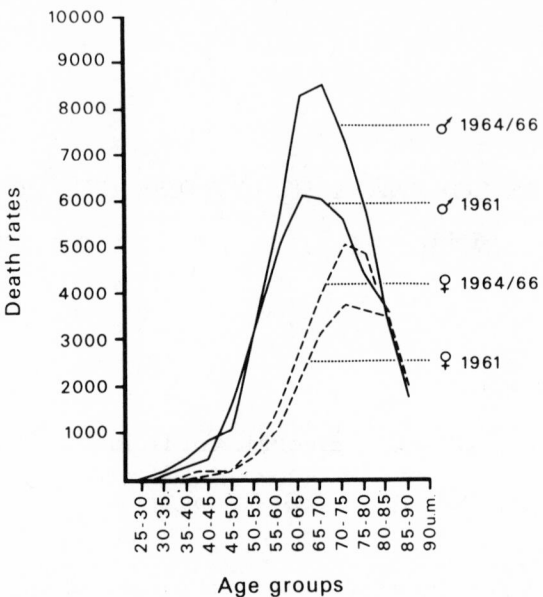

Fig. 1.   Death rates from myocardial infarction in the Federal
Republic of Germany, 1961 and 1964-1966.

suffer from either their first or second myocardial infarction, it
gives us a figure of approximately 600,000.   In addition, we see
an increase of myocardial infarctions for both men and women of
younger ages.   A summary of this is seen in Fig. 1, which com-
pares the death rates due to coronary disease in 1961 with 1964-
1966.   As we expected, there is a higher frequency for men than
for women.

There is a tendency toward a decrease in death rates due to
hypertension in the USA, Great Britain, Sweden, and perhaps in
France.   This is also true for Japan and Italy since 1962-1963.
In the Federal Republic of Germany, however, these rates have
remained constant, with a striking increase in 1967 and 1971.
There is no easy explanation for these discrepancies; in general,
the limit for normal values for blood pressure may be too high in
West Germany.   If we calculate the normal systolic blood pressure
by adding 100 to the age of the patient, this certainly gives us too
high a number.   On the other hand, general control of our patients
suffering from hypertension may not be as strict in Germany as,
for instance, in the USA, Great Britain, or Sweden.

The death rates are frightening, especially since physicians as well as the general population in West Germany know the various methods for preventing myocardial infarction and hypertension. However, we do not yet know which of the known risk factors may be responsible for the high rates.   Studies of primary and secondary prevention of myocardial infarction are under way in West Germany, but are not yet finished.

I would like to report a study of secondary prevention which we began in West Germany in 1965, together with ten medical clinics.   The study was originally done to repeat Engelberg's study on long-term heparin treatment in ischemic heart disease. As you know, Engelberg and coworkers (1) found that by injecting 200 mg of heparin subcutaneously twice a week the survival rate of patients with myocardial infarction was higher than in a control group of untreated patients.   In a period of two years they found that 4 of 105 treated patients had died compared to 21 in the control group of 117 patients.   Lovell (2) and coworkers could not confirm this protective action of the heparin injection in a group of 168 male patients between 30 and 69 years, compared to a group of patients with myocardial infarction receiving lower dosages of anticoagulants (coumarin).   Contrarily, a high dose of anticoagulants did show a protective action.   Böttiger, Carlson, and coworkers (3, 4) did find statistically significant differences between the heparin treated and the placebo group among 91 male patients suffering from myocardial infarction under the age of 65 years. In a follow-up study of three years or more, in the group receiving heparin 7 patients either died or had a second myocardial infarction compared to 14 in the group receiving placebos.   After five years there were 8 such patients in the group receiving heparin and 16 in the placebo group.   Therefore, the authors were slightly positive towards long-term treatment with heparin.

TABLE I

SURVIVAL RATE AFTER LONG-TERM TREATMENT
WITH HEPARIN

	Treatment		Placebo		Total	
	N	%	N	%	N	%
Alive	129	87.2	140	89.2	269	88.2
Dead	19	12.8	17	10.8	36	11.8
Total	148	100	157	100	305	100

TABLE II

REINFARCTION RATE UNDER LONG-TERM HEPARIN TREATMENT

Number of reinfarctions	Treatment N	%	Placebo N	%	Total N	%
0	142	96	150	95	292	96
1	5	3	4	3	9	3
2	0	0	3	2	3	1
3	1	1	0	0	1	0
4 and >	0	0	0	0	0	0
Total	148	100	157	100	305	100

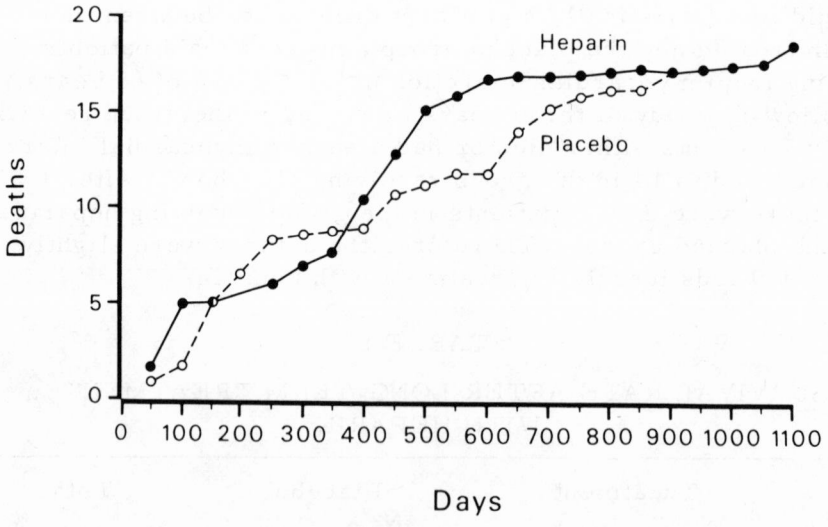

Fig. 2.   Incidence of death under long-term heparin treatment in comparison to a placebo treated control group.

We selected 350 patients out of 1551 males who had suffered a myocardial infarction; there were no limits of age. Of these 350 patients, 54 could not be followed, either because of mistakes during treatment or unreliability of the patient. We were therefore left with 305 patients for the study, the results of which are shown in Table I. The majority (94%) of the patients ranged between 41 and 65 years of age. Most of the patients (70%) were between 51 and 65 years of age. Patients were followed for more than three years, the average follow-up being more than 24 months. The reinfarction rate is shown in Table II. We used the following criteria for estimation of the effects of long-term heparin treatment in patients with myocardial infarction: (1) number of deaths, (2) number of reinfarctions which were registered during the study; the results are shown in Fig. 2. We concluded that the death rate was 2% lower in the group receiving placebos than in the heparin group. Therefore, a significant difference during the time of investigation could not be confirmed. The rate of reinfarctions was approximately the same in both groups.

Our results are very similar to Lovell's data (2) and differ from those reported by the Swedish authors. We do, however, admit that the Swedish study was performed for a period of five years and that differences between control and heparin groups could not be observed before 1-1/2 years of treatment.

TABLE III

INCIDENCE OF DISTRIBUTION OF OVERWEIGHT
IN PATIENTS UNDER STUDY

	Overweight					
	No		Yes		Total	
Age	N	%	N	%	N	%
< 39	24	63	14	27	38	100
40-49	85	62	53	38	138	100
50-59	159	64	88	26	247	100
60-69	190	65	102	35	292	100
> 70	76	69	34	31	110	100
Total	534		291		825	

TABLE IV

TRIGLYCERIDE LEVELS IN THE PATIENTS UNDER
STUDY AT THE TIME OF THEIR FIRST INFARCTION

| | Triglyceride | | | | | |
| | < 200 | | > 200 | | Total | |
Age	N	%	N	%	N	%
< 39	15	63	9	37	24	100
40-49	43	55	35	45	78	100
50-59	62	50	63	50	125	100
60-69	89	62	54	38	143	100
> 69	30	73	11	27	41	100
Total	239		172		411	

When we looked for the known risk factors in a larger group
of our patients, we found data as shown in Tables III to VIII. We
see that in all age groups there was a high incidence of overweight
The number of patients who were overweight at the time of their
first infarction was 291, or 35% of the total sample.   At the time
of the second infarction, 33% of the patients were overweight.

Patients with hypertriglyceridemia were most common in the
age group 50-59 (Table IV).   There were significant differences
between the groups for serum cholesterol levels and for diabetes
and hypertension, but not for elevated levels of uric acid (Tables
V to VIII).

TABLE V

CHOLESTEROL LEVELS OF PATIENTS UNDER STUDY

| | < 250 | | 250-329 | | 330-399 | | > 400 | | Total | |
Age	N	%	N	%	N	%	N	%	N	%
< 39	9	26	17	49	6	17	3	8	35	100
40-49	48	37	64	40	11	9	5	4	128	100
50-59	102	45	110	48	15	7	1	0	228	100
60-69	129	49	109	41	20	8	5	2	263	100
> 70	56	65	25	29	5	6	0	0	86	100
Total	344		325		57		14		740	

TABLE VI

INCIDENCE OF DIABETES IN PATIENTS UNDER STUDY AT THE
TIME OF THEIR FIRST INFARCTION

| | Diabetes | | | | | |
| | Yes | | No | | Total | |
Age	N	%	N	%	N	%
< 39	5	15	28	85	33	100
40-49	23	17	110	83	133	100
50-59	45	19	192	81	237	100
60-69	63	22	229	78	292	100
> 70	34	30	78	70	112	100
Total	170		637		807	

TABLE VII

INCIDENCE OF HYPERTENSION IN PATIENTS UNDER STUDY AT
THE TIME OF THEIR FIRST INFARCTION

| | Hypertension | | | | | |
| | Yes | | No | | Total | |
Age	N	%	N	%	N	%
< 39	8	22	28	78	36	100
40-49	31	25	92	75	123	100
50-59	63	28	164	72	227	100
60-69	100	37	171	63	271	100
> 69	31	34	59	66	90	100
Total	233		514		747	

TABLE VIII

LEVELS OF URIC ACID IN PATIENTS UNDER STUDY

Age	Uric Acid				
	< 7			> 7	
	N	%		N	%
< 39	26	4		4	7
40-49	104	18		9	17
50-59	187	31		13	24
60-69	215	36		17	32
> 70	65	11		11	20
Total	597	100		54	100

In all decades the rate of patients with diabetes was about 7-10% higher than in the normal West German population; this rate continuously increases with age. There were no differences between first and second myocardial infarction. The same tendency could be found for hypertension. At the time of their first infarction, 20% of the men were diabetic; 23% were diabetic when they suffered their second infarction. The percent who were hypertensive at the time of their first and second infarctions were 32% and 31%, respectively. There were significant differences between the numbers of men smoking at the time of their first and second infarction. The highest consumption of cigarettes was found in the youngest patients with myocardial infarction: 85% in the group younger than 45 years of age smoked more than 10 cigarettes per day, while in the group older than 69 years of age only 29% smoked more than 10 cigarettes per day.

In comparing risk factors, we found the following results:

Overweight: No correlation with cigarette smoking, possible correlation with hypertriglyceridemia, positive correlation with hypertension, hypercholesterolemia, and diabetes.

Hypertension: No correlation with hypercholesterolemia and cigarette smoking, positive correlation with diabetes mellitus, positive correlation with hypertriglyceridemia in patients with myocardial infarction who were older than 50 years.

Diabetes mellitus: No correlation with cigarette smoking, positive correlation with hypertriglyceridemia and hypercholesterolemia.

Cholesterol: No correlation with cigarette smoking and elevated levels of uric acid, possible correlation with hypertriglyceridemia.

Cigarette smoking: No correlation with hypertension, diabetes, hyperholesterolemia, slightly positive correlation with hypertriglyceridemia in the age group of 50 years.

When we investigated the significance of the various risk factors in terms of surviving myocardial infarction, we found no positive results from the comparison of the heparin and control groups. Especially there was no positive correlation between hypertriglyceridemia or hypercholesterolemia. During heparin treatment there were no changes in triglycerides, cholesterol, or lipoprotein patterns. Patients with hypertriglyceridemia or hypercholesterolemia were, however, not investigated for their individual lipoprotein pattern. We were not able to demonstrate changes in lipoprotein lipase activity in the group of patients receiving heparin. This is in agreement with results published by Böttiger, Carlson, and coworkers (3, 4).

In a group of 325 patients with their first myocardial infarction, 8% had no risk factors (hypertension, diabetes, hypertriglyceridemia, hyperuricemia, cigarette smoking). If we look at 521 other patients from the same group who also had their first myocardial infarction but in whom triglycerides were not determined, the situation is as follows: 14% had no risk factor, 38% had one, 27% had two, 15% had three, 5% had four, 1% had five, and in no case was there six risk factors altogether.

If we look at different age groups, there was a high rate of risk factors for the group between 39 and 59 years. With increasing age, the incidence of risk factors was lower; the incidence of diabetes, however, increased with age.

In summary, we obtained results very similar to those previously reported in other countries, e.g., the USA. We would like to point out the importance of risk factors, especially of additive risk factors. In a great number of our patients with myocardial infarction, the combination of overweight, diabetes, hypertension, hypercholesterolemia, and hypertriglyceridemia could be demonstrated.   We cannot comment on the important question as to which of these factors plays the greatest role in causing myocardial infarction.   We would, however, like to point out that correcting these risk factors is probably the best method for preventing myocardial infarction.

Just by looking at the incidence of risk factors, we cannot statistically explain the differences in rates of myocardial infarctions between West Germany and the USA.   We also do not have an explanation for the very rapid increase of myocardial infarctions between 1948 and 1956, and the even further increase since 1956. We feel that statistical errors can be excluded because we get similar results when we look at the autopsies during this time. One possible explanation might be the continuous increase of diabetes in West Germany and, secondly, the poor control of hypertension.   Together with cigarette smoking these two diseases probably belong to the most dangerous risk factors.   We have already pointed out the importance of mild hypertension for the development of myocardial infarction.   These international experiences could also be confirmed for West Germany (5).   It could also be demonstrated that by correcting mild cases of hypertension, life expectancy could significantly be improved and the rate of myocardial infarctions could be lowered.   From these data we feel that there is an important difference in treatment with sedation only. Malignant hypertension has to be considered as something else, as we all know that renal and cerebral complications are much more common than myocardial infarction.   The death rates due to diabetes in the USA, Japan and some West European countries show a very similar trend, as already reported for the death rates from myocardial infarction.   We do not know yet exactly how important it is to control diabetes with regard to the development of myocardial infarction.   We have to very carefully check recent data published by Prout (6.7) who found differences in patients treated with diet alone and those treated with insulin or drugs.   From our own autopsies we can confirm that severe cases of coronary arteriosclerosis occur in diabetes and hypertension (8).

The increase in patients with hypercholesterolemia plus hypertriglyceridemia as well as increasing overweight are other risk factors in the Federal Republic of Germany, between 1948 and 1956. We already demonstrated the elevated serum cholesterol levels which are representative for the period from 1942 to 1970. We have to take into account, however, that within this period there

was a time of starvation due to World War II.   So it is possible
that at least some of these elevated cholesterol levels were due
to an altered mechanism in adaptation.   We do not know, however,
why this level is still increasing after 1956.   It may be that since
1948 we have had to deal with very severe forms of atherosclerosis,
and the complicating myocardial infarctions occur now.   There
were a good many coronary thromboses in patients who had died
from myocardial infarctions during a time when food was available
again after the second World War.

Without any doubt, thrombosis plays an important role for the
beginning and prognosis of myocardial infarction.   There are new
ways to treat myocardial infarction and to prevent it.   We cannot
comment on the role which anticoagulants play in this regard.   It
is still the subject of some controversy as to how long anticoagulants should be given in patients with myocardial infarction.   Long-
term treatment with heparin in high doses should not be prescribed,
however.

REFERENCES

1. Engelberg, H. , R. Kuhn, and M. Steinman.   Circulation 13:
   489 (1956).
2. Lovell, R.R.H. , M.A. Denborough, P.J. Nester, and A.J.
   Goble.   Arch. intern. Med. 113:267 (1964).
3. Böttiger, L.E. , L.A. Carlson, L. Engstedt, and L. Oró.
   J. Atheroscler. Res. 5:253 (1965).
4. Böttiger, L.E. , L.A. Carlson, L. Engstedt, and L. Oró.
   Acta Med. Scand. 182:245 (1967).
5. Dengler, H.J. and G. Schettler.   Naturw. u. Med. 7:52 (1965).
6. Prout, T.E. and M.G. Goldner.   Diabetes 19, Suppl. I, 375
   (1970),Suppl. II, 747 (1970).
7. Klimt, C.R. , G.L.Knatterud, C.L. Meinert, and T.E. Prout.
   Diabetes 19, Suppl. II, 747 (1970).
8. Schettler, G.   Deutsch. Med. J. 10:297 (1971).

ROLE OF DIET IN THE PRIMARY PREVENTION OF CORONARY HEART DISEASE

Osmo Turpeinen

Department of Biochemistry, College of Veterinary

Medicine, Helsinki, Finland

For a long time already there has been available a considerable body of evidence favoring the idea that coronary heart disease
(CHD) could, at least partly, be a nutritional disease and hence
susceptible of dietary prevention. I am particularly referring to
the extensive and well-known epidemiological observations and
studies, which have shown that definite associations exist between
dietary fats, serum cholesterol and CHD. However, evidence of
this type alone is, of course, not sufficient to prove the existence
of a cause-and-effect relationship between the diet and CHD and
does not permit us to conclude that a modification of diet would
bring about a reduction in the incidence of the disease. The problem
of dietary prevention of CHD can obviously be definitely solved
only by means of adequately planned intervention studies, that is,
preventive trials in which the diet of a suitable population is deliberately changed and the development of manifestations of the disease
is followed over a sufficiently long period. An otherwise comparable population among which no dietary changes are instituted is
required as a control.

In spite of the obvious difficulties connected with such work, a
few groups of investigators have ventured into this field of study.
Some of the trials are still continuing. The dietary trials aiming
at primary prevention which I am going to review are mainly the
following three: the Anti-Coronary Club Project of New York, which
has been conducted by Rinzler, Christakis and others (1), the Mental
Hospital Study of our group in Helsinki (2), and the clinical trial at

Los Angeles Veterans Administration Center conducted by Dayton and his colleagues (3).

In addition, I wish to mention briefly a fourth, more recently started study, which is being carried out in Minnesota mental hospitals with Dr. Frantz as the principal investigator. This dietary trial involves some 3000 to 4000 subjects, which have been divided by random allocation. No published results are available as yet.

Also, a fifth study may be mentioned. I am referring to the Coronary Prevention Evaluation Program conducted by Stamler and his colleagues in Chicago. This, however, is a multifactorial study involving not only dietary change but also modifications in smoking habits, exercise etc. Since we now are concerned with prevention by diet alone, this trial is not very helpful from our point of view.

But let us return to the trials described in Tables I, II, and III. The subjects in all these three studies have been middle-aged or elderly males. In the New York trial they were free-living men, who were recruited among volunteers. In the Helsinki study they were hospitalized mental patients, and in the Los Angeles trial they were veterans living in a domiciliary unit. The groups in each case contained some hundreds of subjects. As to the age, this was similar in the New York and the Helsinki studies, a little over 50 years, on the average (though the ranges were different), whereas the Los Angeles subjects were considerably older, their mean being about 65 years.

TABLE I

TYPE AND NUMBER OF SUBJECTS IN STUDIES OF PRIMARY
PREVENTION OF CHD

Locality and years of study	Type of subjects	Number of subjects		Age of subjects, years
		Exp	Con	
New York 1957-	Free living men	941	457	40-59
Helsinki 1958-	Mental hospital patients	327	254	34-64 (mean 51.3)
Los Angeles 1959-1968	Domiciled veterans	424	422	54-88 (mean 65.5)

TABLE II

DIETARY FAT, SERUM CHOLESTEROL AND ADIPOSE TISSUE
LINOLEIC ACID IN STUDIES OF PRIMARY PREVENTION OF CHD

| Loc. | Diet | | | | Serum cholesterol mg/100 ml | | Adipose tissue linoleic acid % of total | |
| | Fat content % | | P/S ratio | | | | | |
	Exp	Con	Exp	Con	Exp	Con	Exp	Con
N.Y.	33	40	1.4	0.35	225	250	19	10
Hel.	31	36	1.4	0.25	217	268	27	10
L.A.	39	40	(I.V. 102)	(I.V. 54)	Diff. 30 mg		34	11

In all these studies the diets (Table II) of the experimental
groups were designed with the primary aim of decreasing the serum
cholesterol level. All were relatively high in fat. The dietary
manipulations consisted of increasing the content of polyethenoid
fatty acids and decreasing that of saturated acids. That this was
achieved, is shown by the polyethenoid-saturated fatty acid ratio,
briefly the P/S ratio, which actually was much higher in the experimental diets than in the control diets. In the Los Angeles study
the unsaturation of dietary fats was expressed by the use of iodine
value. Also in this case the fat moiety of the experimental diet
was much more unsaturated than that of the control diet.

In all studies the experimental diet brought about a decrease
in the serum cholesterol values. The mean difference between the
groups was about 25 mg in the New York study, about 50 mg in the
Helsinki study and about 30 mg in the Los Angeles study. These
differences may not seem large, but the experience obtained from
prospective risk factor studies indicates that differences of even
this magnitude are associated with a substantial difference in the
risk of developing CHD.

Another parameter which has proved very useful in long-term
dietary experiments of this type is the fatty acid composition of the
adipose tissue. By now it is well documented that the composition
of human adipose tissue is influenced by the diet. In all experimental groups linoleic acid had considerably increased, in the New

York study to a value about twice and in the two other studies to about three times that found in the control groups. The adipose tissue data constitute valuable evidence for the conclusion that the diets consumed by the experimental and the control groups have indeed been quite different in their fatty acid compositions and also that the adherence to the diets must have been at least fairly good.

TÁBLE III

INCIDENCE OF CHD IN STUDIES OF PRIMARY PREVENTION

Loc.	Number of subjects		Accumulated experience man-years		Coronary events		Incidence per 1000 man-years	
	Exp	Con	Exp	Con	Exp	Con	Exp	Con
N. Y.	941	457	3,954	3,122	17	32	4.3	10.3
Hel.	313	241	1,183	911	17	30	14.4	33.0
L. A.	424	422			54	71		

The incidence rates of CHD in these studies are shown in Table III. From the published material of the Los Angeles study, it does not seem possible to calculate the incidence rates, but since the groups have been of equal size and the mean length of experience in both groups presumably has also been the same, the numbers of coronary events are directly comparable. It is seen that in the New York and the Helsinki studies the incidence rates in the experimental groups have been about 50% lower than in the control groups. If the customary statistical standards are applied, these differences are highly significant. In the Los Angeles study there also was a difference in favor of the experimental group, but it was smaller, about 25%. The difference as such is not significant, but if the coronary events are pooled with cases of cerebral infarction, the difference becomes highly significant. The lesser magnitude of the difference observed in the Los Angeles study could perhaps find an explanation in the fact that its subjects were a great deal older than in the two other studies.

The true comparability of the experimental and the control groups has been of considerable concern in all these studies. In the Los Angeles trial, random allocation of subjects between the groups was used and the follow-up was carried out on a double-

blind basis. Such a design should inspire a great deal of confidence.
In the other two studies the groups have been compared as to
various demographic and risk factor characteristics.   Certain
differences have been found but none was deemed sufficient to
account for the rather marked difference in the incidence of CHD.
Hence the authors of these studies have felt it justified to conclude
that the lower incidence in the experimental groups has been primarily due to the cholesterol-lowering diets.

In order to reduce the possibilities of hidden bias, a cross-over
was done in the Helsinki trial after six years, that means: the
original control hospital was placed on the experimental diet and
vice versa.   In this second phase of the study the serum cholesterol
values became rapidly reversed.   The adipose tissue fatty acid
compositions were also reversed, although this process was much
slower.   The incidence of electrocardiographic changes indicative
of CHD has shown interesting trends: the incidence has decreased
in the new experimental hospital and increased in the new control
hospital.   At this stage of the study, however, we do not yet know
definitely whether the difference in incidence figures will be large
enough to permit statistically valid conclusions.   The trial is continuing and additional data will be available soon.

And now to conclude: what is the evidence for the feasibility of
primary dietary prevention of CHD?   I feel we are justified in say-
ing this: Although the final, irrefutable proof may not yet be at hand,
the intervention studies just reviewed have produced at least substantial evidence in favor of the view that appropriate adjustment of
the fatty acid composition and of cholesterol content of diet has considerable preventive effect.   This conclusion receives further
support from the evidence furnished by epidemiological studies and
animal experiments in many species.

REFERENCES

1.   Rinzler, S. H.   Bull. N.Y. Acad. Med. 44:936 (1968).
2.   Turpeinen, O., M. Miettinen, M. J. Karvonen, P. Roine,
     M. Pekkarinen, E. J. Lehtosuo, and P. Alivirta.   Amer. J.
     Clin. Nutr. 21:255 (1968).
3.   Dayton, S., M. L. Pearce, S. Hashimoto, W. J. Dixon, and
     U. Tomiyasu.   Amer. Heart Assn. Monograph No. 25 (1969).

PROSPECTS WITH MULTIFACTORIAL APPROACHES EMPHA-SIZING IMPROVEMENT IN LIFE STYLE

Jeremiah Stamler, M.D. and David M. Berkson, M.D.

Dept. of Community Health and Preventive Medicine,

and the Dept. of Medicine, Northwestern University

Medical School; the Chicago Health Research Founda-

tion; and the Heart Disease Control Program, Division

of Adult Health and Aging, Chicago Board of Health,

Chicago, Illinois

Ability to Reduce the Current High Mortality Rates from Premature Heart Attack in the U.S.A. -- Evidence from International Studies

The potential for preventing premature death from coronary heart disease (CHD) is abundantly demonstrated by the international vital statistics data (Table I) (1, 2). CHD mortality rates for middle-aged American men are among the highest in the world, and as a result so are mortality rates from all causes. Detailed long-term prospective studies of population cohorts further demonstrate the validity of these differences (Table II) (3, 4). The European countries evaluated in these studies were the principal sources for the immigrants making up the American population. Therefore, the higher mortality rates cannot be due to different gene pools among the populations, with resultant national differences in genetic susceptibility to CHD. The gene pools must be similar. The higher U.S. rates must be due to differences in modes of life, of significance for the etiology of this disease. An essential corollary is that by appropriate improvements in the

TABLE I

1964 Mortality Rates for 22 Countries Ranked
by Mortality Rates for All Causes,
Males, Age 45-54

Country	1964 Mortality Rates per 100,000 Population		
	All Causes	Coronary Heart Disease	All Cardiovascular Diseases
Finland	1120	442	579
U.S.A.*	964*	354*	477*
Scotland	933	359	463
Venezuela	897	131	235
France	863	74	202
Austria	823	159	263
Australia	821	324	425
Belgium	820	159	302
North Ireland	804	324	465
German Fed. Rep.	772	182	275
New Zealand	758	293	386
Canada	752	311	385
Czechoslovakia	738	151	263
United Kingdom – England & Wales	734	254	341
Japan	733	51	251
Italy	717	133	239
Switzerland	658	134	210
Denmark	613	181	248
Netherlands	582	162	222
Israel	572	214	302
Norway	566	164	218
Sweden	522	124	189
Mean	762	212	315
Standard Deviation	± 145	± 103	± 109

*For white males only, mortality rates are: All Causes = 900, CHD = 355, CV = 450.

mode of life, it is possible to control the current epidemic of premature atherosclerotic coronary heart disease. That is, it is possible to reduce the inordinately high rates prevailing in the United States at least to those of other industrialized countries, and even lower.

The quantitative implications of this conclusion merit brief presentation, so that the implications for life-saving are fully appreciated: The mean CHD mortality rate for men 45-54 from the three countries at the top of the list (Finland, U.S.A., Scotland) -- 385 per 100,000 per year – is more than double the median rate for the 22 countries (173/100,000/year) (Table I). To a considerable degree, the high mean rate for these three countries for all causes (1,005/100,000/year) is due to their high CHD rates. The median for the 22 countries for the all causes rate is 755 per 100,000 per year. Reduction in the CHD mortality rate for U.S. middle-aged men to the median level for the 22 countries would be

TABLE II

Five Year Age-standardized Mortality Rates, Coronary Heart Disease and All Causes, Eighteen Cohorts from Seven Countries, Men Originally Age 40-59, All Men and Men CHD-Free at Entry -- International Cooperative Study on Cardiovascular Epidemiology (40)

Cohort	All Men							Men CHD-Free at Entry				
	No. of Men	CHD Mortality			Total Mortality			No. of Men	CHD Mortality		Total Mortality	
		No. of Deaths	Death Rate	Q/E Δ	No. of Deaths	Death Rate	Q/E Δ		No. of Deaths	Death Rate	No. of Deaths	Death Rate
U.S. Railroad--Switchmen	875	13	164	0.73	39	498	0.87	850	13	165	38	483
U.S. Railroad--Sedentary	1,305	37	260	1.08	65	452	0.78	1,235	27	205	51	381
U.S. Railroad--Other	391	12	321	1.26	20	526	0.85	369	6	166	14	372
East Finland	817	29	377	-*	61	777	1.34	775	16	220	47	641
West Finland	860	9	106	-*	50	578	0.96	845	4	44	43	504
Zutphen, Netherlands	878	16	177	0.75	50	556	0.95	864	12	133	46	524
Dalmatia, Yugoslavia	672	3	38	0.17	24	311	0.56	671	3	38	24	311
Slavonia, Yugoslavia	699	7	121	0.38	55	716	1.22	694	7	42	54	704
Velika Krsna, Serbia, Yugoslavia	511	1	16	0.08	23	380	0.73	505	1	16	22	370
Zrenjanin, Serbia, Yugoslavia	516	1	25	0.09	15	280	0.52	508	1	27	13	247
Belgrade Faculty, Serbia, Yugoslavia	538	2	46	0.19	5	96	0.19	532	2	47	5	98
Crevalcore, Italy	993	11	116	0.46	60	607	1.01	982	9	94	56	575
Montegiorgio, Italy	719	5	64	0.30	29	412	0.71	713	3	41	27	392
Rome Railroad, Italy	768	2	31	0.12	24	358	0.57	758	2	31	24	362
Crete, Greece	686	1	12	0.06	10	153	0.26	682	1	12	10	153
Corfu, Greece	529	4	80	0.31	11	219	0.35	526	4	80	11	219
Tanushimaru, Japan	509	4	71	0.32	23	427	0.74	-*	-*	-*	-*	-*
Ushibuka, Japan	504	1	20	0.08	24	482	0.82	-*	-*	-*	-*	-*

All rates are per 100,000 for five years, age-standardized with equal weight for each of the age ranges 40-44, 45-49, 50-54, and 55-59, i.e. they are the arithmetic averages of the rates for the four five-year age groups.

Δ Q/E = observed deaths/expected deaths, expected from a five-year life table based on 1962 vital statistics for age-matched U.S. White men.

*Data not available.

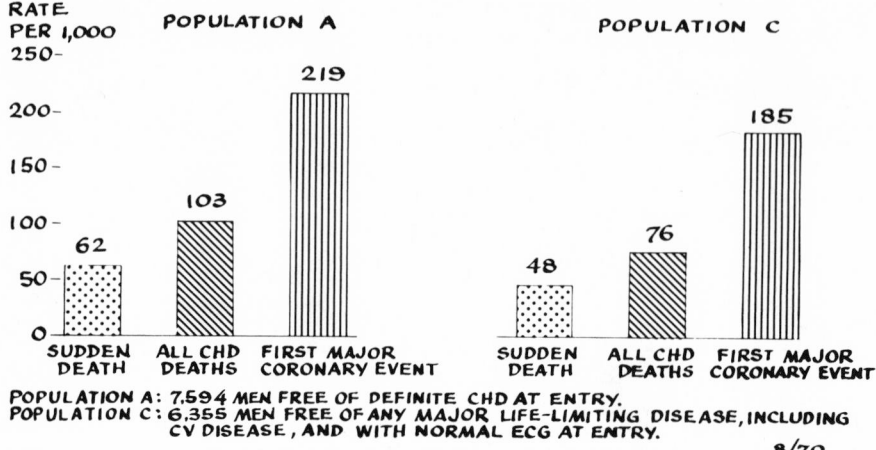

Fig. 1. Risk of experiencing Sudden Death, any Coronary Death, or Major Coronary Event before age 60, U.S. white males age 30-59 at entry; ten year findings, national cooperative Pooling Project (7-19).

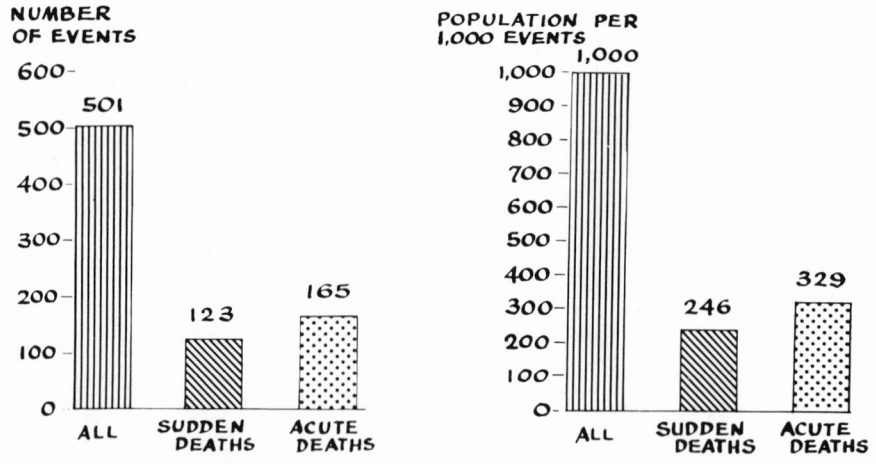

Fig. 2. Sudden Death and Acute Mortality with First Major Coronary Episode; national cooperative Pooling Project, Pupulation A, 7,594 men age 30-59 at entry, ten year experience (7-19).

halfing of this rate, and a reduction in mortality from all causes
of 18.8 percent (from 964 to 783/100,000/year).

Primary Prevention -- The Top Priority in a Sound Strategy
for Controlling the Epidemic of Premature Heart Attacks

The foregoing data indicate theoretical possibilities for reduction in CHD and all causes of mortality.   Before a presentation
of the evidence on means for realizing these possibilities, it is
essential to discuss strategy.   A sound strategy is a necessary
prerequisite for an effective effort to control mass disease.   This
is one of the major lessons from the whole history of modern public health and preventive medicine.   Without a correct strategy
it is entirely possible that over the remaining decades of this
century many expensive battles will be waged against the CHD
epidemic without real progress, i.e., without significantly reducing morbidity and mortality.

Sound strategy for the control of an epidemic must flow from
a detailed, specific analysis of the nature of the disease.   Here
certain cardinal characteristics of CHD must be given central
attention.   They are well illustrated by the experience of the
several U.S. population cohorts whose 10-year findings were
combined in the national cooperative Pooling Project (Figs. 1 and
2) (4,7, 8-19).   Of 7,594 white men age 30-59 and free of coronary
heart disease at entry, 501 experienced a myocardial infarction
or sudden death attributable to coronary heart disease during the
first 10 years of observation (Fig. 2).   Of these incident events,
123 (24.6%) were sudden deaths, here defined as death occurring
within three hours of observed onset of illness.   An additional 42
deaths occurred later in the first acute attack, yielding a total of
165 fatalities, i.e., 32.9 percent of all first episodes terminated
fatally.

As has been amply documented recently by several investigators, well over 50 percent of deaths from acute coronary episodes
occur so rapidly that time is not available to admit the severely
ill patient to a hospital and an intensive coronary care unit.   The
experience of the middle-aged male cohort in the Peoples Gas
Company labor force, under study by our group since 1958, is
presented in Fig. 3.   This high out-of-hospital mortality accounts
largely for the incapacity of coronary care units to achieve a sizeable reduction in overall mortality from acute myocardial infarction.   To this must be added the further problem that coronary

care units thus far have not been able to cope successfully with pump failure as a major cause of death in acute myocardial infarction. For the foreseeable future all indications are that only a limited ability exists for overcoming these two crucial problems for persons already ill with acute coronary episodes.

Moreover, for the approximately 65 percent of middle-aged persons who recover from an acute first episode of myocardial infarction, likelihood of dying in the next 5 or 10 years is much increased, compared with matched persons free of a previous history of myocardial infarction (Fig. 4). Excess mortality is due overwhelmingly to recurrent coronary heart disease frequently manifesting itself as sudden death. The national cooperative Coronary Drug Project in the United States has recorded a similar pattern of mortality in its placebo group of 2,789 middle-aged men with previous proved myocardial infarction (21,22).

These fundamental facts determine the strategy of the effort to control coronary heart disease. For any disease with this natural history, the main strategic thrust must be primary prevention, i.e., treatment before illness, or precoronary care, to achieve prevention of first attacks. The prophylactic effort must begin as early in life as possible, and must be continuous over years and decades. Nothing else has the potential for bringing about a sizeable reduction in the epidemic rate of premature myocardial infarction and sudden death – not cardiac resuscitation, high-powered ambulance services, intensive coronary care units, pacemakers, artificial hearts, cardiac transplantations, etc.

Since treatment before illness is the essential strategy for success in the effort to control the coronary epidemic, this paper focuses on this matter and attempts to review the scientific foundations and experience to date in this area.

Scientific Foundations for Effort to Achieve Primary Prevention of Premature Coronary Heart Disease

The underlying disease process in most persons with heart attack is severe atherosclerosis of the coronary arteries and its complications. The challenge to medicine and public health inherent in the CHD epidemic, therefore, is in essence that of preventing and controlling severe atherosclerosis and its complications.

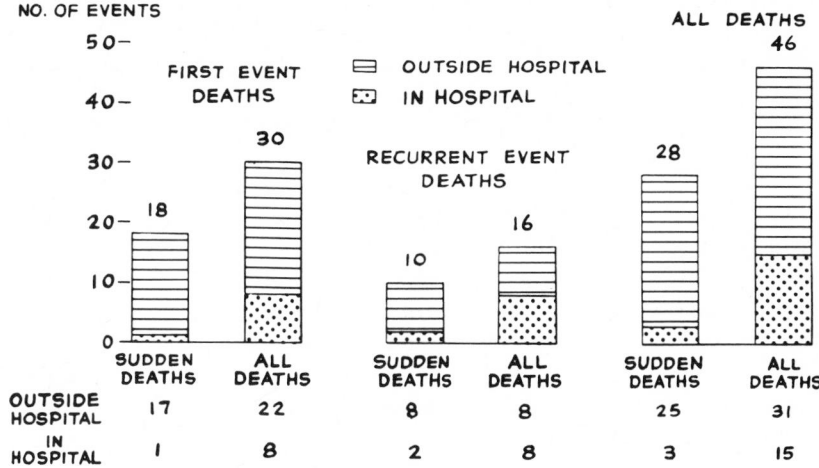

Fig. 3. Hospitalization and mortality with Major Acute Coronary Episodes, First and Recurrent; cohort of 1,329 men age 40-59 in 1958, free of definite CHD, and followed long-term without systematic intervention, Peoples Gas Co. Study, 1958-68 (5,6).

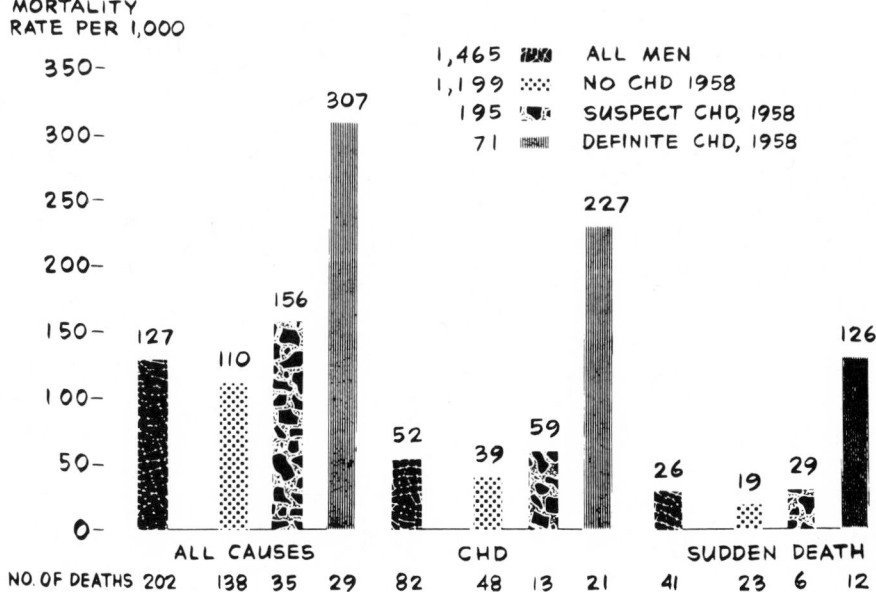

Fig. 4. CHD status and ten year mortality, Peoples Gas Co. Study, 1958-68, 1,465 men age 40-59 at entry; all rates age-adjusted by 5-year age groups to U.S. male population, 1960 (5,6).

Data have been accumulating for decades on the multiple factors involved in the etiology of severe atherosclerosis and its
sequelae, epidemic myocardial infarction and coronary heart
disease.   The accumulated findings constitute a firm foundation
for rational efforts to prevent the disease.

Clinical findings.   Some of the earliest findings, in the 1920s
and 1930s, came from clinical cardiologists.   In the years after
publication of Herrick's classic paper in 1912, as cardiologists
accumulated series of cases of premature myocardial infarction,
certain characteristics of the patients became apparent.   In
particular, it was noted that young and middle-aged adults with
myocardial infarction tended frequently to be hypercholesterolemic,
hypertensive, or diabetic, or all three (23, 24).

Animal experimental findings.   From 1910 on, after the
initial breakthrough in the experimental production of atherosclerotic lesions by feeding rabbits cholesterol and fat, increasing evidence was amassed on the role of dietary lipid in the production of hypercholesterolemia and atherosclerosis in animals.
Particularly after the second world war, lesions were produced
in virtually all species used in the animal research laboratory,
mammalian and avian, herbivorous, carnivorous and omnivorous,
including primates (4-6, 24, 25).   Moreover, as has been clearly
shown in recent work in various species of monkeys, lesions can
be produced by feeding usual table diets of the American type,
diets high in cholesterol and saturated fat, whereas they do not
supervene when these are modified to reduce intake of cholesterol-
fat (26).   In experiments with monkeys, atherosclerotic lesions
were induced with only moderate increases of serum cholesterol,
i. e., without gross organ cholesterolosis and xanthomatosis -- and
they mimicked in their pathology all stages of the human disease,
including severe narrowing of coronary arteries with thrombosis,
occlusion, and myocardial infarction.

Two other sets of key data have emerged from the animal experimental work: firstly, the repeated demonstration that hypertension accelerates the development of lesions when a diet high in
cholesterol and fat is fed, i. e., when the nutritional-metabolic
prerequisites for atherogenesis are present.   Secondly, atherosclerotic lesions are to a considerable degree reversible, particularly by restoration of a diet low in cholesterol.   This has been
repeatedly demonstrated in a wide variety of species, including
most recently in primates (4-6, 24, 25, 27).

The potential importance of this last finding for the primary preventive effort in man cannot be overestimated.   Clearly, for healthy young and middle-aged adults, as yet free of clinical coronary heart disease, the challenge is a relatively modest one, not primarily one of reversing lesions, but – less demanding – stopping or at least slowing progression of atherogenesis, so that lesions severe enough to produce clinical illness are either completely prevented or significantly delayed.   Therefore the demonstration of reversibility in animals, supported by data to the same effect in man (4-6, 24, 25), is indeed most encouraging.

Epidemiological findings -- international comparisons.   Extensive evidence is available from epidemiological research showing that a confluence of sociocultural circumstances is responsible for the emergence of coronary heart disease as the twentieth century epidemic disease of economically advanced countries.   One key circumstance is that the mass of the population in affluent countries is able for the first time in history to enjoy a "rich" diet high in animal products (meats, dairy foods) and is not restricted by harsh economic conditions to cheap starchy foods (bread, potatoes, pasta, oatmeal, cornmeal, etc.).   This modern diet -- excessive in calories in relation to energy expenditure, high in total fat, saturated fat, cholesterol, sugar -- leads to high prevalence rates of hyperlipidemia (hypercholesterolemia, hypertriglyceridemia, hyperbeta- and prebeta- lipoproteinemia) in the adult population, and sustained hypercholesterolemic hyperlipidemia considerably increases risk of premature severe atherosclerotic disease and its clinical sequelae, especially myocardial infarction.

Overwhelming evidence on this matter is available from at least three types of epidemiological research: firstly, there are the repeated analyses making use of data from the U. N. Food and Agriculture Organization and World Health Organization.   These investigations have consistently shown a close relation between habitual intake of saturated fats, cholesterol and calories, and mortality from premature coronary heart disease.   Differences are especially obvious between populations of highly developed and underdeveloped countries, but they are apparent even from analyses limited to economically advanced countries (2-6, 24, 25).   The international data yield other significant correlations as well, e. g. , between per capita use of cigarettes and coronary heart disease mortality, between number of motor cars per 100 persons and coronary heart disease mortality, the multiple aspects of life style

in modern industrial society apparently combining to induce the
epidemic of premature heart attacks.

The conclusion concerning the key role of diet is further
supported by a second set of evidence, represented particularly
by the findings of the International Atherosclerosis Project. This
comprehensive study quantitated atherosclerosis of the aorta and
coronary arteries at necropsy in over 31,000 persons aged 10-69
dying during 1960-65 in 15 cities throughout the world (28). This
massive investigation reported geographic differences in extent
and severity of atherosclerosis. Severity of atherosclerotic
lesions was found to correlate particularly with population intake
of animal fat (saturated fat and cholesterol) and with serum
cholesterol level.

Thirdly, research findings on living population groups are
consistent with these data from vital statistics and necropsy
studies. Especially valuable results are now available from the
International Cooperative Study on Cardiovascular Epidemiology
(3). In this long-term study of 18 population samples in seven
countries -- Finland, Greece, Italy, Japan, The Netherlands,
United States, and Yugoslavia -- approximately 12,000 men originally aged 40-59 have been under investigation for about a decade.
Prevalence, incidence, and mortality rates of these populations
were highly and significantly correlated particularly with saturated
fat intake and serum cholesterol level (Fig. 5) (3,4).

The epidemiological evidence indicates that "rich" diet is involved in the pathogenesis and etiology of the CHD epidemic not
merely because of its tendency to induce frequent hypercholesterolemia. This modern diet also contributes significantly (along
with low levels of energy expenditure) to the current high prevalence rates of obesity in the economically developed countries, and
largely as a consequence, to high prevalence rates of hypertension,
hyperglycemia, hypertriglyceridemia and hyperuricemia, all
implicated as coronary risk factors. Thus diet is related to the
epidemic through several interlinked etiopathogenic mechanisms.

As already indicated, a second aspect of the twentieth century
way of life that has apparently contributed powerfully to the myocardial infarction epidemic has been the development of mass consumption of cigarettes since the first world war. Several sets of
data from developed countries, where the nutritional-metabolic

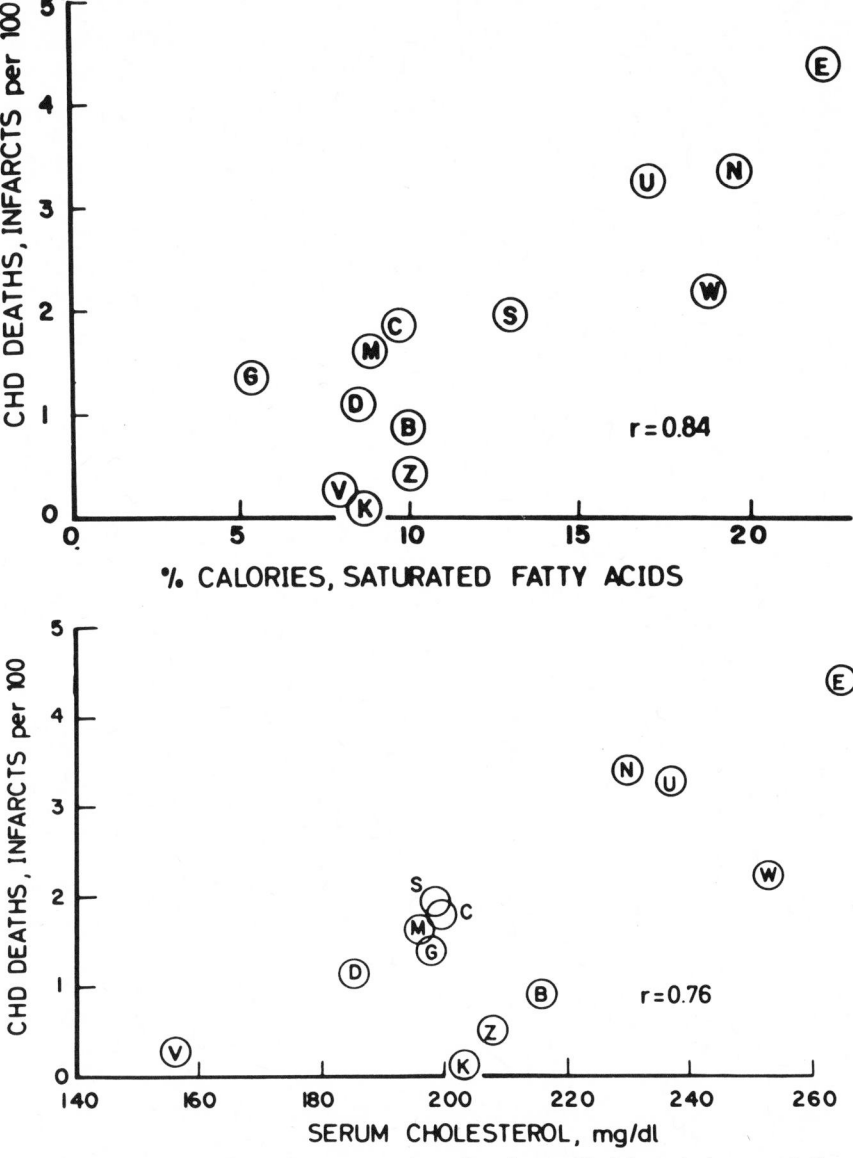

Fig. 5. International Cooperative Study on Epidemiology of Cardiovascular Disease; men originally age 40-59 in seven countries;
upper figure -- age-standardized 5-year incidence rates for fatal
CHD plus nonfatal MI among men CHD-free at entry, plotted
against percentage of total calories provided by saturated fatty
acids in the diet; lower figure -- age-standardized 5-year incidence
rates for fatal CHD plus nonfatal MI among men CHD-free at entry,
plotted against median serum cholesterol concentrations; for
identification of the cohorts (3).

prerequisites for atherogenesis are common, indicate that cigarette smoking adds substantially to risk of premature myocardial
infarction (1-7).

Although the evidence is not entirely air-tight and consistent,
there is reason to believe that lack of exercise -- habitual inactivity
at work and leisure -- may be another important aspect of the
modern mode of life increasing susceptibility to premature myocardial infarction. Finally, data are available showing that the
psychocultural stresses and tensions of modern life in highly
urbanized, competitive society, and their effects on personality
and behavior, may be playing an important contributory part in
the causation of the myocardial infarction epidemic in the developed
countries (4-6).

Epidemiological findings -- coronary risk factors. The basic
thesis summarized above is that socioeconomic and sociocultural
evolution in the twentieth century has led to a way of life for tens
and hundreds of millions in advanced countries that is conducive
to widespread premature coronary disease. Repeated reference
has been made to coronary risk factors and their frequent occurrence in the population of the developed nations. Coronary risk
factors are those habits, traits, and abnormalities associated with
sizeable (100% or more) increases in susceptibility to premature
coronary heart disease, i.e., "rich" diet and diet-dependent hyperlipidemia, obesity, hyperglycemia, hypertension, hyperuricemia;
cigarette smoking; sedentary and stressful living; hypothyroidism,
renal disease; and positive family history of premature vascular
disease (4-6).

Among the variables readily and simply measured in individual
patients, four stand out as cardinal risk factors in view of their
frequency of occurrence, their impact on risk, and their prevent-
ability and reversibility: "rich" diet, diet-dependent hypercholesterolemia, hypertension, and cigarette smoking, particularly
when present in combination. Again, these data from our long-
term prospective study in the People's Gas Company are typical.
Men were classified in 1958 as high or not-high for each of the
three factors (hypercholesterolemia, hypertension and cigarette
smoking), using the cutting points specified. Of the entire cohort
(1,329 middle-aged men, free of definite coronary heart disease
in 1958 and followed long-term without systematic intervention),
284 (21.4%) were classified not-high on all three factors. During

ten years of follow-up (1958-68) no sudden deaths occurred in this group, only one fatal myocardial infarction, 4 cardiovascular-renal deaths, and 13 deaths from all causes. The ten-year mortality rate from all causes was only 42.6 per 1,000. The sizeable group of 621 men with only one risk factor (46.8% of the cohort) exhibited substantially higher mortality rates than the men in the low-risk category with no stigmata. Rates were highest for the group of 420 men (31.7% of the population) with any two or all three risk factors, 17 times higher than the low-risk group for myocardial infarction, four times higher for all causes.

Of these 420 very high-risk men, 67 (5.0% of the entire cohort) manifested all three risk factors. Their ten-year age-adjusted mortality rate from myocardial infarction was 63.4 per 1,000, more than 20 times that of the low-risk group. Their death rate from all causes was 225.9 per 1,000 almost six times that of the low-risk group.

The inference for prevention from the accumulated clinical, animal-experimental, and epidemiological findings is almost self-evident. Major possibilities exist for the prophylaxis of premature myocardial infarction and coronary heart disease through a long-term public health and preventive medicine endeavor, involving the entire population, aiming at the elimination of the harmful living habits generating mass coronary proneness, particularly the harmful habits of "rich" diet, cigarette smoking, and sedentary living. Furthermore, special possibilities exist for immediate successes in prevention by pinpointed, concentrated efforts to detect very high-risk young and middle-aged adults, and to institute effective long-term measures to alter the habits and traits contributing to their marked susceptibility.

As noted, an impressive mass of inferential evidence supports these conclusions about primary prevention. One remaining important question is: What body of direct experience is there concerning the possibility and practicality of this prophylactic approach?

The first prospective data demonstrating relationships between coronary heart disease risk and such traits as hypercholesterolemia and hypertension were presented in October, 1956 and published the following April (29). That report, together with the clinical, pathological, animal-experimental, and epidemiological data then available from other sources, undoubtedly was a key

factor at that time stimulating four research groups to go beyond
descriptive-analytical investigations to experimental studies, i.e.,
field trials on primary prevention.   Three of these "first generation" studies -- begun in the late 1950s -- dealt exclusively with
nutritional intervention, and the ability to achieve primary prevention by altering the composition (quality) of the diet, i.e., by reducing intake of saturated fats and cholesterol, and increasing intake of polyunsaturated fats (30-32).   Their results have been
presented and discussed previously, as well as at this Symposium
(4, 20, 30-35).

Three other long-term primary prevention trials were undertaken in the late 1960s.   Each of these also involves intervention
against only one risk factor, i.e., modification of serum lipids by
diet (36), or by drug (37), or correction of cigarette smoking (38).
No data are available as yet from any of these as to trends of CHD
morbidity and mortality.

Until recent multifactorial intervention studies were launched
in England (38) and Sweden (39), the only investigation involving an
effort simultaneously to control the key major risk factors was the
Chicago Coronary Prevention Evaluation Program (CPEP), designed
by our group in 1957 and begun in 1958 (5, 6, 20, 40, 41).

The Chicago Coronary Prevention Evaluation Program
(CPEP) -- An Effort in Coronary-Prone, Middle-Aged
Men to Achieve Long-Term Control of Major Risk
Factors, Principally by Improving Life Style

This study recruited volunteer participants, chiefly from the
labor force of cooperating Chicago companies, from 1958 to mid-
1968.   The final cohort numbers 519 coronary-prone male volunteers, originally age 40-59 and free of clinical coronary heart
disease and other life limiting diseases.   Criteria for the high
risk designation generally included combinations of hypercholesterolemia, hypertension, cigarette smoking, overweight, and
fixed minor T-wave abnormalities on the baseline resting electrocardiogram (low voltage, flat, or diphasic T-waves) (Figs. 6 and
7).   In addition to these criteria, a few men with severe hypercholesterolemia, in the range 325 mg/100 ml or greater, were
accepted based on this risk factor alone.

Unlike other "first generation" studies, dealing exclusively
with diet, the Coronary Prevention Evaluation Program undertook

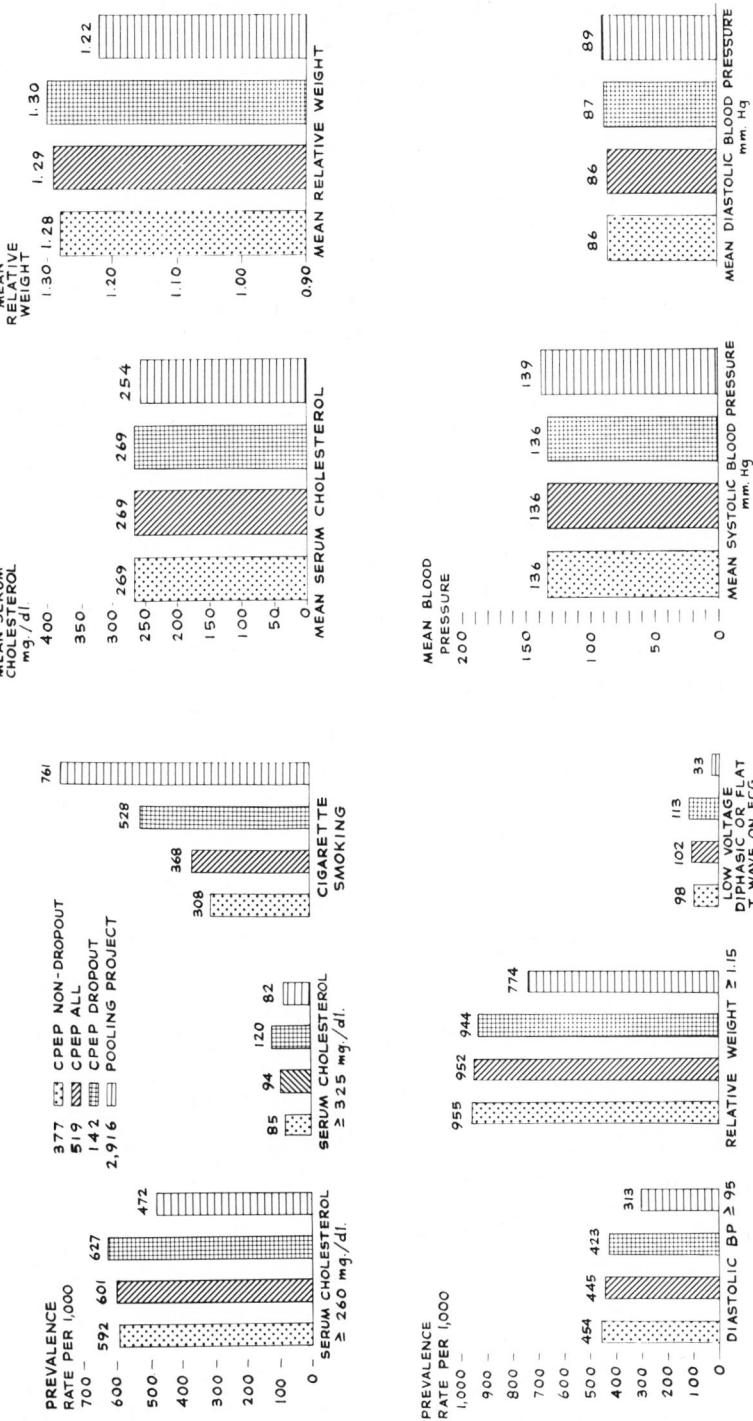

Fig. 6. Comparability in risk factor status at entry, national cooperative Pooling Project (7-19) and Coronary Prevention Evaluation Program cohorts; prevalence rates and mean values for risk factors considered singly, i.e., independently of each other.

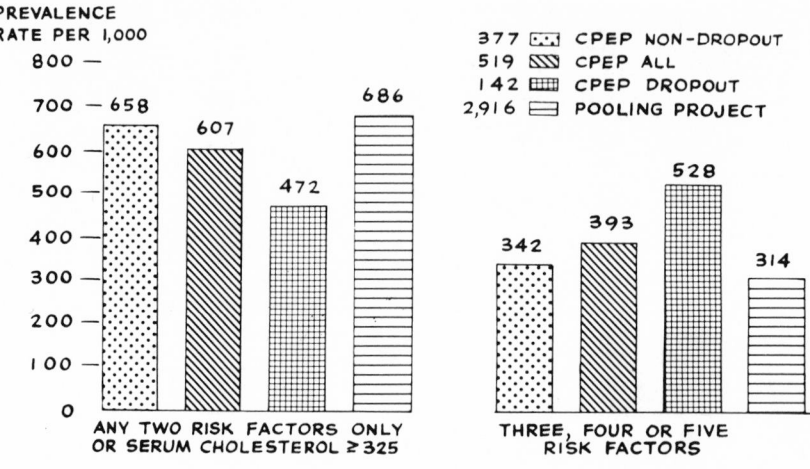

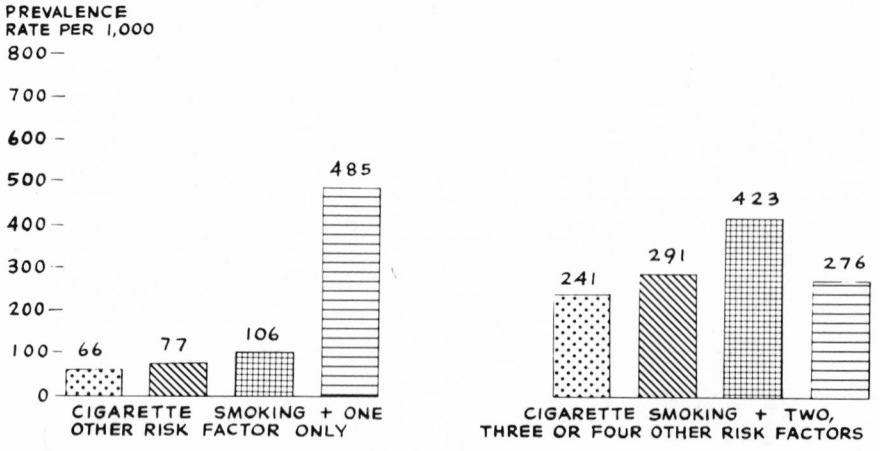

Fig. 7. Comparability in status at entry for combinations of risk factors (see Fig. 6), national cooperative Pooling Project (7,8-19) and Coronary Prevention Evaluation Program cohorts.

to assess combined nutritional-hygienic means for the correction of five coronary risk factors: hypercholesterolemia, obesity, hypertension, cigarette smoking, and physical inactivity. The deliberate decision was made to intervene against all these, to test the general hypothesis that primary prevention of myocardial infarction and coronary heart disease in high-risk middle-aged men could be achieved by controlling several major coronary risk factors. A nutritional-hygienic approach was from the beginning the cornerstone of the effort, in keeping with the basic theoretical conclusion that the coronary heart disease epidemic is a result of socioeconomic evolution leading frequently to a pattern of faulty living habits that act synergistically to intensify risk. The hypothesis, then, was that the key to prevention must be the establishment and maintenance of sound living habits, leading to correction and control of coronary risk factors. In this context drugs were viewed only as adjuvant tools by and large, not of central and decisive importance for mass prevention of disease. Therefore the control of hypertension in the Coronary Prevention Evaluation Program investigation was limited to nutritional means, principally correction of overweight and moderate salt restriction -- and any indicated drug therapy was left to the judgment of the participant's personal physician.

Modification of nutritional habits has been the primary and major effort of the program, for the control chiefly of hyperlipidemia and obesity, but also for its role in the management of hypertension. The cornerstone of the nutritional program is to work for a permanent change in eating habits in order to effect and maintain correction of diet-related risk factors. The diets are moderate in calories, moderate (not low) in total fat and carbohydrate, low in saturated fat, cholesterol and simple sugars, moderate (not high) in polyunsaturated fat. Changes in nutrient intake were accomplished by altering habits with regard to ingestion of all five major sources of saturated fat and cholesterol in the U.S. diet: meats, dairy products, commercial baked goods, eggs, and table and cooking fats. A systematic and sustained process of education and motivation was carried out for this purpose (5,40).

During initial months in the study attention of participants and their wives was focused on the effort to change eating habits. Attention was turned only during subsequent months to correction of cigarette smoking and sedentary living habits, and the data suggest that the program has been less successful in controlling these risk factors than those related to nutrition (see below).

Recruitment of middle-aged healthy male volunteers for this study was readily accomplished, principally through the cooperation of several industrial firms in Chicago. A key concern throughout has been the maintenance of maximal effective long-term participation. All men were asked to volunteer for a period of at least five years. The original protocol of the study set a goal of keeping the five-year dropout rate under 50 percent, since it was appreciated that failure to attain this minimum objective would negate any possibility of an effective field trial.

Each year the program "closes book" as of 31 March, and makes a detailed evaluation of the status of all participants. In this way, no men have been lost to follow-up. Data as of 31 March 1970 reveal overall cumulative dropout rates (calculated by life table method) (42) considerably less than 50 percent at five years -- actually only 22.6 percent, with a seven-year dropout rate of only 37.1 percent. Dropout rate has been conspicuously higher, almost double, in men with the cigarette smoking habit at entry, compared with non-cigarette smokers (see below).

As a result of the recommended nutritional alterations, men in the Coronary Prevention Evaluation Program experienced a highly significant decline in weight, serum cholesterol, and triglycerides. Detailed findings have been reported elsewhere (41). In brief, once weight and serum lipids were reduced, changes were generally maintained for years by active participants. Thus for hypercholesterolemic men in the program for at least five years, fall in serum cholesterol averaged 15 percent, from a control value of 307 mg/100 ml to 260 (range over the years 247-269). Weight reduction averaged about 7 percent. In association with this change in caloric balance and the alteration in dietary composition, serum triglycerides of hypertriglyceridemic men fell by approximately 30 percent from a baseline level of 213 to 149 mg/100 ml.

These reductions in serum lipids were effected by Coronary Prevention Evaluation Program nutritional recommendations without utilizing jiggers of oil, special oil allotments, or fat-modified foods. Such dietary measures were not required to achieve the desired alterations in quantity and quality of ingested nutrients. Ordinary foodstuffs generally sufficed, particularly since the main emphasis for most participants was not on achieving high intake of unsaturated and polyunsaturated oils. Rather it was on assuring a low saturated fat, low cholesterol, moderate calorie intake, with consumption of polyunsaturated fats in moderate amounts as adjuvant.   This nutritional emphasis of the Chicago Program was clearly somewhat different from that of the Helsinki and Los Angeles studies, with their major efforts to increase considerably the intake of polyunsaturates.   The Chicago program approach has been premised on the mass experience of populations with low serum cholesterol levels, and low rates of mortality from coronary heart disease and all causes among middle-aged persons.   In all these populations, e. g., Dalmation, Greek, Japanese, southern Italian, intake of saturated fat and cholesterol is much lower than among Americans, but polyunsaturated fat intake does not differ. In particular, it is not higher, in fact in some populations (e. g., Japanese) it is lower.   And no population habitually consumes more than 10 percent of calories from polyunsaturates (2, 3, 5, 6). No clear-cut population or experimental evidence is extant on the lifespan safety of diets very high in polyunsaturates (e. g., 15% or more of total calories).   There is no real need for such diets and therefore no real reason to "push hard" for them.   They are best avoided.   The sound approach is to emphasize control of saturated fat, cholesterol, and calorie intake.

The Chicago nutritional effort was associated with a significant sustained fall in blood pressure of hypertensive men, from a base-line mean level of 101 mm Hg to an average of 92 over a five-year period of active participation (range 91-94).   Almost certainly this was largely a byproduct of control of overweight in these obese hypertensive men.

Of the 519 participants, 191 were cigarette smokers at entry. As already indicated, dropout rate was sizeable in this group. Of the 116 cigarette smokers at entry who were still active participants in the program as of 31 March 1970, only 43 (37. 1%) met study criteria for effective cessation of cigarette smoking -- no consumption of cigarettes for at least one year.   Thus, as already noted, the relatively limited endeavors to cope with this habit, compared with the major attention to changing nutritional habits, achieved only limited success.   This experience is of considerable relevance in relation to the long-term preventive goals of the program (see below).

With respect to exercise, interview data suggest that a majority of active participants have made a transition from an essentially sedentary living habit to one of light activity.   Fitness evaluation by quantitative graded exercise tests on a subgroup of men entering the study in 1967-68 suggests a modest improvement in fitness.

Mortality is the decisive endpoint under assessment in this program. The mortality experience in Coronary Prevention Evaluation Program participants is being evaluated in comparison with findings for men in the national cooperative Pooling Project, selected from its data tape to meet the entry criteria of the Coronary Prevention Evaluation Program with respect to age, and medical and risk factor findings. The mortality analysis presented below deals with seven year follow-up for the cohort, as of 31 March 1970, and corresponding data from the Pooling Project (7-19). Of the several thousand men with data in the Pooling Project, 2,916 were identified who met the age, and medical and risk factor criteria. Age-adjusted semi-annual and cumulative mortality rates were calculated by the life table method (42) for the first seven years of experience for the cohorts of Coronary Prevention and Pooling Project men, and appropriate subgroups (as indicated below). As of 31 March 1970, the mean duration of follow-up for the Coronary Prevention Evaluation Program cohort was almost five years. Of the 519 men, 244 (47.0%) had completed five years of participation and 161 (31.0%) had completed seven years of participation. Since numbers of Coronary Prevention Evaluation Program men at risk are small beyond the seventh year of follow-up, data are presented only through this period.

Overall data on mortality are presented in Fig. 8 for seven years of follow-up. For the key endpoints, total mortality, coronary heart disease mortality, and sudden death, the seven year cumulative mortality rates indicate a trend in favor of the Coronary Prevention Evaluation Program participants, compared with the Pooling Project men. This is particularly ture for the 377 continuing active participants (non-dropouts) in the Coronary Prevention Evaluation Program. For this latter group, total mortality at seven years is 46.0 percent lower compared with the experience of the 2,916 Pooling Project men; coronary heart disease mortality and sudden death mortality are 75.0 and 86.7 percent lower, respectively. For all 519 CPEP men (continuing participants and dropouts combined), total mortality is 40.0 percent lower than that of the Pooling Project men, and coronary heart disease mortality and sudden death rates are 40.0 and 73.3 percent lower, respectively. No sizeable difference is present for mortality from malignant neoplasms.

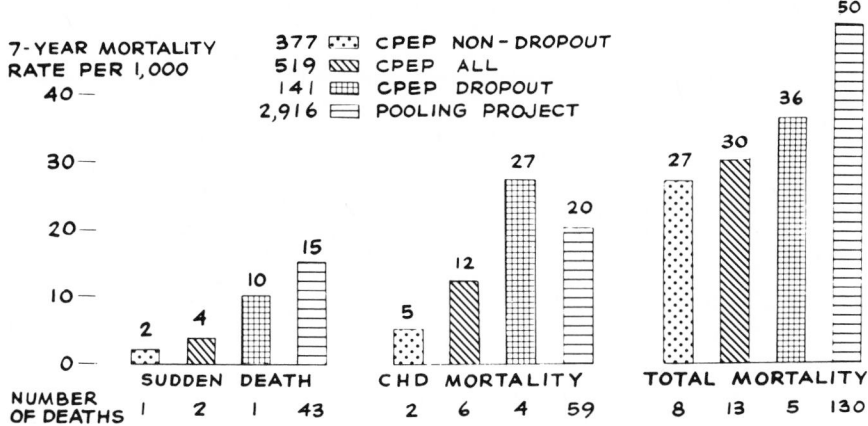

Fig. 8. Seven-year cumulative mortality rates, high-risk disease-free men age 40-59 at entry; national cooperative Pooling Project (7-19) and Coronary Prevention Evaluation Program men stratified by dropout status, as of March 31, 1970; all rates calculated by life table method, with age-adjustment by 5-year age groups to U.S. male population, 1960.

The generally favorable trend of the mortality rates for Program men for all causes and coronary disease is further evident from the data on proportionate mortality. Thus, for the high risk men of the Pooling Project, coronary heart disease mortality rate at seven years was 40.0 percent of total mortality rate. In contrast, for the 377 active participants in the Program, the corresponding statistic is 18.5 percent. Similarly, for the Pooling Project cohort, sudden death rate was 30.0 percent of total mortality rate, whereas for the CPEP non-dropouts it was only 7.4 percent. These seeming benefits from long-term active participation in the Coronary Prevention Evaluation Program are further suggested by the data showing that, for the 142 men dropping out of the program, findings for these rates and ratios were generally similar to those of the Pooling Project men.

The mortality rates for the CPEP men were further compared with those for the individual cohorts of the Pooling Project. Seven-year cumulative mortality rates for coronary heart disease and sudden death in the total CPEP cohort of 519 men were lower than those of any of the individual comparison cohorts. Mortality rate

for all causes for this Program cohort was lower than the rate
for all but one of the Pooling Project cohorts.   The contrast was
similar and even more conspicuous for the cohort of 377 CPEP
active participants (non-dropouts).

Further, the seven-year age-adjusted cumulative total mortality rates of 30 per thousand for all 519 CPEP men -- and 27 per
thousand for the 377 continuing active participants -- are unusually
low by any standard for men at this age.   They are considerably
lower than the rates for all U.S. men and all U.S. white men of
this age (43).   Thus the 1967 age-adjusted mortality rate for U.S.
white men age 40-59 -- lower in average age than the Coronary
Prevention Evaluation Program cohort over its seven years of
follow-up -- was 9.4 per 1,000, or 65.8 per 1,000 over seven years
(without adjustment to account for higher death rates with greater
age).   Of greater importance, in terms of valid comparison, these
rates are lower than those reported for male standard life insurance risks of like age (44).   Thus for standard life insurance
risks originally age 45 and 55, ten-year mortality rates were 79
and 159 per 1,000, respectively, or 54.3 and 111.3 per 1,000
over seven years.   Moreover, the rates for the CPEP men are
almost identical with the calculated seven-year age-adjusted mortality rate from all causes for the approximately 20 percent of
men of the same age at greatly lower risk, i.e., not high for either
serum cholesterol, blood pressure, or cigarette smoking -- in the
People's Gas Company study.   Is this pure chance, or a true shift
from higher to lower risk status of the Coronary Prevention Evaluation Program active participants as a result of the prophylactic
regimen?

Several additional analyses were done in an attempt further to
evaluate this question.   First, a detailed tabulation was obtained
of the main information about the 13 men who died during the first
years of the Coronary Prevention Evaluation Program study (Table
III).   Four facts stand out.   Firstly, 11 of the 13 decedents (84.6%)
had three or more coronary risk factors at entry, whereas only
39.3 percent of the entire CPEP cohort manifested this pattern at
entry, the remainder (60.7%) having only two factors or severe
hypercholesterolemia only (Fig. 7).

Secondly, 10 of the 13 men (76.9%) were cigarette smokers at
entry, so that there was a disproportionately high percentage of
cigarette smokers among decedents compared with the overall

TABLE III

Detailed Data on Thirteen Men, Non-Dropouts and Dropouts,
Dying During the First Seven Years of Follow-up --
Coronary Prevention Evaluation Program,
Total Cohort of 519 High Risk Men, as of March 31, 1970

Case No.	Age at Entry	Risk Factors at Entry	Cigarette Status Prior to Death	Months, Dropout to Death	Months, Entry to Death	Cause of Death
			Non-Dropouts			
1045	59	C + W + S	Current Smoker	-	18	Carcinoma of Lung
3202	51	C + H + W	*	-	9	Carcinoma of Stomach
5094	56	H + W + S	Current Smoker	-	31	Carcinoma of Pancreas
6403	47	H + W + S	Current Smoker	-	15	Homicide
6821	58	C + W + S	Current Smoker	-	7	Carcinoma of Liver
1020	53	C + H + W + S	Current Smoker	-	36	CHD
2971	47	C + H	Non-Smoker	-	19	CHD
6162	52	W + H	Non-Smoker	-	62	Subarachnoid Hemorrhage
			Dropouts			
0131	58	C + H + S	No Information	12	33	Hypertensive Encephalopathy
1018	51	C2+ H + W + S	Current Smoker	25	26	Coronary Heart Disease (CHD)
1037	50	C2+ W + S	Current Smoker	19	41	CHD
2117	53	H + W + S	Current Smoker	57	65	CHD
3109	40	C + W + S	No Information	8	29	CHD

```
C  is hypercholesterolemia, 260-324 mg./dl.
C2 is marked hypercholesterolemia, 325 mg./dl. or greater.
W  is overweight, relative weight of 1.15 or greater.
S  is any regular current use of cigarettes.
H  is hypertension, diastolic blood pressure 95 mm.Hg or greater.

*  Current cigar smoker.
```

Program cohort (36.8%). Thirdly, these cigarette smokers who died all had two or more other risk factors at entry (rather than one only), whereas only 29.1 percent of the overall CPEP cohort showed this very high risk factor pattern at entry.

Fourthly, at least 8 of the 10 cigarette smokers, possibly as many as 12, were still smoking cigarettes at the time of death, i.e., the Program had been ineffective in convincing them to quit this habit. Even though the number of decedents was small, these data strongly suggest that continued cigarette smoking is associated with very high risk of premature death for very coronary-prone

men and that other preventive measures are by themselves of
limited value for them as long as they fail to give up cigarette
smoking.

These detailed data highlighted an important problem, the
comparability of the various groups being evaluated -- first and
foremost in regard to cigarette smoking status at entry, but also
in terms of other risk factors considered singly and in various
combinations. Were the trends toward lower mortality rates of
the total CPEP cohort and the CPEP non-dropouts due to lower
risk at entry, especially in regard to cigarette smoking status at
entry? Extensive tabulations have recently been completed in an
effort to clarify these problems. One of these involved a detailed
analysis of the comparability of the cohorts in regard to risk factor status at entry. Prevalence rates per 1,000 were computed
for each of the six risk factors individually -- hypercholesterolemia
(260-324 mg/dl), overweight, hypertension, cigarette smoking,
severe hypercholesterolemia (325 mg/dl or greater), fixed minor
T-wave abnormalities on initial resting electrocardiogram, and
for every possible combination of these. The findings are summarized in Figs. 6 and 7.

This matter of comparability of the Coronary Prevention
Evaluation Program and Pooling Project cohorts is a critically
important one for this study. While identical criteria were utilized
for their acceptance into the two cohorts of 519 and 2,916 men,
respectively, the possibility remains of disparate risks, based on
detailed patterns of risk factor combinations. This is also a problem with respect to the two subgroups of CPEP men, non-dropouts
and dropouts. In fact, as long as the method of random assign-
ment was not used in setting up these comparison groups, i.e.,
as long as they do not represent true experimental versus control
groups in terms of optimal research design, this problem must be
of the utmost concern.

Comparison of the total Pooling Project and CPEP cohorts of
2,916 and 519 men respectively reveals the following: in regard
to prevalence rates of each of the six risk factors considered
separately, rates were considerably higher for the CPEP cohort
for four of them (hypercholesterolemia, hypertension, obesity,
minor T-wave abnormalities) compared with rates for the Pooling
Project cohort (Fig. 6). The Pooling Project cohort had a far
higher proportion of cigarette smokers than the total Coronary

Prevention Evaluation Program cohort. These Pooling Project men were predominantly cigarette smokers with one other risk factor only, whereas CPEP cigarette smokers were predominantly men with at least two or more other risk factors (Fig. 7). For such combinations of cigarette smoking plus two or more other factors, the two studies were generally well matched. With respect to all combinations of three or more risk factors, the cohort of 519 CPEP men generally had sizeably higher proportions of such very high risk men compared with the Pooling Project cohort.

When the CPEP continuing participants (377 non-dropouts) were compared with the Pooling Project cohort, results similar to the foregoing were obtained (Figs. 6 and 7). As to the 142 CPEP dropouts, their prevalence rates were higher than those of the Pooling Project for five of the six risk factors considered singly, and for all but one of the very high risk (three, four, or five factor) combinations. Although, as already noted, a disproportionate number of CPEP dropouts were cigarette smokers, the prevalence rate of cigarette smoking at entry for this group was still below that of the Pooling Project cohort.

Finally, comparison of the CPEP non-dropout and dropout groups shows them to have generally similar prevalence rates for five of the six individual risk factors (Figs. 6 and 7). As already noted, prevalence rate of cigarette smoking was much higher in the dropouts than in the non-dropouts. Largely as a consequence of this phenomenon, the dropouts also showed higher prevalence rates for combinations of three, four, or five factors, i.e., dropouts as a group tended to be higher risk at entry than non-dropouts.

These detailed data on comparability of groups and limitations therein, especially the differences in prevalence rates of cigarette smoking at entry, underscored the need for the additional data analyses, presented in Tables IV and V, stratifying the groups based on cigarette smoking experience (see Table III).

For non-cigarette smokers all mortality rates were low, and no clear-cut differences are apparent between the Pooling Project and Coronary Prevention Evaluation Program men (Table IV). While the trend of mortality from coronary heart disease and all causes favors the CPEP cohort, further assessment is needed based on longer follow-up, e.g., the ten-year life table data. These findings will be forthcoming in the next years.

TABLE IV

Seven Year Cumulative Mortality Rates for Non-Cigarette
Smokers at Entry, Pooling Project and CPEP Groups

| | Pooling Project Non-Cigarette Smokers | CPEP Non-Cigarette Smokers | | |
| | | All – 328 Men | Non-Dropout – 261 Men | Dropout – 67 Men |
	697 Men			
Total Mortality	14* 24Δ ± 7**	3 11 ± 7	3 18 ± 11	0
CHD Mortality	4 6 ± 3	1 2 ± 2	1 3 ± 3	0
Sudden Death	1 1 ± 1	1 2 ± 2	1 3 ± 3	0
Malignant Neoplasm Mortality	3 5 ± 3	1 2 ± 2	1 3 ± 3	0

*Number of Deaths.

ΔAge-adjusted rate per 1,000.

**Standard error of the rate.

TABLE V

Seven Year Cumulative Mortality Rates for Cigarette
Smokers at Entry, Pooling Project and CPEP Groups

	Pooling Project Cigarette Smokers	CPEP Cigarette Smokers				
				Non-Dropout		Drop-out
		All	All	Quit Cigarettes	Didn't Quit	
	2,219 Men	191 Men	116 Men	43 Men	73 Men	75 Men
Total Mortality	116* 60Δ ±6**	10 73±22	5 75±31	0	5 150±52	5 68±31
CHD Mortality	55 25 ±4	5 25±11	1 8±8	0	1 15±14	4 45±22
Sudden Death	42 20 ±3	1 6± 5	0 0	0	0 0	1 15±14
Malignant Neoplasm Mortality	26 14 ±3	3 32±17	3 60±29	0	3 124±49	0 0

*Number of events.
ΔRate/1,000 age-adjusted.
**Standard error of the rate.

As to the cigarette smokers (Table V), mortality rates were much higher overall than for non-cigarette smokers. Total mortality rate for CPEP men smoking cigarettes at entry was slightly higher overall than this rate for Pooling Project men. Coronary heart disease mortality rate was the same for the two groups. Sudden death rate was lower for CPEP than for Pooling Project men. For the 116 CPEP non-dropouts, both coronary heart disease and sudden death rates were lower than for the Pooling Project men, despite the fact that the former had a far higher proportion of very high risk men, men with cigarette smoking plus two or more other risk factors. The CHD mortality rate for these Coronary Prevention Evaluation Program men was only one-third that of the Pooling Project men, and they had had no sudden deaths. Moreover, of these men remaining active in the Program, all the deaths occurred among the 73 who did not quit cigarettes. Of the five deaths among these 73 continuing participants who did not quit cigarettes, 3 were cancer deaths, of liver, lung, and pancreas, respectively, occurring relatively early in the study (7, 18, and 31 months after entry, respectively) (Table III).

No deaths from cardiovascular or neoplastic causes occurred among the 43 CPEP men who stopped smoking cigarettes (Table V). Obviously there is a problem here owing to the small size of groups. Nonetheless, the data certainly lend support to the concept that multifactor intervention to control several risk factors, including cigarette smoking as well as diet-dependent factors, is effective in preventing fatal coronary heart disease and in reducing mortality rate from all causes in highly coronary-prone middle-aged men. They are also consistent with the concept that low saturated fat, low cholesterol, moderate calorie, and moderate polyunsaturated fat diets are without risk of excess morbidity and mortality from non-cardiovascular causes, specifically carcinomata (32-34). These data further suggest that nutritional prophylactic measures may be of only limited value for very high risk cigarette smokers unless cessation of cigarette smoking is also accomplished as a key part of the multifactor prevention effort. Obviously all these inferences are tentative, since the mortality rates leading to them were based on a small group of men, randomization into experimental and control groups was not done, and the study remains to be completed.

Conclusion : Perspective

This "first generation" study on primary prevention of coronary heart disease -- like the New York Anti-Coronary Club, the

Finnish mental hospital study, the Los Angeles Veterans Administration Domiciliary Center Study -- has recorded findings indicating that change in living habits, particularly diet and cigarette smoking habits, is associated with decreased incidence or mortality, or both, from coronary heart disease. This study -- like the others -- was not foolproof or perfect in design, methodology, or results. It was handicapped first and foremost by relatively small numbers, an unavoidable difficulty because of the small resources available when it was undertaken in 1957-58. It has other problems as well, e. g. , lack of a proper randomly assigned control group. Nevertheless, the findings are encouraging, and assume added significance in view of their consistency with other studies as well as their agreement with expectation in terms of findings from clinical, pathological, animal-experimental, and descriptive epidemiological research. Certainly they cannot be dismissed or ignored.

Clearly, "second generation" trials are urgently needed, based on the earlier studies and learning from them, including primary prevention trials of multifactorial intervention against the major risk factors. Fortunately, the recent request for contract proposals for such a study from the National Heart and Lung Institute now gives reasonable assurance that the effort will proceed. But no results will be forthcoming for years.

Practitioners of preventive and therapeutic medicine cannot and should not "sit on their hands" in the interim, especially in view of the coronary heart disease epidemic confronting them. As the experiences of the Chicago Coroncary Prevention Evaluation Program clearly show, large numbers of middle-aged men and their families are prepared to respond eagerly to effective professional leadership to combat this epidemic by changing life style. Wisdom and responsibility call for widespread professional implementation now of reasonable, safe nutritional-hygienic approaches to primary prevention (1, 4).

Acknowledgments

It is a pleasure to acknowledge the cooperation and support of Eric Oldberg, M. D. , President, Chicago Board of Health, and Chairman, Board of Directors, Chicago Health Research Foundation. It is also a pleasure to pay tribute to the entire staff of the Heart Disease Control Program, Division of Adult Health and Aging, Chicago Health Department, and of the Chicago Health

Research Foundation, aiding in this research, especially the authors' senior colleagues in the long-term investigations presented here: Yoland Hall, M.S., Howard A. Lindberg, M.D., Louise Mojonnier, Ph.D., Richard Shekelle, Ph.D., Rose Stamler, M.A.; also Howard Adler, Ph.D., Donald B. Cohen, M.D., Morton B. Epstein, Ph.D., George Farah, M.D., Jerome Frankel, M.D., S. Grujic, M.D., Louis Kolokoff, M.D., William MacIntyre, M.D., C. R. Paynter, M.D., Quentin D. Young, M.D., Stevie Catchings, Roberta Crawford, Nancy Dalton, Wanda Drake, Celene Epstein, Elise Fuente, W. Jackson, Dana King, Cecelia Kohorst, W. H. McAtee, Wilda A. Miller, Dorothy Moss, Joy Nelson, Gail Pacelli, Frances Petersen, Peggy Powell, Margie Shores, W. Sime, Betty Stevens, Eka Tomashewaky, June Wallace, T. Whipple, and Carol Zehnle. We are also grateful to P. Meier, Ph.D., of the Department of Statistics and the Biological Sciences Computation Center, University of Chicago. It is also a pleasure to express appreciation to the several Chicago organizations giving invaluable cooperation in this research effort, particulaly the People's Gas, Light and Coke Company, its Chairman, R. McDowell and its Medical Director, Howard A. Lindberg, M.D.; the Newspaper Division of the Field Enterprises, particularly Wilbur Munnecke, formerly Vice-President and General Manager, John G. Trezevant, Vice-President and General Manager, and Jacques Smith, M.D., Medical Director; the Medical Department of the American Oil Company, particularly Gilbeart Collings, M.D., and John Malia, M.D.; Armour and Company, particularly William Wood Prince, former Chairman of the Board; Illinois Bell Telephone Company and its Medical Director, Robert R. J. Hilker, M.D.; the Internal Revenue Service and its former Medical Director, Michael W. Langello, M.D.; and Mr. Donald J. Erickson, of Arthur Andersen and Company.

The author is most grateful to the principal investigators of the studies of Albany civil servants, Chicago Western Electric Company employees, Framingham community residents, and Minneapolis-St. Paul business and professional men and to the coordinators of the national cooperative Pooling Project for making data available from these major U.S. prospective studies for comparison with the findings of the Coronary Prevention Evaluation Program. It is a pleasure to acknowledge the cooperation and aid of our colleagues in this endeavor, Drs. John M. Chapman, Thomas R. Dawber, Joseph T. Doyle, Frederick H. Epstein, William B. Kannel, Ancel Keys, Felix J. Moore, Oglesby Paul, and Henry L. Taylor.

This research has been supported by the American Heart Association, Chicago Heart Association, Best Foods Research Center, A Division of C. P. C. International, Inc. , and the National Heart Institute, National Institutes of Health, United States Public Health Service.

References

1. Arteriosclerosis--Report by National Heart and Lung Institute Task Force on Arteriosclerosis, Vol. I, U.S. Department of Health, Education, and Welfare Public Health Service, DHEW Pub. No. (NIH) 72-137, Washington, D. C. , June (1971).

2. Stamler, J. , R. Stamler, and R.B. Shekelle, in Ischaemic Heart Disease. (Eds.) J. H. deHaas, H. C. Hemker, and H. A. Snellen, Leiden University Press, Leiden, the Netherlands (1970) p. 84.

3. Keys, A.   Circulation 41: Suppl. 1 (1970).

4. Atherosclerosis Study Group and Epidemiology Study Group-- Report of Inter-Society Commission for Heart Disease Resources.   Circulation 42: A55 (1970).

5. Stamler, J.   Lectures on Preventive Cardiology, Grune and Stratton, New York, N.Y. (1967).

6. Stamler, J. , D. M. Berkson, and H. A. Lindberg, in Pathogenesis of Atherosclerosis. (Eds.) R. W. Wissler and J. C. Geer, Williams and Wilkins, Baltimore, Md. (1972) in press.

7. Data from the Pooling Project, Council on Epidemiology, American Heart Association -- a national cooperative project for pooling data from the Albany civil servant, Chicago People's Gas Company, Chicago Western Electric Company, Framingham community, Los Angeles civil servant, Minneapolis-St. Paul business men, and other prospective epidemiologic studies of adult cardiovascular disease in the United States.   The following are representative references (8-19) on the individual studies and on the results of the Pooling Project to date.

8. Doyle, J. T.   New York J. Med. 63: 1317 (1963).

9. Stamler, J.   Amer. J. Cardiol. 10: 319 (1962).

10. Paul, O. , M. H. Lepper, W. H. Phelan, G. W. Dupertuis, A. MacMillan, H. McKean, and H. Park.   Circulation 28: 20 (1963).

11. Dawber, T.R., W.B. Kannel, and P.M. McNamara. Trans. Assoc. Life Insur. Med. Dir. Amer. 47: 70 (1964).

12. Chapman, J.M. and F.J. Massey. J. Chron. Dis. 17: 933 (1964).

13. Keys, A., H.L. Taylor, H. Blackburn, J. Brozek, J.T. Anderson, and E. Simonson. Circulation 28: 381 (1963).

14. Moore, F.E. Conf. on Cardiovasc. Disease Epidemiology, Council on Epidemiology, Amer. Heart Assn., New Orleans, Louisiana, March (1969).

15. Doyle, J.T. and S.H. Kinch. Amer. Heart Assn., 42nd Scientific Sessions, November (1969).

16. Epstein, F.H. and F.E. Moore. Progress Report to Natl. Heart Inst. on the Natl. Cooperative Pooling Project (1968).

17. Paul, O. Brit. Heart J. 33: (Suppl.) 116 (1971).

18. Doyle, J.T. and W.B. Kannel. VI World Congress of Cardiology, London, England, September (1970).

19. Berkson, D.M., J. Stamler, H.A. Lindberg, W.A. Miller, E.L. Stevens, R. Soyugenc, T.J. Tokich, and R. Stamler, in Atherosclerosis, Second International Symp. (Ed.) R.J. Jones, Springer-Verlag, New York, N.Y. (1970) p. 382.

20. Stamler, J. Brit. Heart J. 33: (Suppl.) 145 (1971).

21. The Coronary Drug Project Research Group. JAMA 214: 1303 (1970).

22. The Coronary Drug Project Research Group (1972) in press.

23. White, P.D. Heart Disease, 3rd Ed., Macmillan, New York, N.Y. (1944) p. 478.

24. Katz, L.N. and J. Stamler. Experimental Atherosclerosis, Charles C. Thomas, Springfield, Illinois (1953).

25. Katz, L.N., J. Stamler, and R.P. Pick. Nutrition and Atherosclerosis, Lea and Febiger, Philadelphia, Pa. (1958).

26. Wissler, R.W. Progr. Biochem. Pharmacol. 4: 378 (1968).

27. Armstrong, M.L., E.D. Warner, and W.E. Connor. Circ. Res. 27: 59 (1970).

28. McGill, H.C., Jr. (Ed.) Geographic Pathology of Athero-sclerosis, Williams and Wilkins, Baltimore, Md. (1968).

29. American Public Health Association Symposium.   Amer. J Public Health 47: No. 4, Pt. 2 (1957).

30. Rinzler, S. H.   Bull. N. Y. Acad. Med. 44: 936 (1968).

31. Turpeinen, O., M. Miettinen, M. J. Karvonen, P. Roine, M. Pekkarinen, E. J. Lehtosuo, and P. Alivitra.   Amer. J. Clin. Nutr. 21: 255 (1968).

32. Dayton, S., M. L. Pearce, S. Hashimoto, W. J. Dixon, and U. Tomiyasu.   Circulation 40: Suppl. 2 (1969).

33. Ederer, F., P. Leren, O. Turpeinen, and I. D. Frantz, Jr. Lancet 2: 203 (1971).

34. Dayton, S., in Pharmacological Control of Lipid Metabolism, Proc. Fourth International Symp. on Drugs Affecting Lipid Metabolism.   (Eds.) W. L. Holmes, R. Paoletti and D. Kritchevsky, Plenum Press, New York, N. Y. (1972) p. 245.

35. Turpeinen, O., in Pharmacological Control of Lipid Metabolism, Proc. Fourth International Symp. on Drugs Affecting Lipid Metabolism.   (Eds.) W. L. Holmes, R. Paoletti and D. Kritchevsky, Plenum Press, New York, N. Y. (1972) p. 207.

36. Frantz, I.   Personal Communication.

37. Oliver, M.   Personal Communication.

38. Rose, G.   Personal Communication.

39. Tibblin, G.   Personal Communication.

40. Stamler, J.   Progr. Cardiovasc. Dis. 3: 56 (1960).

41. Stamler, J., in Modern Trends in Cardiology.   (Ed.) A. M. Jones, Buttersworths, London (1969) p. 88.

42. Cuttler, S. J. and F. Ederer.   J. Chronic Dis. 8: 699 (1958).

43. Vital Statistics of the United States, 1967, Vol. II, Part A, Mortality, U. S. Department of Health, Education and Welfare, PHS, Washington, D. C. (1969).

44. Lew, E. A., in The Epidemiology of Hypertension.   (Eds.) J. Stamler, R. Stamler and T. N. Pullman, Grune and Stratton, New York, N. Y. (1967) p. 392.

CHOLESTEROL-LOWERING IN MAN

Seymour Dayton

V. A. Hospital (Wadsworth) and U. C. L. A. School of

Medicine, Los Angeles, California

Discussions of the question before this panel frequently take a disturbingly illogical course. I refer to the following common argument: the cholesterol hypothesis, we are told, has been before us for decades, and the possibility of prevention has been under study in man for twelve or fifteen years. These studies have not proved that dietary cholesterol-lowering can prevent coronary heart disease (CHD), and therefore, it is alleged, we should abandon this hypothesis.

Abandonment of the hypothesis on the basis of currently available data would be patently inappropriate. Let us remember that the total literature on tests of primary prevention by diet consists of three trials. To be sure, individually or jointly, they do not provide totally convincing evidence that cholesterol-lowering prevents clinical complications of atherosclerosis. However, in each trial, the observed decrement of CHD incidence in treated subjects was at least as great as that predicted from observational data. The inconclusive nature of these trials has not been due to failure to produce the predicted outcome, but rather it has been due to limitations in size or design. There is clearly no scientific reason whatsoever for abandonment of the hypothesis that we can prevent heart disease by a modified diet. Our present need is for better designed and larger trials, unless we believe that these are unfeasible or potentially more costly than our society can bear.

Let us review a few of the relevant facts.

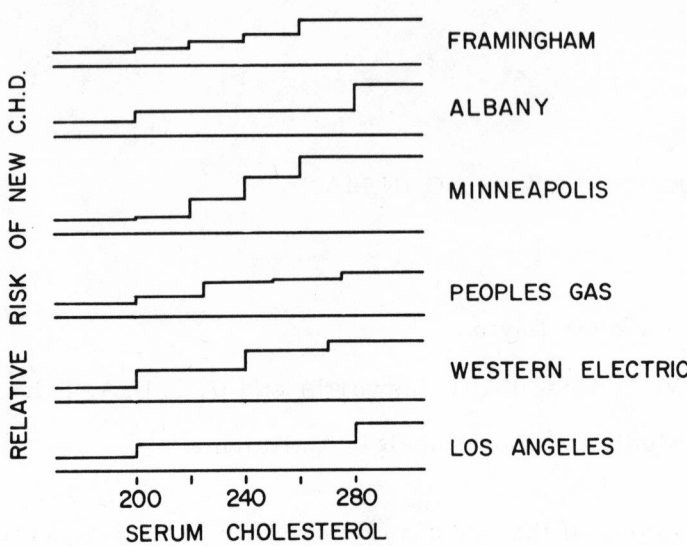

Fig. 1.   Relative incidence of CHD at different levels of initial
serum cholesterol concentration in U.S. males, as observed in six
prospective epidemiologic studies.   Incidence among men with
serum cholesterol < 200 mg/dl was given the same arbitrary value
in each study, and rates among men with higher levels were plotted
in relation to that group.   From data assembled by Stamler (1).

Figure 1 will serve to refresh our memory as to the strength
of the relationship between serum cholesterol concentration and
risk of CHD in man.   The figure summarizes the results of half a
dozen major prospective epidemiological programs.   In each
instance, the relative risk of CHD is plotted along the ordinate at
various increments of serum cholesterol concentration.   Without
exception, there is a stepwise rise of risk, of substantial magnitude,
as serum cholesterol concentration rises.   Moreover, as serum
cholesterol rises, risk rises disproportionately fast.

We worry a good deal, with some justification, about how early
in life lipid-lowering must be undertaken in order to be effective.
It is sometimes alleged that serum cholesterol ceases to be predic-
tive of CHD beyond the age of 60, but the Framingham data usually
cited in support of this allegation do not truly bear it out.   Note

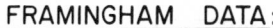

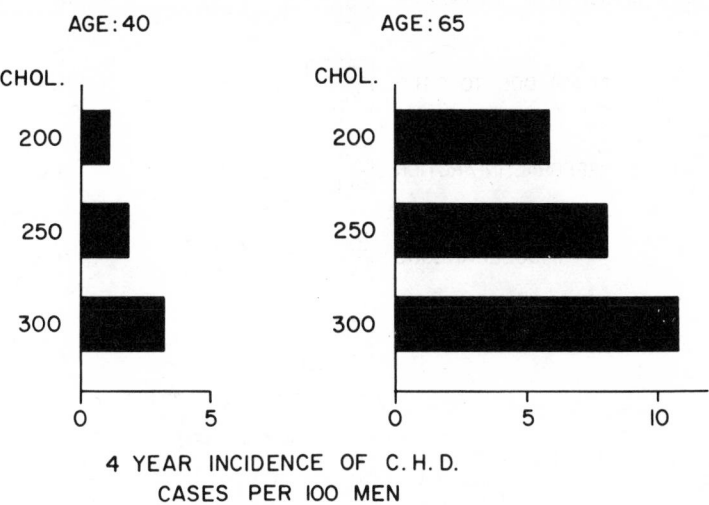

Fig. 2.   Relationship of CHD incidence in the Framingham study
to serum cholesterol concentration, in men at ages 40 and 65.
Derived from data in the Framingham Monograph (2).

Figure 2.   Viewed percentage-wise, the gradient of risk with rising
cholesterol concentration is higher in Framingham men at age 40
than at 65.   However, if we consider the gradient in absolute terms,
i.e., numbers of men per year, rather than in relative terms, it is
plain that at age 65 there is actually a greater theoretical potential
for salvage than at age 40.   Of course, I do not mean to imply by
these remarks that we ought deliberately to delay dietary change
until late in life, but rather that we should not consider cholesterol-
lowering a futile exercise in the older individual.

The three clinical trials of primary prevention to which I have
alluded include the Anti-Coronary Club in New York City (3), the
trial conducted by Dr. Turpeinen and his colleagues in Helsinki (4),
and our own trial in Los Angeles (5,6).   This trial was a double-
blind endeavor in randomized middle-aged and elderly veterans.
The mean test period was six and a half years.   The experimental
diet was rich in polyunsaturated fatty acids, and lean with respect
to saturated fat.   It induced a 12.7% decrease in serum cholesterol
concentration.

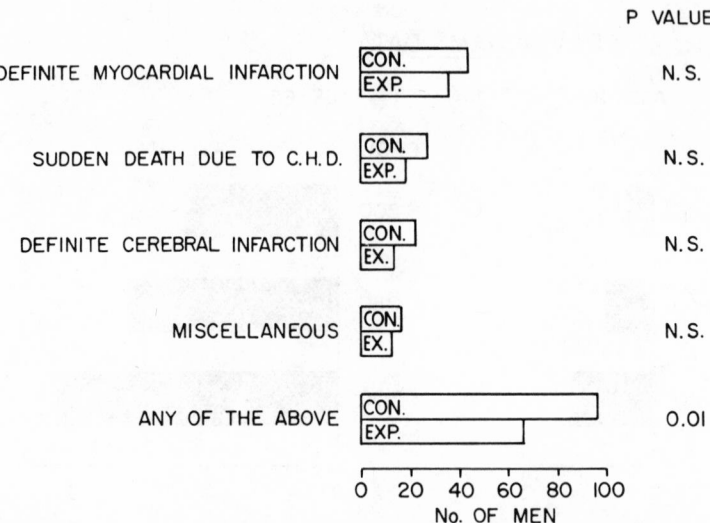

Fig. 3.   Numbers of major clinical events in the Los Angeles
Veterans Administration dietary trial.   Total group size was 422
men in the control group and 424 in the experimental group.   For
each category of event and for the pooled data at the bottom, a man
having multiple events within the category was counted once only.
P values were estimated by the chi-square test.

        Figure 3 describes the outcome in summary fashion, insofar
as principal end points were concerned.   The experimental group
sustained fewer definite myocardial infarcts, fewer instances of
sudden cardiac death, fewer definite brain infarcts, and fewer episodes in miscellaneous categories.   For each of these end points
taken individually, the difference between experimental and control
groups was not significant, but when they were pooled, we had 96
such events in the control group and 66 in the experimental, yielding a p value of 0.01 by chi-square.

        Deaths due to acute atherosclerotic events were less numerous
in the experimental group.   However, on stratification of the subjects into two groups above and below the median age of 65-1/2
years (Figure 4), we found that practically all the effect occurred
in the younger stratum.

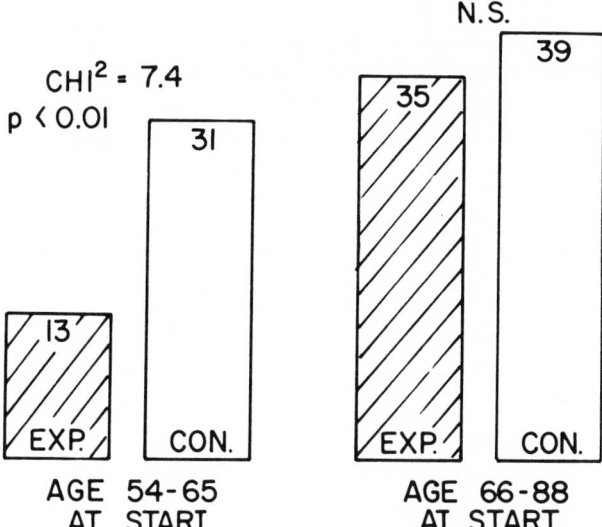

Fig. 4. Numbers of fatal atherosclerotic events in the Los Angeles Veterans Administration dietary trial, stratified by age at start of trial above and below the median level. Numbers of cases are shown on the bars.

Despite these encouraging results, we did not have nearly a convincing effect insofar as total mortality was concerned. Note in Figure 5 the upper pair of curves showing cumulative numbers of deaths by year. For the first four or five years, there were fewer total deaths in the experimental group, but toward the end of the study, the curves converged so that the final totals were 178 control deaths and 174 experimental deaths. Presumably, there were compensating causes of death in the experimental group, and we examined the data for these. As shown in Figure 6, most of the difference in non-atherosclerotic deaths was due to a surplus of cancer deaths in the experimental group. This was not quite a significant difference by chi-square.

There are two mitigating considerations which apply to these data. First of all, if this augmented incidence of cancer were diet-related, we would expect to find a relationship between adherence to diet and the incidence of cancer. In fact, no relationship was found. Furthermore, in these elderly men, suppression of one

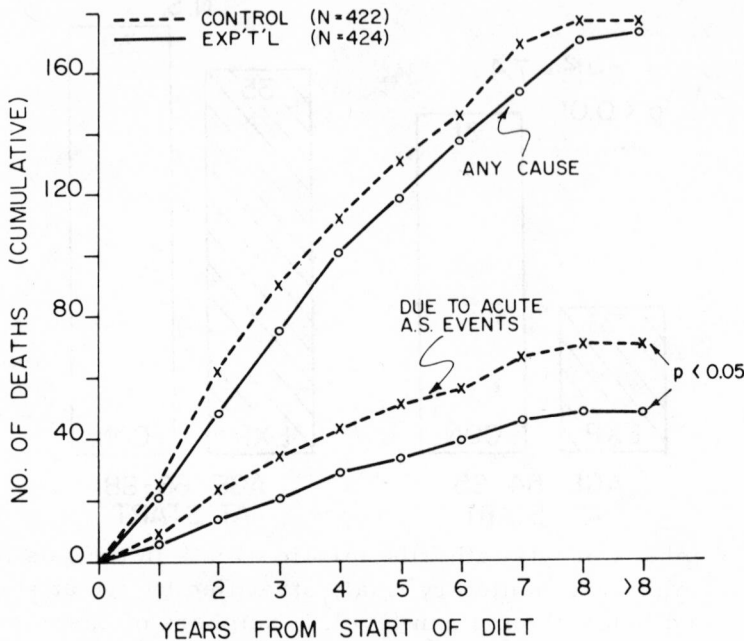

Fig. 5. Cumulative numbers of total deaths and deaths due to acute atherosclerotic events in the Los Angeles Veterans Administration trial.

lethal disease would be expected to augment the emergence of other causes of death, and perhaps this was what was being observed. Nonetheless, it is important not to take these observations too lightly. There have been a number of experiments in animals which provide clear evidence of co-carcinogenicity on the part of highly unsaturated vegetable oils in various models (7, 8).

Ederer and others have reported that the combined experience in four other trials with similar diets failed to provide evidence of a co-carcinogenic effect (9). We find this report encouraging but not totally reassuring. The four studies combined accounted for less than half as many cancer deaths as did the Los Angeles trial; most of the other studies contributing data to this report were briefer than the Los Angeles trial; and some of the reported cancers in the other studies were unconfirmed.

Instinctively, the scientist in us says we should now test the diet-cancer hypothesis in man. But surely that is out of the question. As difficult as it is to achieve a definitive answer on the diet-heart question, it is certainly hopeless to provide an answer for a disease of substantially lower incidence.

It is plain that our experimental subjects <u>as a group</u> were not hurt insofar as longevity was concerned by the experimental diet, but it is not clear that the experimental diet is capable of prolonging life. I believe that new, larger, and more meticulous trials should be mounted, but that they should concentrate on a diet of somewhat different composition.

The prospective epidemiologic observations of Keys and his colleagues (10) provide us with the suggestion that a diet rich in monounsaturated acids might prove more salubrious. Figure 7 shows Keys' mortality figures for population groups in seven countries. In common with Italy and Japan, the Greek islands of Crete and Corfu are favored by a very low incidence of CHD. But unlike Italy and Japan, they also enjoy unusually low mortality rates from other causes. Indeed, the total mortality in these areas is 35% of the U.S. rate. The Greek population in this study consumes

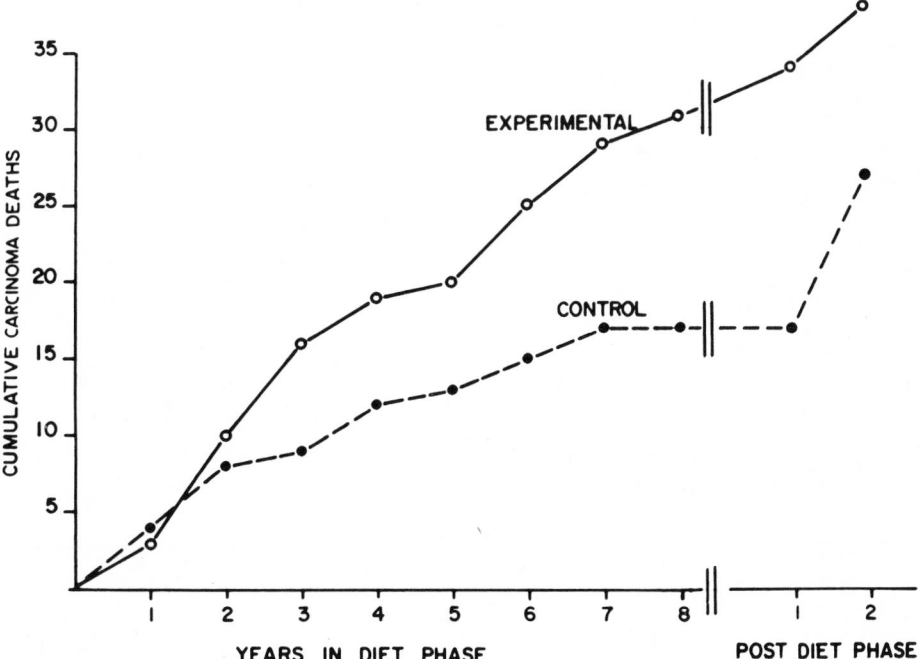

Fig. 6. Cumulative numbers of deaths due to carcinoma in the Los Angeles Veterans Administration trial. Reproduced, with permission, from Lancet (6).

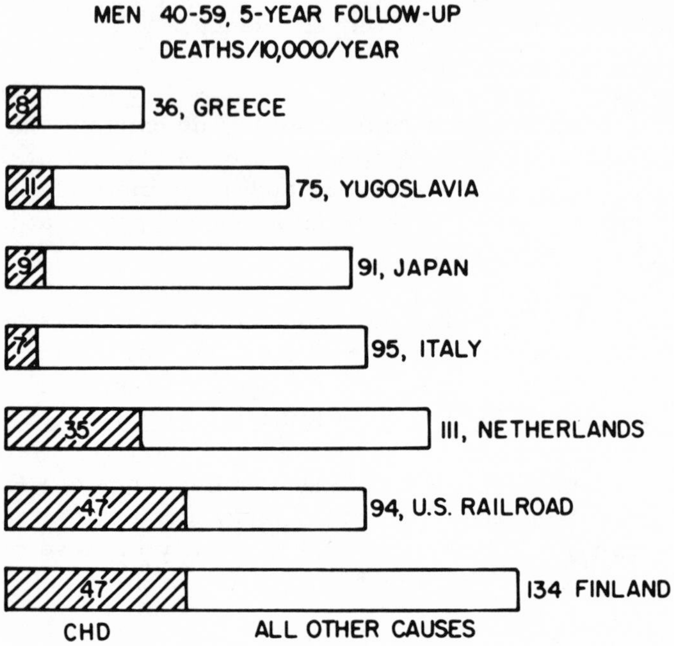

MEN 40-59, 5-YEAR FOLLOW-UP
DEATHS/10,000/YEAR

CHD   ALL OTHER CAUSES

Fig. 7.   Age-standardized average yearly death rates in studied population groups in seven countries.   Reproduced, with permission, from the report of Keys (10).

a diet nearly as high in fat as in the United States, but it is mostly monoenoic fatty acid derived from olive oil (Figure 8). We believe that the next test of a cholesterol-lowering diet should study a ration comparable to this one.   If it is both therapeutic and nontoxic, it ought to be possible to demonstrate a decrease in total mortality, the most unassailable and meaningful end point of them all.

In summary, we can cite support for the hypothesis that cholesterol-lowering by a diet rich in polyunsaturated fatty acid abates the incidence of complications of atherosclerosis, though we cannot support the hypothesis that it prolongs life.   We believe that more definitive tests need to be undertaken and that they should involve study of a diet commended to us by recent epidemiological observations.

AVERAGE % CALORIES FROM FATS

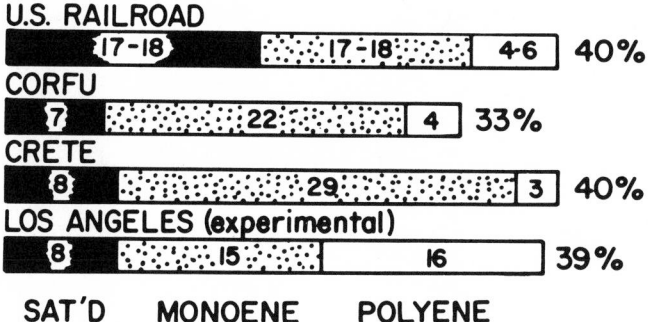

Fig. 8. Amount and type of fat in a U.S. diet, in Crete and Corfu (10), and in the experimental diet of the Los Angeles Veterans Administration trial.

REFERENCES

1. Stamler, J., in Lectures on Preventive Cardiology. Grune & Stratton, New York (1967), p. 109.

2. Gordon, T., and J. Verter, in The Framingham Study, Section 23. Serum cholesterol, systolic blood pressure, and Framingham relative weight as discriminators of cardiovascular disease. National Institutes of Health, (1969).

3. Rinzler, S. H. Bull. N.Y. Acad. Med. 44:936 (1968).

4. Turpeinen, O. Atherosclerosis. Proceedings of the Second International Symposium on Atherosclerosis. Springer-Verlag, New York (1970), p. 572.

5. Dayton, S., M. L. Pearce, S. Hashimoto, W. J. Dixon, and U. Tomiyasu. American Heart Association Monograph No. 25, (1969).

6. Pearce, M. L., and S. Dayton. Lancet 1:464 (1971)

7. Gammal, E. B., K. K. Carroll, and E. R. Plunkett. Cancer Res. 24:1737 (1967).

8. Carroll, K. K., and H. T. Khor. Cancer Res. 30:2260 (1970).

9. Ederer, F., P. Leren, O. Turpeinen, and I. D. Frantz, Jr. Lancet II:203 (1971).
10. Keys, A. (Ed.) American Heart Association Monograph No. 29, (1970).

ISCHEMIC HEART DISEASE: A SECONDARY PREVENTION

TRIAL USING CLOFIBRATE (ATROMID-S)

M. F. Oliver[*]

Department of Cardiology, Royal Infirmary

Edinburgh, Scotland

When the initial clinical trials of clofibrate had been completed and when it seemed fairly certain that this drug had no toxic effects and only minimal side effects, a formal trial was established to determine whether reduction of elevated serum cholesterol levels would be associated with a lower morbidity and mortality rate in patients with established ischemic heart disease. This was begun in 1965 and was completed in 1970.

DESIGN OF THE TRIAL

The trial was conducted in 19 hospitals in Scotland. The following categories of patients were admissible:

1. Men and women, aged 40-69 years.

2. Patients with their first myocardial infarct between 8 and 16 weeks prior to the date of admission to the trial. Patients who had had a previous myocardial infarct were not admissible to the trial.

3. Patients with angina of not more than 2 years and not less than 3 months duration, provided certain ECG categories of

---

[*] On behalf of a Research Committee of the Scottish Society of Physicians.

ischemia were present in the resting record or after exercise.
Patients with angina and normal electrocardiograms were <u>not</u>
admitted to the trial.

    4.   A combination of (2) and (3).

The electrocardiograms were coded according to the WHO criteria
by one observer (MFO) who was unaware of the "treatment" group
to which patients had been allocated and unaware of the clinical
history.

END POINTS

    The end points assessed in this study were:

    1.   Sudden death - defined as death occurring within one hour
of the onset of symptoms, or death within one hour of being seen
alive.

    2.   Fatal myocardial infarction - defined as death occurring
from 1 hour - 28 days after the onset of symptoms.

    3.   Definite myocardial infarction - defined as an ECG change
sufficient to meet the WHO criteria of myocardial infarction.

    4.   Probable myocardial infarction - defined as elevation of
serum enzyme levels and a clinical history suggestive of myocardial infarction in the absence of a codable ECG change.

RESULTS

    The duration of the trial was four years.   A total of 593 male
and 124 female patients with ischemic heart disease were admitted
to the study;   288 males were allocated to treatment with clofibrate
and 305 males to the placebo group: there were 62 females in the
treated group and 62 in the placebo group.   These patients were
grouped under five categories:

    1.   Myocardial infarct only.

    2.   Angina only.

    3.   Angina plus myocardial infarct - this category comprised

patients with recent myocardial infarction (8-16 weeks earlier)
who also had experienced angina of a duration of not less than 3
months and not more than 2 years.

4.   All infarcts - categories (1) and (3).

5.   All anginas - categories (2) and (3).

While random allocation of patients between the clofibrate and
placebo groups was satisfactory, there was a lower initial mean
serum cholesterol level in males in the clofibrate-treated group
(259 mg/100 ml) compared with males in the placebo group (272
mg/100 ml).   The number of withdrawals from the trial was equal
in the clofibrate and placebo groups and the reasons for withdrawal
were the same.

The principal results are summarized in Table I from which
it can be seen that there was significant reduction in the sudden
death rate in the "all angina" group and in all events.   Within the
"all angina" group, the category "angina and myocardial infarct"
showed the greater difference between the clofibrate and placebo
groups, and in this subcategory there was also a significant reduction in fatal and nonfatal myocardial infarcts.   While in the "all
infarct" group there was no significant difference in the events
between clofibrate and placebo treated groups, in fact there were
significantly more fatal infarcts in the "infarct only" group treated
with clofibrate compared with the placebo group.   When consider-
ing these figures it is relevant to point out that the death rates in
the placebo groups were appreciably lower than those reported in
the literature where the range is between 4-11% per year.

When this trial was initiated in 1965, serum lipoprotein
analysis and serum triglyceride estimations were not generally
available and the only serum lipid which was estimated at regular
intervals was serum cholesterol.   The chief points to emphasize
are that (1) the response of serum cholesterol to treatment with
clofibrate was less in patients with events compared with those
who did not experience any incidents during the trial,   (2) the reduction in events in the "all angina" subcategory was independent
of the initial serum cholesterol level, and (3) such reduction in
the event rate which did occur in the "all infarct" subcategory was
only in patients with an initial serum cholesterol level of more
than 260 mg/100 ml.   It would be unwise to assume that the bene-

TABLE I

SECONDARY PREVENTION OF IHD WITH CLOFIBRATE

SCOTTISH SOCIETY OF PHYSICIANS TRIAL

4-YEAR FIGURES

First clinical presentation	Regime	No.	Deaths		All deaths Rate/1200 patient mos.	Non-fatal M.I.		All Events	
			Sudden death	Fatal M.I.		No.	Rate/1200 patient mos.	No.	Rate/1200 patient mos.
Angina > 3 and < 24 mos. duration	Clofibrate	147	3**	5	1.50**	11	2.13	19	3.63***
	Placebo	167	14	9	3.97	20	3.78	43	7.75
Myocardial infarction	Clofibrate	260	13	16	3.40	20	2.43	49	5.73
	Placebo	263	15	11	3.21	33	3.95	59	6.82
All Cases+	Clofibrate	350	15	19	2.89	25	2.20	59	5.09
	Placebo	367	21	14	2.97ƚ	41	3.45	79ƚ	6.42ƚ

+ Patients who were classified as having 'Angina + Myocardial Infarction' on entry into the trial are represented in both sub-categories. The figures for 'All cases' are therefore less than the totals obtained by adding the two sub-categories.

ƚ Includes three deaths from CHF.

Asterisks against a figure in the placebo group indicate a significant difference from the corresponding figure in the clofibrate group.

** $p < 0.02$ *** $p < 0.01$

ficial effects reported here are necessarily a result of reduction of elevated serum cholesterol levels by clofibrate, which has a more profound effect in reducing elevated plasma triglycerides and also reduces elevated free fatty acids, increased fibrinolysis, abnormal platelet stickiness, and elevated fibrinogen levels.

Comparable findings have emerged from another secondary prevention trial conducted in England. This trial was designed and conducted independently of the Scottish study. In those treated with clofibrate, there was significant reduction in sudden death and all deaths and all events in the "all angina" subcategory and a favorable trend for fatal and nonfatal myocardial infarct. There was also a favorable but not significant trend in the "myocardial infarction" subcategory treated with clofibrate. When the "all angina" and "all myocardial infarct" subcategories were considered together, there was overall significant reduction in the death and the all event rate in those receiving clofibrate. These positive results from the English trial were also independent of the starting levels or degree of response in serum cholesterol.

CONCLUSION

It is concluded from the Scottish trial that clofibrate has a beneficial effect in reducing mortality, and to a lesser extent morbidity, in patients with angina and that this effect is independent of initial serum cholesterol levels or the degree of response to the drug. Clofibrate also has a small beneficial effect in patients with a myocardial infarction with initially high serum cholesterol levels. The drug appears to be of no value in patients with myocardial infarction with initially normal serum cholesterol levels.

ADDENDUM

The definitive results of these trials were published in the British Medical Journal in December 1971, as follows:

1. Report by a Research Committee of the Scottish Society of Physicians, "Ischaemic Heart Disease: A Secondary Prevention Trial using Clofibrate." Brit. Med. J. 4:775 (1971).
2. Five year study by a group of physicians of the Newcastle upon Tyne region, "Trial of Clofibrate in the Treatment of Ischaemic Heasrt Disease." Brit. Med. J. 4:767 (1971).
3. Dewar, H. A. and M. F. Oliver. A Joint Commentary on the Newcastle and Scottish Trials. Brit. Med. J. 4:784 (1971).

CLOSING SESSION

ANTILIPEMIC DRUGS AND THE POSITION OF THE FDA

Marion J. Finkel

Food and Drug Administration

Rockville, Maryland

The U.S. Food and Drug Administration is charged with the responsibility of assuring safety and efficacy of marketed drugs and safe conditions for clinical investigation of drugs.

The antilipemic agents, and to a lesser extent, the hypoglycemic agents, are in a different class with respect to efficacy than the vast majority of drugs, since the antilipemics are largely employed to ameliorate asymptomatic laboratory findings.

Since the ultimate efficacy, namely, amelioration or delay in onset of atherosclerotic complications, has yet to be demonstrated convincingly with any of the antilipemic drugs currently in use, a large measure of safety should be inherent in these drugs prior to approval for marketing.

Another consideration, however, has been discussed in the past two years, precipitated by the findings in the University Group Diabetes Program (UGDP). As most of you know, this is a study which has encompassed a period of 9 years to date. The purpose of the study was to determine whether various anti-hyperglycemic regimens are of more value in preventing complications of adult-onset diabetes mellitus than is diet alone. The patients were divided into six treatment groups, all of which received diet in addition to: (1) fixed dose of insulin; (2) variable dose of insulin; (3) fixed dose of tolbutamide; (4) fixed dose of phenformin; (5) tolbutamide placebo; (6) phenformin placebo. During the course of the study it was apparent that a statistically significant high incidence of deaths due to cardiovascular disease occurred in the tolbutamide and phenformin groups, whereas the incidence in the insulin groups was similar to placebo. Whether the increased risk

Of cardiovascular death in the two oral hypoglycemic agent groups
is drug-related cannot be stated with certainty. Nevertheless,
prudence dictated discontinuance of the tolbutamide and phenformin
portions of the study by the UGDP. The FDA, as well as the AMA
Council on Drugs and the American Diabetes Association recommended
that in adult-onset diabetes uncontrolled by diet alone, insulin
be used for control unless in the judgment of the physician this is
not feasible, in which case the oral agents are to be used.

With respect to altering the appearance of, or progression of
the less severe vascular complications, none of the drug treatment
groups, including the insulin groups, demonstrated any significant
advantage over diet alone, although the study is still ongoing and
some advantage for tight control of blood sugar may eventually be
demonstrated.

The UGDP study has, at least, shaken our beliefs that the oral
hypoglycemic agents are rather innocuous for long-term use, and,
in addition to relief of signs and symptoms of adult-onset diabetes,
might possibly have a salubrious effect on vascular complications
of diabetes. Further, a possibly stronger belief, namely, that
insulin may be beneficial in delaying vascular complications has
been brought into question, at least insofar as adult-onset diabetes
is concerned.

To return to the topic at hand, namely, antilipemic agents, in
the past few years, the Food and Drug Administration has approved
for marketing two drugs for the treatment of hyperlipemia:
clofibrate and dextrothyroxine. These drugs were approved solely
on the basis that they lowered serum lipid levels. However, the
considerations of long-term safety and the necessity for establish-
ing a more meaningful benefit/risk ratio has led the Food and Drug
Administration to the belief that postmarketing studies should be
performed following approval by the FDA of an antilipemic agent.
An Ad Hoc Advisory Committee to the FDA, convened one year ago,
affirmed the desirability of this course of action.

As you are well aware, much thought is necessary before
instituting such a requirement. Who will design and execute the
studies; who will fund them; what drugs are to be tested as controls;
what patient population is to be employed? If one agent, which,
e.g., primarily affects serum cholesterol, is found to be effective
in delaying the onset of, or ameliorating existing, atherosclerosis,
can this be extrapolated to other cholesterol-lowering agents,
regardless of mechanism of action? And, even if one decides that
extrapolation is reasonable, what about the unknown safety of another
compound given for prolonged periods? Since all drugs eventually
capable of being approved for marketing cannot and will not be
subject to intense studies of 5-10 years duration, should the FDA

limit its approval only to those drugs which appear, from the hypo-lipedemic standpoint, to have an advantage over other available agents?

Meetings between members of the National Heart and Lung Institute of NIH and the FDA have led the FDA to await results of the ongoing NIH-sponsored "Coronary Drug Project," the WHO-sponsored trial in myocardial infarction prevention,and the proposed NIH-sponsored primary and secondary prevention trials in Type II (Fredrickson-Lees-Levy classification) hyperlipoproteinemia, before requesting extensive post-marketing studies for antilipemic agents not included in the above trials. We have been assured that NIH will consider inclusion of important new agents in their ongoing trials.

In the interim, we will proceed as follows:

(1) The FDA, as part of its program to develop clinical guidelines for testing of various categories of drugs has, in conjunction with the Pharmaceutical Manufacturers' Associa-tion and an Ad Hoc Advisory Committee, devised a set of guide-lines for antilipemic agents. These guidelines have also been sent to various specialty and pharmacology societies for comment. They provide only for short-term testing of up to two years duration and only for measurement of serum lipids for efficacy. They will, of course, require revision as newer techniques are devised. They represent the minimal requirements for approval for marketing and will be available to anyone who wants them. They will provide some uniformity of basic clinical design among drug companies testing antilipemic agents, but they will also allow for innovation with respect to new agents.

(2) FDA will approve new entities for marketing if they are safe and effective as lipid-lowering agents.

(3) FDA will ask for certain postmarketing clinical trials directed primarily to questions of safety. Precedent for this includes the post-marketing studies requested by FDA for L-Dopa, approved for marketing in 1970.

It will, of course, require at least several more years of large-scale clinical trials before reasonable conclusions can be drawn with respect to efficacy of lipid-lowering techniques. Until such knowledge is forthcoming, the FDA believes it has taken an appropriate stand with respect to investigational and marketing requirements for these drugs.

CONCLUDING REMARKS

Hugh Sinclair

Magdalen College, Oxford, England

INTRODUCTION

When William Penn founded this City as a haven of refuge, he named it with the Greek word for "brotherly love", Philadelphia. Not surprisingly therefore the smooth waters of lipid metabolism have during this excellent symposium been ruffled only occasionally, as when Bernstein and Oliver had a disagreement about the necessity of controls in clinical trials. Even the Panel of six experts from four different countries under the experienced chairmanship of Dr Irvine Page produced only about half-a-dozen different views. This equanimity is also to be expected since we have been meeting in what is officially called a "Rose Garden" (though without roses) with superb arrangements for which we must thank the hard work of Dr Bill Holmes, his assistant Mr Hollerorth and his secretary Mrs Carolyn Hyatt. For so excellent a programme we are indebted to Dr Dave Kritchevsky. We may reasonably assume that the other seven members of the International Organizing Committee were more decorative than effective, but it was delightful to see the two fathers of these Symposia (first held in Milan in 1960), Professor Garattini and the ubiquitous Professor Paoletti who in this electronic age still obtains results with a smoked kymograph. We are grateful to the twenty-three commercial firms for financial support, and to the projectionists for skilled surgery in removing impacted slides. As an aside on slides, may I suggest that the three men in a boat, depicted in a slide from Bethesda that we see several times a year, should now be sunk or sent to Cuba.

ECONOMY OF CHOLESTEROL

This is the fourth Symposium, and the first was held eleven

years ago. In concluding remarks during that one at a time when
triparanol was being used, I asked whether we needed to lower
cholesterol and what else we were doing if we did lower it. During
the present Symposium in which we have very properly passed from a
consideration of the cell to epidemiological studies, we have had
excellent discussions of the economy of cholesterol. Its synthesis
is increased by cholestyramine (Myant) and decreased by clofibrate
(Ahrens); we need to know more about the 7α-hydroxylase that initiates
oxidation to bile acids and may be the rate-limiting reaction (Boyd).
Faecal excretion continues to be extensively studied, with diminished
reabsorption in the gut caused by cholestyramine, β-sitosterol,
cholestane-triol or neomycin. Although only about 1 mg is excreted
daily in human urine, 80 mg is excreted by the skin (Connor).
Passage into and egress from tissues continues to receive high
priority, and Ahrens suggested that the main determinant of plasma
cholesterol might be saturation of the tissues : daily feeding of
cholesterol to man (20 g over 16 days) could lead to storage without
any change in plasma cholesterol, and in his opinion polyunsaturated
fatty acids removed cholesterol from plasma to tissues. It is generally
agreed that unesterified cholesterol passes into cells, and clofibrate
prevents this (Robertson). Two interesting papers (Bjorkerud &
Bondjers) reported on the passage of cholesterol in and out of the
rabbit intima in relation to endothelial integrity: when the endothelium is intact the amount of unesterified cholesterol is fifty
times the esterified but the two uptakes are correlated; there is no
correlation in areas denuded of endothelium (eg at branching points)
where probably lipoproteins enter; the free cholesterol is rapidly
esterified and removed so that only a small part of it remains.

Of course accumulation of cholesterol could be caused by decreased infiltration (or increased local synthesis). Cholesteryl
linoleate and arachidonate are easily mobilised, but cholesteryl
oleate is not, and this is the predominant ester in early atheromatous
plaques (fatty streaks). As I discussed at the end of the first
symposium in 1960, such accumulation tends to occur in avascular
tissues. Tendon is one such, and Carlson has told us that 6 g daily
of nicotinic acid can remove xanthoma tendinosum. Casdorph stated
that arcus senilis is always accompanied by hypercholesterolaemia,
but Mishkel believed it could occur in persons under thirty years of
age with normal plasma cholesterol, and in persons over fifty years
it had no meaning. I have studied an interesting form of arcus which
occurs on the cornea in association with a dermoid cyst at the lim-
bus, and disappears when the arcus is removed; we are trying to
produce this experimentally by obstructing the flow of tissue fluid
from the conjunctival capillaries to the cornea which may be the
only way in which essential fatty acids can reach the cornea.

The economy of cholesterol should be elucidated by converting

pools A and B into factual rather than mathematical concepts, and
recent techniques of biopsy will assist this. Carlson studied the
effects of hypolipidaemic compounds on lipid pools by repeated
biopsies of skeletal muscle and adipose tissue. Though these
techniques are now standard, it might be worth studying "non-living"
erythrocytes and "living" leucocytes, since these are still the
easiest tissue to biopsy.

LIPOPROTEINS

Since all cholesterol in plasma is present in lipoproteins,
these properly received due emphasis; obviously the amount of cholesterol in plasma depends on the amount of lipoprotein available to
carry it. The hepatic parenchymal cells and the absorptive cells of
the gut make VLDL (density less than 1.006) which is metabolised
through an intermediate (1.006 to 1.019) to LDL. In a characterist-
ically excellent review of the apoproteins (of which there are six
major ones) Fredrickson struck an optimistic note : "Who knows, the
lipoproteins may sometime have some relevance to atherosclerosis";
and he even pronounced them correctly with a short "i". The Bethesda
work was carried further by Levy who described the action of drugs
on lipoprotein metabolism but emphasised that diet is often sufficient
treatment and always should come first. Formation of lipoproteins
in the endoplasmic reticulum and Golgi apparatus was discussed by
Hamilton, and their metabolism by Havel. We now have six types of
hyperlipoproteinaemias, and the importance of their differentiation
is obvious : for instance, cholestyramine (16 to 32 g daily) is the
drug of choice for Type II but may make worse Type III in which clofibrate (2 g daily) is indicated; nicotinic acid is not good in
heterozygotes of Type II but excellent combined with cholestyramine
in homozygotes. There is now a clear sequence. Free fatty acids
in the liver form triglycerides which are incorporated into VLDL;
formation of VLDL is increased by clofibrate (Eder), and in nephrosis and von Gierke's disease; its metabolism is decreased in myx-
oedema. VLDL forms the intermediate (1.006 to 1.019), splitting off
HDL which is decreased by clofibrate. LCAT converts the intermediate
to LDL whose catabolism is increased by cholestyramine or D-thyroxine
and diminished by nicotinic acid or possibly clofibrate. Perhaps
it was not surprising that Edman degradations with the automated
Beckman sequencer had been used (Brewer) to determine the sequence
of the 79 aminoacids in human apoLP-ala, which forms 30% of VLDL
and 5 to 10% of HDL. By the time of the next Symposium we may
expect synthetic lipoproteins, and we shall probably be lowering
plasma cholesterol by specific antibodies.

PLATELETS

Mention was made (Stamler) of the rise in reported deaths from ischaemic heart disease in certain European countries as soon as the Second World War ended. But a very interesting fact about these deaths in Great Britain is that the pre-war rise was resumed in 1943 when diet changed but many other factors such as petrol-rationing did not. If a sudden change in the national diet can cause an almost immediate change in the incidence of deaths attributed to ischaemic heart disease, the relevant factor is likely to be thrombosis rather than a chronic process such as athersclerosis.

This Symposium was unusual in that very little discussion took place about the effect of drugs on lipid metabolism and of this on platelets and hence thrombosis. It has often been shown that unusually "sticky" platelets are found after a coronary thrombosis or in persons at unusual risk of this (such as Type II hyperlipoproteinaemia). As Paoletti mentioned in his interesting discussion of cyclic-AMP and prostaglandins, PGE is extremely effective in making such sticky platelets normal. Paoletti mentioned also that in deficiency of essential fatty acids FFA are raised in plasma and intravascular thrombosis may occur; it is well known that saturated fatty acids increase thrombosis with increasing efficiency with chain-length up to C18, but unsaturated fatty acids do not affect it.

DIET

There were clearly many participants who thought that diet was the most important factor in controlling atherosclerosis and coronary heart disease, and discussion of this rightly centred on fats with almost no mention of carbohydrate. A small contingent, led by Oliver, appeared to believe that the pathological conditions arose from dietary deficiency of clofibrate.

The Panel discussion, under the able direction of Irvine Page, represented these opposing views. Turpeinen, reminding us that Scandinavian countries had recommended some years ago that a change should be made in the national dietaries from saturated to polyunsaturated fats, urged that recommendations should be made in the light of existing knowledge; Page agreed that we were not in a position to make final recommendations, but "in public health work we cannot always wait for irrefutable proof". Perhaps by the time of the next Symposium, in Milan in September 1974, the definitive trial we all hope to see conducted in the USA will be well advanced, and we may even be in a position to make final recommendations. That is a hope for the future.

CONCLUSION

Looking instead back into the past, we may note that three centuries ago William Penn was an undergraduate at Christ Church, Oxford, a contemporary of Sir Thomas Browne - wise old Sir Thomas who said he preferred the discovery of the circulation of the blood to the discovery of America. William Penn was sent down by Christ Church because he failed to attend chapel. A couple of centuries later, chapel was regularly attended by the mathematics tutor at Christ Church, the Reverend Charles Lutwidge Dodgson, who told stories to little girls (before Freud said one should not do this) and published them under the name of Lewis Carroll. He taught mathematics to someone who was a friend and colleague of mine, and had he lived to be present today he might have modified Jabberwocky as follows:

Atherosclerocky

'Twas Saturday.   The Congressmen
        Were tired and slumbered in their rows,
All sludgy were their platelets then
        As each atheroma grows.

Bill Holmes, now lacking stamina,
        Had an alarming dream:
That he was in the intima
        And heard the cells blaspheme.

"I like God's sludge I slither in"
        Said a young fibroblast;
"Some saline, glucose, lecithin
        And protein's my repast.

My membranous caveolae
        Imbibe these as they will;
So I'll grow large and multiply
        Without becoming ill."

"Beware cholesterol, my son!"
        Advised an old smooth muscle cell,
"Beware triglyceride, and shun
        A saturated hell!

Beware a mural thrombus as
        Von Rokitansky once advised -
Though I don't believe one ever has
        Got endothelialized."

He watched his sons increase in size;
   Long time some EFA they sought
For membranes, since they utilize
   These lipids - or they ought.

For if some saturated fat
   Becomes incorporated in
The cell, then compounds enter at
   The membrane lecithin.

Type III! Type II! so through and through
   The lipoproteins enter in,
Bringing cholesterol like glue,
   And some triolein.

The frumious plaques increase in size;
   Then swell and burst smooth muscle cells;
Cholesteryl esters crystallize,
   Sounding death's knells.

For when the plaques then ulcerate
   Anoic fatty acids fuse
The platelets, which then aggregate
   And a thrombus ensues.

"Beware cholesterol, you men!"
   Commercial congressmen made clear,
And Oliver. "Take drugs and then
   Your plaques will disappear!

Take neomycin, heparin,
   And compounds like amphetamine,
Take oestrogens and thyroxine,
   And cholestyramine.

Take nicotinate, clofibrate,
   And prostaglandins F and E,
Have no concern for what you ate;
   Drink and smoke lazily."

'Twas Saturday. The Congressmen
   Were tired and slumbered in their rows,
At Dave Kritchevsky's call, they came
   And solved what? Who knows?

ABSTRACTS OF SUBMITTED PAPERS

MECHANISM OF ETHANOL-INDUCED HYPERLIPEMIA

E. BARAONA, R. PIROLA and C.S. LIEBER

Department of Medicine, Mount Sinai School of Medicine (CUNY)
and Section of Liver Disease & Nutrition, Veterans Administration
Hospital, Bronx, New York

The mechanism of alcoholic hyperlipemia was studied in
rats fed liquid diets with 36% of calories as ethanol or
carbohydrate (controls). ^{3}H-palmitate was given intragastrically
and ^{14}C-lysine injected intravenously with or without Triton.
Ethanol increased serum lipid concentration several fold,
mainly in the very low density lipoprotein fraction (VLDL) with
enhanced specific activities of both lipid and protein moieties.
VLDL labeling was also increased in alcohol fed rats after
injecting labeled chylomicrons (^{14}C-palmitate, ^{3}H-glycerol),
and the ^{14}C/^{3}H ratio tripled, incriminating increased production
of serum lipids rather than decreased removal of dietary
chylomicrons. Furthermore, blocking serum lipid removal with
Triton did not prevent the lipemic effect of ethanol. To
investigate the source of increased serum lipids, intestinal
lymph was diverted. Ethanol still increased significantly the
incorporation of ^{14}C-lysine into serum lipoproteins, but not
into chylous lipoproteins, indicating a non-intestinal
(probably hepatic) site of increased lipoprotein production.
However, ethanol also increased lymph lipid output and
incorporation of dietary ^{3}H-palmitate into lymph lipids. This
may be explained by the findings that ethanol in vitro, or
previous ethanol feeding in vivo, inhibited ^{14}C-palmitate
oxidation by intestinal slices. Thus alcoholic hyperlipemia
may result from both enhanced hepatic lipoprotein production
and decreased intestinal fat oxidation.

THE EFFECT OF PROBUCOL (DH-581) ON CHOLESTEROL METABOLISM

J.W. BARNHART, J.D. JOHNSON, D.J. RYTTER and R.B. FAILEY

The Dow Chemical Company, Human Health Research and Development
Laboratories, Post Office Box 10, Zionsville, Indiana 46077

Probucol is an effective hypocholesterolemic agent in
animals and man. Studies in mice have shown that it can act as
quickly as four hours after either oral or iv administration.
The administration of cholesterol-4-^{14}C in conjunction with
probucol results in the absorption of similar quantities of
cholesterol-^{14}C in liver when compared to controls, but lesser
quantities in serum. This fact, along with the rapidity of
action, suggests an inhibition of transport of cholesterol. An
inhibition of free fatty acid release from adipose tissue of
rats has also been observed; however, this may not be involved
in the mechanism of action in man.

The administration of a single dose of Probucol to human
subjects results in peak plasma concentration of the drug in
24 hours. There is a subsequent disappearance from plasma in a
manner which would suggest that a two compartment model is
operative.

D,L-α-METHYLTHYROXIN-ETHYLESTER (CG 635), A NEW LIPID-LOWERING AGENT

R. BECKMANN, G. HILLMANN, F. LAGLER, W. LINTZ and W. VOLLENBERG

Chemie Gruenenthal GMBH, 519 Stolberg im Rheinland, Zweifaller Strasse 24, Germany

Among the numerous derivatives of α-methylthyroxin which were investigated as to their lipid-lowering activity, the compound CG 635 was shown to possess the optimal therapeutic index (lipid lowering activity/basal metabolism increasing activity). In comparison to L-Thyroxin (= 100) in rats, the relative potencies of CG 635 in regard to its antihypercholesterol-emic activity, oxygen consumption increase, goiter prevention, increase of heart frequency, and heart weight increase, were 3 - 7, 0.1, 0.1, 0.05 - 0.1, and 0.1 - 0.4, respectively. The therapeutic index is 30 - 70. In acute and long term studies in dogs, rats, and mice it could be demonstrated that the toxicity of the substance is remarkably low.

The average half-life of the compound in the rat, and in man was shown to be 16 hrs., and 6.3 days, respectively. Following an intravenous injection of ^{125}I labeled CG 635 to the rat, most of the radioactivity is excreted by the feces, via the bile. Little radioactivity (approx. 10%) is found in the urine. In man, following multiple administrations of 40 mg CG 635, maximal plasma concentrations (0.6 - 0.9 μg/ml), are reached within 25 - 30 days.

CLINICAL EXPERIENCES WITH MK-185, A NEW HYPOLIPIDEMIC AGENT

DONALD BERKOWITZ, M.D.

245 North Broad Street, Philadelphia, Pennsylvania 19107

MK-185, 2-acetoamidoethyl (4-chlorophenyl) (3-trifluoro-methyl phenoxy) acetate is a new hypolipidemic agent with the additional ability to decrease blood uric acid levels. Preliminary studies have indicated that doses of 500 mg. to 1500 mg. are most effective and may be administered once daily.

This regimen has been used in an on-going study with 34 type IV hyperlipoproteinemic subjects, 19 males and 15 females, with ages ranging from 25 to 66 years. No dietary restrictions were used.

After 3 months of treatment there was a significant reduction in the serum triglycerides in 28 patients (83%), the mean decrease for the group being 45% (p < 0.01). Cholesterol levels were irregularly affected, the mean decrease being 11%. The serum uric acid level was reduced in each patient, the mean reduction being 3.6 mg%. Toxicity tests performed during this period showed no significant alterations.

The triglyceride and uric acid lowering ability of MK-185 suggests that it may have potential value in the treatment of type IV hyperlipidemic subjects in whom hyperuricemia is frequently present.

THE EFFECT OF SODIUM DEXTROTHYROXINE ON SERUM CHOLESTEROL AND

MORTALITY RATES IN CARDIAC PATIENTS

ARTHUR BERNSTEIN, M.D. and FRANKLIN SIMON, M.D. and
WILLIAM WARNER, M.D.

2130 Millburn Avenue, Maplewood, New Jersey   07040

Of major concern to the practicing clinician at this
stage in the assessment of the value of lipid therapy is
whether or not the results of studies such as those by Leren
and Dayton can be duplicated under clinical conditions. To
answer this question for ourselves we treated a group of our
own patients with CHOLOXIN (sodium dextrothyroxine) in
individualized doses for periods up to 9 years. During this
time serum cholesterol levels were reduced 15 to 20% over
initial levels, and there was no escape from this effect.
Side effects were minimal, and from all stand points dextrothyroxine was judged to be a perfectly satisfactory substitute
for the diet when, for whatever reason, diet is ineffective
as lipid-lowering therapy.

Cumulative percent survivals were calculated for our
patients and were compared with similar data for previously
published studies using the life-table method. The survival
rate for dextrothyroxine-treated patients were comparable to
those of diet-treated patients, and markedly greater than
groups receiving no hypocholesteremic therapy.

BIPHASIC RATE OF GLUCOSE UTILIZATION BY ADIPOSE TISSUE OF RATS

TREATED WITH NICOTINIC ACID AND 5-CARBOXY-3-METHYL-PYRAZOLE (5C3MP)

A. BIZZI, A.M. CODEGONI, A. MEDEA and S. GARATTINI

Istituto di Ricerche Farmacologiche "Mario Negri", Via Eritrea, 62,
20157 Milan, Italy

The rate of utilization of glucose _in vitro_ by epididymal
adipose tissue from fasted rats pretreated with lipolysis
inhibitors, such as nicotinic acid and 5C3MP, follows a
biphasic response.

During the first 30' after administration of the drug,
the rate of glucose utilization (measured as CO_2 formation and
triglyceride incorporation) by incubated adipose tissue from
treated rats was higher than in control rats, while beginning
1 hr to 6 hr post-drug, it was sharply reduced.

The sensitivity of adipose tissues from 5C3MP-treated rats
to noradrenaline and to insulin was not affected; however, 10
times the usual dose of insulin was necessary to produce a
similar rate of glucose incorporation in adipose tissue from
normal and pretreated rats. Corticosterone, given to rats kept
under the same experimental conditions, elicited like responses;
adrenalectomy reduced, but did not abolish the effect of

nicotinic acid and 5C3MP on glucose utilization by adipose
tissue.

ENDOTHELIAL INTEGRITY AND PERMEABILITY OF PLASMA CHOLESTEROL IN

NORMAL RABBIT AORTA

S. BJORKERUD AND G. BONDJERS

Departments of Histology and Internal Medicine I. University of
Goteborg, S-400 33 Goteborg, Sweden

     The integrity of the aortic endothelium in normal rabbits
was evaluated with a specific perfusion staining procedure. A
large proportion of the aortic surface was covered with
immature endothelium or was devoid of endothelial lining. Such
areas with decreased endothelial integrity were related to
branching points.

     The concentration and uptake in vivo of free and esterified
cholesterol was determined in regions with intact and defective
endothelium. The cholesterol content and the uptake of free
and esterified cholesterol was higher in the latter regions.
These results indicate that the heavy hemodynamic strain
normally present at branching points may decrease the integrity
of the endothelium and thereby cause increased permeability of
plasma cholesterol and biochemical changes in the underlying
aortic wall. A high incidence of atherosclerosis in the same
regions indicates that changes in the endothelial lining may
either be a primary atherogenic factor or a factor facilitating
the development of atherosclerosis.

SPLANCHNIC SECRETION RATE OF BLOOD PLASMA TRIGLYCERIDES IN

PATIENTS WITH HYPERTRIGLYCERIDAEMIA

J. BOBERG, L.A. CARLSON, U. FREYSCHUSS, B. LASSERS AND M. WAHLQVIST

Department of Geriatrics, Box 641, S-751 27 Uppsala, Sweden

     Splanchnic secretion rate of blood plasma triglycerides
(TG) have been determined in fourty-two men with a wide range of
fasting plasma TG concentration from 0.53 to 16.5 mmol/l. A
constant infusion of albumin-bound H^3-labelled palmitate was
given and blood was simultaneously sampled from the hepatic
vein and an artery for determination of hepatic venous-arterial
differences of labelled and unlabelled plasma TG. Furthermore
plasma TG clearance was measured.

     Similar figures were obtained for plasma TG "turnover
rates" by the splanchnic chemical TG secretion and the plasma
TG clearance methods. The values for these two methods were
principally between 3 and 80 mol/min and m^2 body surface
area with the same range for both normo- and hypertriglyceridaemic
subjects. The splanchnic isotope TG secretion method resulted
in lower values probably due to that this method only measures

the splanchnic plasma TG secretion derived from plasma free
fatty acids.

No correlations were found among normotriglyceridaemic
subjects between plasma VLDL-TG concentration and plasma TG
"turnover rates". However, for patients with hypertriglyceridaemia significant, positive correlations were found between
these two parameters.

All patients with hypertriglyceridaemia had decreased
"fractional turnover rates" of plasma TG suggesting decreased
removal capacity. This might explain why their plasma TG
concentrations in contrast to normotriglyceridaemic subjects
were more dependent on the splanchnic secretion rates of plasma
TG.

CHOLESTEROL ACCUMULATION AND REMOVAL IN DEFINED REGIONS OF

ATHEROSCLEROTIC LESIONS IN RABBIT AORTA

G. BONDJERS and S. BJORKERUD

Departments of Histology and Internal Medicine I, University of
Goteborg, Fack, S-400 33 Goteborg, Sweden

The focal accumulation of cholesterol and cholesteryl
ester is one characteristic of atherosclerotic lesions.
Information concerning local mechanisms for the accumulation
and its relationship to structural changes is scarce. --- The
uptake in vivo and the concentration of free and esterified
cholesterol was determined in morphologically defined regions
of mechanically induced atherosclerotic lesions. --- The
content of free cholesterol was increased in regions devoid of
endothelium or covered with immature endothelium. The uptake
of labelled cholesterol in these regions was 10 - 16 times
greater than into regions with mature endothelium. These
results indicate that defective endothelium may be an important
factor for the accumulation of cholesterol. --- The specific
activity of free cholesterol was higher in the intima than in
the corresponding media indicating a direction of transfer of
cholesterol from lumen to the adventitia. The specific
activity of esterified cholesterol was similar in intima and
media suggesting a more rapid transfer of esterified than of
free cholesterol, since the rate of esterification in these
tissues is similar. The specific activity of esterified
cholesterol was higher than that of free cholesterol in
reendothelialized regions suggesting that increased turnover of
esterified cholesterol may be related to removal of cholesterol
from atherosclerotic tissue after reendothelialization.

PHYSICAL AND CHEMICAL CHARACTERIZATION OF THE LIPOPROTEINS IN

RABBITS ON ATHEROGENIC DIET

VIRGILIO BOSCH,*HALINA C. MENDEZ*and GERMAN CAMEJO

Centro de Biofisica y Bioquimica, Instituto Venezolano de
Investigaciones Cientificas (IVIC), Apartado 1827, Caracas,
Venezuela.

In rabbits addition of 1% by weight of cholesterol to a
regular diet induces hypercholesterolemia and formation of
atheromatous lesion. To investigate this process, we studied
the physical and chemical characteristics of the plasma lipoproteins of rabbits subjected to an atherogenic diet. Four
days after the beginning of the diet analytical centrifugation
showed the increase in VLDL and LDL fractions above the levels
of control rabbits. The level of VLDL and LDL reached 250 to
1658 mg/100 after 3 weeks of diet as compared to 15 - 34 mg/100
for the controls. The percentage composition of LDL and HDL was
similar in control and experimental animals, but the VLDL of
the hypercholesteremic animals contained aprox. 50% of cholesterol
esters as compared to a 10% in VLDL of controls. Gel electrophoresis indicated that the proteins of VLDL, LDL and HDL were
similar to the respective fractions in control and experimental
animals and that the abnormal VLDL contained the same protein
as LDL. Analysis of liver lipids showed that there was 10 times
more cholesterol ester in experimental animals. Studies attempting
to elucidate the metabolic phenomena leading to the hyperlipoproteinemia will be discussed.

* Universidad Central de Venezuela (UCV), Instituto de Medicina
  Experimental, Catedra de Bioquimica, Caracas, Venezuela

THE COMPLETE AMINO ACID SEQUENCE OF AN APOLIPOPROTEIN OBTAINED

FROM HUMAN VERY LOW DENSITY LIPOPROTEIN (VLDL)

H.B. BREWER, JR., R. SHULMAN, P. HERBERT, R. RONAN and K. WEHRLY

National Heart and Lung Institute, Bethesda, Maryland

The delipidated lipoprotein (carboxyl terminal-alanine)
apoLP-ala constitutes 30% of the protein component of the
human VLDL particle. ApoLP-ala is a single chain 79 amino
acid polypeptide containing 1 or 2 residues of neuraminic
acid, and 1 each of galactose and galactosamine. The complete
covalent structure of apoLP-ala was determined by sequential
Edman degradations of the intact and desialated apoprotein,
and its tryptic peptides. Edman degradations were performed
by the manual technique, and with the automated Beckman
sequencer. The complete amino acid sequence is as follows:
Ser-Glu-Ala-Glu-Asp-Ala-Ser-Leu-Leu-Ser-Phe-Met-Gln-Gly-Tyr-
Met-Lys-His-Ala-Thr-Lys-Thr-Ala-Lys-Asp-Ala-Leu-Ser-Ser-Val-
Gln-Ser-Gln-Gln-Val-Ala-Ala-Gln-Gln-Arg-Gly-Trp-Val-Thr-Asp-
Gly-Phe-Ser-Ser-Leu-Lys-Asp-Tyr-Trp-Ser-Thr-Val-Lys-Asp-Lys-
Phe-Ser-Glu-Phe-Trp-Asp-Leu-Asp-Pro-Glu-Val-Arg-Pro-Thr-Ser-
Ala-Val-Ala-Ala. The single carbohydrate side chain is
attached to threonine, residue 74. ApoLP-ala represents the
first apolipoprotein to be sequenced. The primary structure
of the apolipoproteins undoubtedly contains the information
requisite for lipid binding. Studies on peptide fragments, and
synthetic analogues of apoLP-ala and comparison with amino acid
sequences of the other apolipoproteins may provide information
of great importance in defining the mechanisms of lipid transport
and possibly even of atherogenesis.

SERUM TRIGLYCERIDES, BETACHOLESTEROL PERCENTAGE, CHOLESTEROL IN

HEALTHY SUBJECTS AND IN PATIENTS SUFFERING FROM CAD IN ISRAEL

D. BRUNNER, S. ALTMAN, and K. LOEBL

Donolo Institute of Physiological Hygiene, Tel Aviv University,
P. O. Box 93, Jaffa, Israel

Serum cholesterol, beta-cholesterol percentage and
triglycerides were determined in 130 males and 58 females
suffering from CAD and 3082 males and 2021 females, all
between 35-74 years, without clinical and electrocardiographical
signs of CAD. No statistical significant difference in
cholesterol levels were found in the four 10-years sub-groups
of men 35-74 years old and in the two female sub-groups
35-54 and 55-74 years old. The only exception was in the
youngest male group 35-44. However, in all age sub-groups,
men and women, significant differences between healthy subjects
and coronary patients in respect to triglycerides and betacholesterol % were found. In male subgroups with cholesterol
levels less than 200 mg%, 200-224, 225-249 and over 250 mg%,
significant differences between healthy and coronary groups
in triglycerides and betacholesterol % were found, In male
subgroups with triglyceride levels less than 120 mg%, 120-179,
180-249 and over 250 mg%, no differences in cholesterol levels,
but highly significant differences in respect to betacholesterol %
were found. Similar results were detected in female subjects.
In another study no differences were found between lipoprotein
values in the non-acute stage of post-myocardial infarction
patients and their lipoprotein values in the pre-disease period.

It is concluded that under conditions prevailing in
Israel cholesterol value determinations are of small importance
determination of triglycerides and betacholesterol percentage
of great importance in the detection of high risk subjects
for CAD. It seems that triglycerides and betacholesterol
percentage determinations are particularly important in
relatively young subjects without increased cholesterol.

FRACTIONATION OF ANTIBODIES FROM A POLYVALENT ANTI-CHYLOMICRON +

VLDL SERUM

M. BURSTEIN and H.R. SCHOLNICK

Centre National de Transfusion Sanguine, 6 Rue Alexandre
Cabanel, Paris XV, France

Antisera of rabbits immunized with chylomicrons + VLDL
isolated from lipemic human sera precipitate not only the
lipoproteins injected but also LDL, the abnormal lipoprotein
of jaundiced sera (Abn-Lp), and a small fraction of HDL.
Following addition of pure HDL to the antiserum, antibodies
were isolated from the washed specific precipitate by a
technique based on the adsorption of the HDL by barium sulfate
after dissociation of the antigen-antibody complex at acid pH.

The antibodies precipitate only a fraction of HDL, but completely precipitate VLDL, and the Abn-Lp. This demonstrates that the fraction of HDL precipitated by the immune serum contains peptides in common with VLDL and the Abn-Lp.

After adsorption with HDL the antiserum was subsequently adsorbed with LDL. By immunodiffusion techniques with lipid stain, the antiserum adsorbed by HDL and LDL reacts with VLDL. This lipid stained precipitin line is very pronounced in sera with elevated VLDL and is not present either in the 1.006 bottom or in the serum after intravenous injection of heparin.

In summary, in addition to anti-LDL antibodies, the anti-chylomicron + VLDL serum contains antibodies against an antigenic site unique for VLDL, and against antigenic sites common to VLDL, Abn-Lp and a fraction of HDL.

THE AGGRESSIVE THERAPY OF TYPE II HYPERLIPIDEMIA (FAMILIAL

HYPERCHOLESTEREMIA)

H. RICHARD CASDORPH, M.D., Ph.D.

Lipid Research Foundation, Long Beach,
University of California, Irvine, College of Medicine,
1729 Termino Avenue Suite A, Long Beach, California 90804

The agressive therapy of type II hyperlipidemia will normalize the blood lipids in 95 to 99% of patients. The basic therapy consists of cholestyramine (Ctyr) administration in doses of 12-24 g.d. In more severely affected individuals combined therapy with the addition of nicotinic acid or dextrothyroxine is necessary.

Longitudinal studies on the hypolipidemic effect of cholestyramine have been conducted on 129 hyperlipidemic patients representing 2,031 patient-months of therapy.

Out-patient studies: The average serum cholesterol (C) for the 129 patients was reduced from 322.7 to 254.5 mg per 100 ml, an average reduction of 68 mg (-21.1%). 79 type II patients obtained a -19.4% reduction; 2 type III patients, -20%; 32 type IV patients, -22% and 16 untyped hypercholesteremic patients, -23.1%. Statistical significance at the P .01 level. No significant change in triglyceride levels has been observed.

In-patient studies on 15 hospitalized type II patients under steady state conditions treated with Ctyr produced a reduction in the serum cholesterol ranging from 26 to 57% with a mean of -42%.

There is no evidence of malabsorption of vitamins A, D or E. There is evidence of mild impairment of vitamin K absorption.

Side effects consisted of constipation in 30 patients (24%), epigastric distress in 6, acute pancreatitis in 5 patients.

EVALUATION OF DEXTROTHYROXINE IN THE CARDIAC PATIENT

H. RICHARD CASDORPH, M.D., Ph.D., ROBERT AUSMAN, M.D. and
THOMAS H. SCHMITZ, Ph.D.

1729 Termino Avenue Suite A, Long Beach, California 90804

To ascertain the effect of sodium dextrothyroxine (DT_4)
in patients with pre-existing heart disease, a number of studies
have been performed by many different investigators. Information
is available from 6,605 patients, representing persons with all
varieties of cardiac difficulties. Some of the studies were of
the double blind crossover design with active drug and placebo.
Since DT_4 is a thyroxin compound and as such may induce hyper-
metabolism, a condition thought to be detrimental where cardiac
function is impaired by disease, a careful analysis has been
carried out to determine the effect of the drug on asymptomatic
and symptomatic patients. Particular attention has been directed
at persons with arhythmias and conduction defects, angina,
hypertension, and congestive heart failure.

Results of these analyses will be reported and comment
will be made about the use of DT_4 in the cardiac patient.

CLOFIBRATE: DURATION OF TREATMENT AND EFFECT ON CHOLESTEROL

BIOSYNTHESIS

M.N. CAYEN and D. DVORNIK

Department of Biochemistry, Ayerst Research Laboratories,
P. O. Box 6115, Montreal 101, Quebec, Canada

Male albino rats were fed a diet containing 0.25%
clofibrate (CPIB) from 1 to 14 days. Liver homogenates and
intestinal sections were prepared and the incorporation of
^{14}C acetate and ^3H mevalonate into cholesterol was measured.
In the liver, cholesterol synthesis from acetate was reduced
by 50% after only 24 hours and by 95% after 7 days of CPIB
feeding; 7-day treatment with CPIB was required to significantly
suppress (40%) mevalonate incorporation into cholesterol. In
contrast, intestinal cholesterol synthesis from either acetate
or mevalonate remained unchanged even after 14 days of feeding
CPIB. At least 2 days of treatment were required to lower
serum triglycerides as well as cholesterol and phospholipid
levels in serum lipoprotein fractions obtained with dextran
sulphate; maximal reduction of serum lipid levels was reached
after 4 days of CPIB treatment.

The results show that while 24 hour feeding of CPIB is
sufficient to suppress cholesterol synthesis in the liver, in
the intestine no effect was noted even after 14 days of
treatment. The finding reflects the difference between the
mechanisms involved in the control of hepatic and intestinal
cholesterol synthesis.

THE HYPOCHOLESTEROLEMIC ACTION OF CHOLESTANE-3β,5α,6β-TRIOL IN

SPONTANEOUSLY HYPERCHOLESTEROLEMIC PIGEONS AND IN RABBITS WITH

DIETARY HYPERCHOLESTEROLEMIA

CONNOR, W.E., A. WARTMAN, and D. WITTIAK

The Clinical Research Center and the Department of Internal
Medicine and the College of Pharmacy, University of Iowa,
Iowa City, Iowa

Cholestane-3β,5α,6β-triol, a cholesterol analogue, was
incorporated into the diets of 11 rabbits made hypercholesterolemic
with 0.5% cholesterol and 2.5% peanut oil added to the chow, and
into the diets of eight White Carneaux pigeons fed a cholesterol-
free chow. Hypercholesterolemia was successfully treated in the
cholesterol-fed rabbits. The terminal values for triol (T) and
control (C) rabbits were: serum: 118$\pm$31 (T), 1733$\pm$248 (C) mg%;
liver: 16.96$\pm$4.4 (T), 130$\pm$12 (C) mg/gm; intestine: 19.1$\pm$1.3 (T),
21.4$\pm$2.4 (C) mg/gm; and aorta: 3.32$\pm$0.05 (T), 69.14$\pm$16.38 (C)
mg/gm. Aortic atherosclerosis was virtually absent in triol
rabbits (grade 0.08) and severe (grade 2.48) in controls.

Although other drugs have not decreased the endogenous
hypercholesterolemia of the White Carneaux pigeon, cholestane-
triol had a great effect on the serum cholesterol levels and
the cholesterol balance. The addition of 0.5% of this compound
to the diet decreased the mean serum cholesterol levels from
348$\pm$27 (S.D.) mg% to 255$\pm$33.5 mg%. Both fecal neutral sterol
and bile acid excretion increased. Raising the dose of
cholestane-triol to 1% caused no additional decrease in serum
levels but caused a further rise in fecal steroid output which
suggested augmented cholesterol biosynthesis.

Cholestane-triol acts by preventing the absorption of
cholesterol through the intestinal mucosa. This was documented
by the oral administration of cholesterol-4-C^{14} and fecal sterol
analyses. Most of the labeled sterol was found in the stool.
Cholestane-triol-4-C^{14} was poorly absorbed. Only small quantities
were found in the tissues. The three hydroxyl groups of
cholestane-triol were important for its activity.

LONG TERM TREATMENT WITH CLOFIBRATE IN HYPERLIPIDEMIC PATIENTS

CREPALDI, G., FEDELE, D., FELLIN, R., BAGNARIOL, G., BRIANI, G.

Clinica Medica Generale, Universita di Padova, Via Giustiniani-
Padova (Italy)

Thirty hyperlipidemic patients have been treated with
1,5-2,0 g of clofibrate for periods of 10 to 22 months. During
treatment no dietary variations were made. Nineteen were of
Fredrickson's type II and had pretreatment cholesterol levels
of 394 mg/100 ml; they showed a mean maximum decrease of serum
cholesterol of 36%, with a mean total decrease of 20%. The
mean monthly percent decrease was: 14 after one month, 17
after two months, 20 after 6 months, 28 after one year, and
25 at the end of the trial. Three patients (brothers) were type

III and their pretreatment serum triglyceride levels were
850 mg/100 ml, their cholesterol 479 mg/100 ml. All three
displayed a normalization of serum lipid levels after 1-2
month's therapy. During two intervening placebo periods of
one month each rebound effects were observed, the serum lipid
values returning to pretreatment levels. Eight patients were
of type IV and their pretreatment triglyceride and cholesterol
values were 1326 mg/100 ml and 344 mg/100 ml respectively. In
all eight serum triglyceride values were normalized in a few
months: their mean maximum percent decrease of triglycerides
and cholesterol were 87 and 34 respectively.

This trial confirms the particular efficaciousness of
clofibrate treatment in types III and IV. It furthermore
proves its effectiveness in type II to reduce serum cholesterol.

RELATIONSHIP OF SERUM TRIGLYCERIDE LOWERING TO HEPATIC ULTRA-

STRUCTURAL CHANGES INDUCED BY DIFFERENT CLASSES OF DRUGS

COLIN DALTON and HERBERT SHEPPARD

Hoffmann-La Roche Inc., Research Division, 340 Kingsland Street,
Nutley, New Jersey 07110

Phenobarbital (I), 5,5'-diphenyl-2-thiohydantoin (II)
and chlorcyclizine (III) are potent microsomal enzyme inducers
which, in common with the hypolipidemic agents, clofibrate
(IV), SaH42-348 (V), and Su-13437 (VI) cause liver hypertrophy
in the rat. Chronic oral hypolipidemic doses of I-VI were
positively correlated with hepatomegaly, and liver protein and
phospholipid content. I, II and III caused a dose related
increase in liver microsomal N-demethylase activity accompanied
by an increase in protein and phospholipid which was marked in
the hepatic microsomal fraction and small in the mitochondrial
fraction. On the other hand IV, V and VI caused an increase
in phospholipid and protein which was large in the mitochondrial
fraction and small in microsomal fraction. N-demethylase
activity was increased only at the higher doses. It would
appear that these drugs increase the synthesis and amount of
lipoprotein associated with both microsomal and mitochondrial
membranes. It is postulated that the increased formation and
maintenance of the structural lipoprotein results in a deficit
in the production of secretory lipoprotein. This would be
followed by a decreased secretion of lipoprotein into the
plasma and a consequent decrease in serum lipid level.

ANALYSIS OF THE BIOLOGICAL EFFECTS OF SU 13,437 (AN ARLOXYBUT RIC

DERIVATIVE WITH BLOOD LIPID LOWERING PROPERTIES)

J.L. de GENNES, G. TURPIN, and J. TRUFFERT

Clinique Endocrinologique Hopital de La Pitie, 83, Boulevard
de l'Hopital, 75 Paris 13, France

Hundred and twenty-six patients (86 males and 40 females) presenting with Hereditary Hyperlipemia were included in this study. Seventy-seven had a familial hypercholesterolemic tendinous xanthomatosis (X.T.H.F., type II), twenty-one an essential hypercholesterolemia (H.C.E., type II), twenty-eight a mixed hyperlipemia (type III or II + IV).

SU 13437 was given for 3 to 18 months at a dose of 200 mg, 3 times daily with a standard restricted cholesterol diet. A 3 months period study with placebo alone was performed both before and after treatment.

Clinical tolerance to the drug has been satisfactory. Treatment had to be withdrawn in only 8 cases, 4 of which developed frank or wild jaundice of unknown mechanism.

Biological results were as follows:

- In X.T.H.F. patients, usually shown to resist to hypercholesterolemic drugs, blood cholesterol returned in the normal range in 6, close to normal in 21 (P 0,001). The lowering was less but significant (P 0,05) in the remainder of the cases.

- Similar results were obtained in the H.C.E. and the mixed hyperlipemia groups. The earliest fall were found in the latter group, often starting within the first month of therapy and increasing thereafter.

For the whole group of patients, the best results were obtained in subjects following strictly the diet. A relapse occured in all cases when placebo was given alone.

INTERACTION OF CHOLESTEROL SYNTHESIS INHIBITORS WITH THE

SQUALENE AND STEROL CARRIER PROTEIN (SCP)

MARY E. DEMPSEY, MARY C. RITTER, and DONALD T. WITIAK

Department of Biochemistry, University of Minnesota Medical School, Minneapolis, Minnesota, and Division of Medicinal Chemistry, College of Pharmacy, Ohio State University, Columbus, Ohio

In earlier work (e.g., Ritter and Dempsey, J. Biol. Chem., 246, 1536 (1970)) we described the properties of a squalene and sterol carrier protein (SCP) essential for conversion of water insoluble precursors to cholesterol by liver microsomal enzymes. We also showed that apo-SCP (M.W. 16,000) specifically binds cholesterol precursors and that a component of serum high density lipoprotein may be identical to SCP. The purpose of this report is to present evidence that inhibitors of specific steps in cholesterol synthesis block formation of the activated conformation of SCP (a high molecular weight aggregate of SCP and sterol substrate) and also interfere with the interaction of microsomal enzymes with a sterol substrate-SCP complex. Our data show that the most effective inhibitors are tightly bound to both SCP and microsomal enzymes. Structure-action comparisons indicate the requirement for highly polar as well as bulky hydrophobic groups in the inhibitor molecules. An intriguing finding is that often slight structural modifications (e.g., esterification of a hydroxyl or replacement with an oximino group) renders a compound an activator rather than inhibitor of cholesterol synthesis. Compounds we studied are various oxygen, nitrogen, or sulfur containing derivatives of cholestane and cholesterol; clofibrate, its free acid, and various open chain and cyclic analogs; AY-9944 (gift of Dr. D. Dvornik); phenformin and related biguanide analogs (gifts of Dr. H. S. Sadow). (Supported by USPHS grants HE-8634 and HE-6314)

THE EFFECT OF A-METHYL-THYROXIN (CG-635) ON THE LIPOPROTEINS OF

HUMAN BLOOD

DITSCHUNEIT, H., H.H. DITSCHUNEIT, H.U. KLOR, D. RAKOW and
P. SCHWANDT

Zentrum fur Innere Medizin und Kinderheilkunde der Universitat
Ulm, 79 Ulm/Donau, Steinhavelstr. 9

The effect of a-methyl-thyroxin on the lipoproteins was tested in normals without obvious metabolic disease and in hyperlipemic patients. In a short time study for 4 weeks 40 mg of CG 635 were administered daily to 10 normals, while another ten were given placebos. The sex- and age-matched group (8 males, 12 females, age 27 ± 16 years) had a body weight which was in average 4.3% above the ideal weight. During the study a diet which consisted of 65% carbohydrate was given in order to induce a hyperlipemia. The following parameters were measured every week: Triglycerides, total cholesterol, FFA, glucose and basal and reactive levels of IMI. The VLDL and LDL were prepared by zonal ultracentrifugation. Then their lipid composition and electrophoretic mobility was determined. The results show that CG 635 is able to reduce the carbohydrate-induced hyperlipidemia.

In a long time study CG 635 was given in a dosage of 40 mg daily to 42 hyperlipemic patients. 27 patients had a hyperlipemia Type IV, 7 patients had Type II, 6 patients had a mixed hyperlipidemia Type II and IV, and 2 had a hyperlipidemia Type V. Side effects on skin, liver, kidney or blood were not observed. There were no clinical signs of hyperthyroidism, though the PBI rose to values of 50-80 gr%. In hypertrigly-ceridemia as well as in hypercholesterolemia we could observe a good lipid-lowering effect of CG 635.

PROPERTIES OF DIFFERENT ADENOSINETRIPHOSPHATASE ACTIVITIES FROM

PLASMA MEMBRANE OF RAT EPIDIDYMAL ADIPOSE TISSUE

P. DORIGO and G. FASSINA

Institute of Pharmacology, University of Padua, 35100 Padua, Italy

A highly active Mg^{++} and/or Ca^{++} adenosinetriphosphatase activity, has been detected in rat epididymal fat cell ghosts. This bivalent cation-dependent ATPase was significantly inhibited by oligomycin, by ethacrinic acid and by sodium fluoride. 2,4-Dinitrophenol did not affect the reaction, whilst an ouabain inhibition was evident only in the presence of sodium azide, a preferential inhibitor of Mg^{++} ATPase. The specific activity of the ouabain-sensitive ATPase corresponds only to 36% of the cation-dependent ATPase activity.

A sodium iodide purification procedure of fat cell ghosts was performed according to Nakao et al., as reported by Matsui and Schwartz. The Na^+, K^+ ATPase activity was not found in the purified enzyme, instead the Mg^{++} and/or Ca^{++}-dependent activity was increased about 5-fold. The purified enzyme was affected by oligomycin to a stronger degree, on the contrary DCCD (N,N'-dicyclohexylcarbodiimide), an inhibitor of oxidative phosphorylation and of mitochondrial-stimulated ATPase activities (in contrast with oligomycin, whose activity is on protoplasmic membrane too), was not active on the purified enzyme. Therefore in adipose tissue, as in other tissues, the action of the oligomycin is not confined to mitochondrial level.

The results also show: (1) the existence of different ATPase activities in membrane of epididymal adipose cells, (2) that the movements across the plasma membrane of bivalent cations (Ca^{++} and Mg^{++}) are mediated by an energy-requiring process. Thus, it seems that in the adipocytes plasma membrane the Na^+ and K^+ transport may be correlated with variations in Mg^{++} and Ca^{++} movements. Such a correlation could have metabolic consequences, since Mg^{++} and Ca^{++} ions are effective modulators of various enzyme activities and of different hormonal actions on adipose tissue metabolism.

STRUCTURE-ACTIVITY RELATIONSHIPS OF VARIOUS STEROIDS RELATIVE

TO LIPID METABOLISM IN HUMAN BLOOD CELLS

GREGORY S. DUBOFF, M.S., D.Sc., (Edin.)

Department of Medicine, University of Michigan, Ann Arbor, Michigan

Numerous C_{18}, C_{19}, and C_{21} steroids are used as drugs. The aim of this study was to determine the effect of the ketonic (KS) and non-ketonic species of these compounds on human blood cell lipid metabolism. Incubation of whole blood (WB) or platelet-rich-plasma (PRP) with $1\text{-}^{14}C$-acetate affords an opportunity to determine the pattern of biosynthesis of fatty acids (FA) and the major lipids characteristic of each class of hemocytes. Introduction of the individual steroids into the incubation system enables one to detect any deviation from the normal characteristic pattern of incorporation of the labeled acetate into the individual FA and their esterification with major lipids by employment of various separation techniques including gas-chromatography (GC). Radiometry of the GC effluent peaks revealed a strikingly consistent alteration in the formation and turnover of FA, markedly significant decrease in total uptake of the 2-carbon precursor, and a distortion of the normal ratio of short to long chain FA. Non-keto steroids had no effect on the system. Evidence will be presented indicating that this hitherto unrecognized function of KS on hemocytes in vitro and in vivo, appears to act directly on the cells as a result of the presence, number and location of ketones on the steroids.

SERUM CHOLESTEROL AND TRIGLYCERIDE LOWERING ACTIVITY OF

5-(4-biphenylyl)-3-methylvaleric acid (W2531)

CHARLES H. EADES, JR., E. SCHWARTZ and D. ABRUTYN

Warner-Lambert Company, 170 Tabor Road, Morris Plains, New Jersey 07950

Lowering both serum cholesterol and triglycerides may be of value in the treatment of cardiovascular disease and atherosclerosis. In our laboratories W2531 has been found to inhibit liver cholesterol biosynthesis in dogs and rats and to lower serum cholesterol in normal and hypercholesterolemic rats. (Med. Pharmacol. exp. 14: 234-240, 241-245 (1966). To determine what effect W2531 has on serum triglycerides of rats, 3 groups of 30 adult male CFN rats each were fed a chow diet, a thrombogenic diet, or a chow diet with 10% fructose as drinking fluid ad libitum for 14 days. Ten animals in each group then received the same diets containing 0.3% W2531 for 7 days while the other 20 animals of each group continued on the original diets as controls. At the end of the study blood was obtained for serum cholesterol and triglyceride analyses. W2531 significantly lowered serum cholesterol values in all three dietary groups. It also significantly reduced the serum triglyceride levels in the rats on the chow and thrombogenic diets but only slightly in the chow-fructose group. In an additional study the concentration of W2531 was varied in the chow and thrombogenic diets to cause an intended daily drug intake of 20, 100, or 500 mg/kg by the rats. Again W2531 lowered the serum cholesterol values significantly at all dose levels on both diets. Also the serum triglyceride levels were significantly reduced in all the chow fed groups receiving W2531; however, only the high dose caused a significant decrease in rats on the thrombogenic diets. These studies show that W2531 significantly lowers both serum cholesterol and triglycerides in normal adult male rats fed chow or thrombogenic diets.

THYROXINE, RIBOFLAVIN AND TRYPTOPHAN METABOLISM IN NEPHROTIC

HYPERLIPIDAEMIA

K. DAVID G. EDWARDS and MARGARET R. HAWKINS

Keith Kirkland Renal Unit, Medical Research Department, Kanematsu Memorial Institute, Sydney Hospital, Sydney 2000 Australia

Because chlorophenoxyisobutyrate (Atromid-S) and similar drugs (betabenzalbutyrate and MK-185) are able to control acute

puromycin aminonucleoside (PA) induced nephrotic hyperlipidaemia
in rats, it is proposed that the causes of the lipid disorder
may be inversely related to actions of the drug (Biochem.
Pharmacol., 1970, 19:2719). In the rat, Atromid-S is known to
induce lipoprotein lipase and block free fatty acid (FFA)
mobilization peripherally, and to increase hepatic thyroxine
and NAD levels and decrease hepatic FFA uptake centrally. In
nephrosis, it is already known that lipoprotein lipase activity
is decreased and FFA mobilization increased, so that these
defects may be expected to be corrected by Atromid-S. In the
present study it has been found in mild to moderate PA-nephrosis
(single injection of 75 to 100 mg PA/kg i.p.) in 27 rats that
localized hepatic hypothyroidism, hyporiboflavinaemia and
hypotryptophenaemia (tryptophan being the precursor of NAD)
occur concurrently with the hyperlipidaemia. Hepatic thyroxine
concentration was 74% serum tryptophan 68%, albumin 86%,
total cholesterol 130%, triglycerides 170%, and total phospholipids 120% of normal in mild nephrosis ($p < 0.05$ in each
case). In moderate nephrosis, hepatic thyroxine was 70%,
serum tryptophan 33%, albumin 58%, riboflavin 70%, and the
lipids 330%, 1660% and 250% of normal, respectively ($p < 0.01$).
The degree of hypoalbuminaemia correlated significantly with
hepatic thyroxine, serum tryptophan and serum riboflavin levels.
Preliminary studies suggest minor falls in serum thyroxine
(88% of normal) and in liver content of tryptophan (88%),
NAD (89%), NADH (80%) (NAD/NADH ratio, 106%), NADP (74%) and
NADP/NADPH ratio (73%) in nephrosis. The finding of hepatic
hypothyroidism, hyporiboflavinaemia and hypotryptophanaemia in
nephrotic hyperlipidaemia supports the concept that albumin-
bound compounds (thyroxine, riboflavin and tryptophan, in
addition to FFA) may be controlling factors in hepatic lipogenesis, and that these may be disturbed in hypoalbuminaemic
states such as the nephrotic syndrome (Progr. Biochem. Pharmacol,
1971, vol. 7: in press, Karger/Basel).

VITAMIN A's INFLUENCE ON CHOLESTEROLGENESIS

C.D. ESKELSON and L.A. MEEKS

Veterans Administration Hospital, South 6th Street,
Tucson, Arizona 85723

An elucidation of vitamin A's activity on cholesterol
metabolism is confused since both increased and decreased
cholesterolgenesis have been reported in animals treated with
the vitamin. To determine the role this vitamin plays in
cholesterol metabolism rat liver homogenates were subjected to
the various forms of the vitamin. It was observed that
retinoic acid, retinyl acetate and retinal are the most potent
in vitro cholesterolgenic inhibitors from both ^{14}C-acetate
and ^{14}C-mevalonate substrates. This inhibition was elicited
only at 10^{-3} M vitamin A concentrations, however, if the
vitamin was added to triad or tetrad mixtures of the fat
soluble vitamins an in vitro inhibition of cholesterolgenesis
was elicited at 3.3×10^{-6} M vitamin concentration, but only
when acetate was substrate.

Liver homogenates from rats pretreated with triad and
tetrad-vitamin A-containing mixtures of the fat soluble

vitamins, also had decreased cholesterolgenesis from acetate substrate. Phillips reported a greater cholesterolgenesis from mevalonate substrate in rats on a normal diet as compared to rats on vitamin A-deficient diets. These results have been confirmed, and, additionally, cholesterolgenesis in liver homogenats from vitamin A-deficient rats was increased by the in vitro addition of 10^{-5} to $5X10^{-6}$ M Retinol. This increased cholesterolgenesis was not sufficient to return the cholesterol-genic activity to that of liver homogenates from vitamin A intact animals. It is deduced from these studies that: vitamin A is an inhibitor of cholesterolgenesis from acetate; functions as a cofactor in cholesterolgenesis beyond the mevalonate stage; and possibly is required for the synthesis of a protein necessary for cholesterol metabolism.

EFFECTS OF CLOFIBRATE AND BETABENZYLBUTYRATE ON HEPATIC

TRIGLYCERIDE BIOSYNTHESIS

R.G. LAMB, L.L. ADAMS, and H.J. FALLON

Departments of Medicine and Pharmacology, University of North Carolina School of Medicine, Chapel Hill, North Carolina 27514

Clofibrate and betabenzylbutyrate promptly lower serum triglyceride levels in man and animals. Clofibrate reduces the incorporation of ^{14}C-glycerol into hepatic and serum triglyceride 6 hours after ingestion of chow containing 0.25% clofibrate. There was a simultaneous fall in serum triglyceride. These changes preceded a decline in serum glycerol and hepatic sn-glycerol-3-P. No change in liver triglyceride occurred. Addition of clofibrate and betabenzylbutyrate (1-10 M) to homogenate and microsomal preparations inhibited diglyceride and triglycerid formation from ^{14}C-sn-glycerol-3-P. The first reaction in this pathway, the acylation of sn-glycerol-3-P, was inhibited by both agents in vitro. Both drugs displace albumin bound acyl CoA onto microsomes without increasing free acyl CoA levels. Increasing microsomal bound acyl CoA accounts in part for the inhibition of esterification by these drugs. However, inhibition also occurs in the absence of albumin and without changes in microsomal bound acyl CoA. None of the other microsomal reactions in triglyceride biosynthesis were inhibited by either drug. It is concluded that both drugs inhibit hepatic triglyceride biosynthesis in vivo, possibly by a direct inhibition of the acylation of sn-glycerol-3-P. This effect occurs promptly, is sustained, and precedes many of the other metabolic changes produced.

EFFECT OF GLYCOLYSIS INHIBITORS ON CYCLIC AMP SYNTHESIS IN RAT

ADIPOSE TISSUE

G. FASSINA and P. DORIGO

Institute of Pharmacology, University of Padova, Largo E. Meneghetti, 2, 35100 Padova (Italy)

The effect of monoiodoacetic acid and of sodium fluoride on cyclic AMP in rat epididymal fat and in its incubation medium, was investigated using cyclic nucleotide-dependent protein kinases (1).

The concentration of cyclic AMP was strongly decreased by monoidoacetic acid (0.001 M) and by sodium fluoride (0.04 M), in the presence of noradrenaline plus theophylline.

The antagonistic action by the inhibitors of glycolysis on hormone-stimulated lipolysis, was previously demonstrated (2,3). The fact that these drugs inhibit to the same extent, both lipolysis as well as cyclic AMP synthesis, could suggest that the glycolytic pathway is strictly related with adenyl-cyclase activity, and, particularly, that the ATP necessary for cyclic AMP synthesis is essentially furnished by the glycolytic process. This would agree with data (1,4,5) indicating that, unexpectedly, the alteration of energy equilibrium at the level of oxidative phosphorylation is, in contrast, not essential for cyclic AMP synthesis.

References:
  (1) J.F. Kuo and P. Greengard, J. Biol. Chem. 245, 4067 (1970)
  (2) B. Mosinger, Handbook of Physiology: Adipose Tissue, (Eds. A.E. Renold and G.F. Cahill Jr.) p. 601 (1965)
  (3) G. Fassina, I. Maragno and P. Dorigo, Biochem. Pharmacol. 16, 1439 (1967)
  (4) J.F. Kuo, Biochem. Pharmacol. 18, 757 (1969)
  (5) G. Fassina, P. Dorigo, R. Badetti and L. Visco, Abs. Physiology and Pharmacology of Cyclic AMP, an international Conference, Milan, Italy, 20-23 July (1971)

INTESTINAL CHOLESTEROL SYNTHESIS AND ABSORPTION: EFFECTS OF

D- AND L-THYROXINE

ELAINE B. FELDMAN, CHARLES Y. CHENG and DOLORES H. HENDERSON

Department of Medicine, State University of New York, Downstate Medical Center, 450 Clarkson Avenue, Brooklyn, New York 11203

Intestinal cholesterol biosynthesis from acetate was measured in hamsters given L- or D-thyroxine (T_4), 0.125 mgm, 7 doses (thrice weekly - "chronic"), or 4 daily doses ("acute").' Chronic administration increased acetate incorporation into intestinal cholesterol: L-T_4: 20%, D-T_4: 50% ($p < 0.01$). Intestinal cholesterol concentration was unchanged (L-T_4), or decreased 20% (D-T_4) ($p < 0.02$). L-T_4 and D-T_4 increased specific activities 28%, and 80% respectively ($p < 0.01$). Acute L-T_4 increased intestinal cholesterol radioactivity 150%, specific activity 100%; D-T_4 increased both 400%. Both drugs decreased plasma cholesterol 10%. Chronic D-T_4 increased luminal cholesterol 67%. Recirculation studies using radio-labeled micellar cholesterol (Nembutal, jejunum) showed lesser absorption of radioactivity with acute L-T_4 (30%) than with D-T_4 (80%), compared with control absorption. Non-labeled sterol absorptions were 67% and 50% respectively. Chronic L-T$_4$ treatment gave lesser changes. Brush border sterol uptake in vitro was unaffected by added 10-100 µg D- or L-T$_4$, while uptake in vivo was decreased 50%. Pretreatment acutely with L- or D-T$_4$ resulted in 30% decrease in brush border sterol uptake. Jejunal mucosal cholesterol and ester radio-activity, after 2 hour recirculation, increased 2 to 5-fold with drug treatment, or addition. These data suggest that hypocholesterolemic effects of thyroid isomers via intestinal mechanisms result from increased "secretion" of sterol into the gut lumen and hold-up in mucosa as well as decreased brush border uptake.

TREATMENT OF HYPERLIPIDEMIAS WITH A TETRALIN DERIVATIVE

FELLIN, R., FEDELE, D., BAGNARIOL, G., CREPALDI, G.

Fellin, Renato - Clinica Medical Generale Universita Padova - Via Giustiniani, Italy

Ten hyperlipidemic patients (2 type I^O, 4 type II°, 4 type IV°-V^O of Fredrickson) were treated with Su-13'437 - 2-methyl-2 p-(1,2,3,4 tetrahydro-1-naphthil) phenoxy - propionic acid - (300-500 mg/daily) for one year. Placebo was given during the 1st month and again for 3 weeks after 4 month's therapy. No dietary restrictions were adopted. Type I^O patients displayed a definite reduction of triglycerides during treatment, although normalization was not reached. During the intermediate placebo period, triglycerides returned to pretreat-ment levels. In type II° patients a mean cholesterol decrease of 27% was observed after 3 months of Su-13'437, followed by a return towards pretreatment values during intermediate placebo and a minor decrease (20%) in the second period of treatment. The best results were obtained in patients with types IV°-V^O, both triglyceridemia and cholesterolemia being normalized. During the first placebo period a marked decrease in serum lipid values was observed, followed by normalization during the first period of treatment. In the second placebo period a rebound effect was registered, all patients displaying a marked increase of serum lipids, even up to pretreatment values. The 2nd period of treatment brought serum triglycerides back to normal in all patients. Su-13'437 was well tolerated by all patients; liver functional tests and haematological parameters did not vary during one year's therapy.

INVESTIGATIONS WITH THE SCAN ELECTRON MICROSCOPE INTO THE EFFECTS

OF DISTURBANCES OF FAT METABOLISM ON THE ARTERIAL WALL AND THE

EFFECT ON DRUGS ON THEM

H. FROST

Medizinische Poliklinik der Universitat Munchen, 8 Munchen 15, Pettenkoferstrasse 8a, Germany

Investigations with the scan electron microscope have shown that feeding a rabbit for 2-3 weeks with fodder containing 2% cholesterol produces numerous thrombocytic adhesions on the arterial wall. This raises the consideration that the adherent thrombocytes are laden with fat and are being incorporated into the vessel wall along with the fat. In addition to thrombocytes, drop-like adhesions with a diameter of about 0,5 to 1,0 μ were found here and there. Since these structures were never seen in control animals with normal serum fat levels, nor in the preparations which were dehydrated in increasing concentrations of alcohol, it is probable that they were droplets of fat. Feeding with cholesterol enriched diet for eleven wks produced an excessive increase in the serum cholesterol levels (over 1200 mg%). However, while after this long feeding period the thrombocyte adhesions were only rarely found, other structures adhering to the wall appeared which could be identified as cholesterol crystals. These crystals are found also in the subendothelium in clefts in the thickened intima. These adhesions to the vessel wall do not appear to be solely dependent on the pathologically high cholesterol levels. Investigations with substances which did produce falls in the cholesterol levels, although these levels still lay pathologically high, showed no clear thrombocyte adhesions in a short term test, and in a long term test considerably fewer adhesions of cholesterol crystals on the arterial wall.

SEPARATION OF MOLECULAR SPECIES OF LIPOPROTEIN LIPASE FROM ADIPOSE

TISSUE

ARLENE S. GARFINKEL and MICHAEL C. SCHOTZ

Research, Veterans Administration Hospital (Wadsworth), Los Angeles, California 90073 and Department of Biological Chemistry, UCLA School of Medicine, Los Angeles, California 90024

One of the key regulators of lipid deposition in adipose tissue is lipoprotein lipase. This enzyme was extracted from rat, epididymal fat tissue and separated by gel filtration chromatography (Biogel A - 1.5 M) into two fractions (LPL_a and LPL_b). LPL_b had a molecular weight of approximately 2×10^5 whereas LPL_a was greater than 1.5×10^6. Both fractions were shown to have the characteristics of lipoprotein lipase, i.e., an alkaline pH optimum, inhibition by NaCl, and requirement for activation of the substrate by serum. However, when assayed for lipase activity in the presence of heparin, the activity of LPL_a was enhanced whereas that of LPL_b was inhibited. On rechromatography these species do not appear to be interconvertible. We have concluded that LPL_a and LPL_b fraction represent two distinct species of lipoprotein lipase.

DRUGS AFFECTING UPTAKE OF FREE FATTY ACIDS IN THE IN VIVO CANINE

MYOCARDIUM

V.V. GLAVIANO and T.N. MASTERS

Department of Physiology and Biophysics, Chicago Medical School/ University of Health Sciences, 2020 W. Odgen Avenue, Chicago, Illinois 60612

The intracoronary administration of norepinephrine
(.02 μg/Kg/min) leads to stimulation of myocardial free fatty
acid (FFA) uptake in anesthetized open-chest dogs. Prior
treatment with the β-adrenergic blocking drug, dl-propranolol
(1 mg/Kg), caused a marked inhibition of norepinephrine (NE)
stimulation of myocardial uptake of FFA. To clarify the
inhibitory mechanism of propranolol on extraction of FFA,
analysis of cardiac muscle subcellular organelles showed that
an increase in TGFA and a decrease in FFA occurred almost pre-
dominately in the supernatant faction. The rise in levels of
TGFA pointed to a decrease during β-blockade in intracellular
utilization of FFA. These studies were supported by the finding
that intracoronary administered Na-palmitate-1-^{14}C was readily
incorporated into the TGFA cytoplasmic faction. In other dogs
treated with propranolol, dibutyryl cyclic AMP was found to
reverse the blockade to uptake of FFA. Another study involving
the intracoronary infusion of prostaglandin E$_1$ (PGE$_1$) showed
the antilipolytic action of PGE$_1$ to be similar to propranolol.
In these experiments, PGE$_1$ increased myocardial levels of TGFA
while decreasing levels of cyclic AMP, uptake of FFA and lipolytic
activity of heart muscle. Arterial levels of FFA or myocardial
physical performance were not found to be sufficiently altered
to account for changes in FFA uptake observed with NE, propranolol, PGE$_1$ or dibutyryl cyclic AMP. The decline in cardiac
extraction of FFA and rise in myocardial levels of TGFA with
propranolol or PGE$_1$ indicate a close relationship between the
uptake of FFA by the heart, its subsequent utilization, and
the adenyl cyclase system. (Supported by ONR, Contract
Nonr 3502(01).

ESTROGEN INDUCED PANCREATITIS IN FAMILIAL TYPES IV AND V

HYPERLIPOPROTEINEMIA

CHARLES J. GLUECK M.D.

General Clinical Research Center, Cincinnati General Hospital,
234 Goodman Street, Cincinnati, Ohio   45229

Recurrent acute and sub-acute pancreatitis in 4 post-
menopausal women and 1 man post prostatectomy followed
administration of potent estrogens: Diethylstilbesterol (3 mg/day),
Premarin (1.25 mg/day), Chlorotriasene (25 mg/day). Index
triglycerides on estrogens, measured well after resolution of
clinical symptoms were 5850, 5970, 5825 and 385 mg% in the
women, and 2800 in the man. Fourteen days after estrogens were
stopped, triglycerides fell to 1060, 482, 1154, and 200 mg% in
the women, 478 in the man. Familial type V hyperlipoproteinemia
was subsequently documented in 3 women; one man and woman had
Familial type IV. Mean post-heparin lipolytic activity was
depressed on estrogens to .18, range .13-.35 Eq FFA/ml/min,
and rose 78% to normal levels (.33, range .28-38) after estrogen
was discontinued. On therapy with the progestin Norethindrone
Acetate (5 mg/day) or the anabolic compound Oxandrolone
(7.5 mg/day) pancreatitis has not recurred. Mean triglycerides
in the 3 women with type V have fallen further to 229, 347, and
343 mg%, and are 135 in the woman with type IV. Mean postheparin lipolytic activity on progestational-anabolic therapy

was .40.   Previously covert familial hyperglyceridemia may
become overt when post menopausal or prostatectomy estrogen
"therapy" exacerbates hyperglyceridemia, impairs triglyceride
clearing enzymes, and causes pancreatitis.

RED BLOOD CELL AND PLASMA PHOSPHOLIPIDS IN AGED HUMANS

MARTIN GOLD and HENRY ALTSCHULER

Philadelphia Geriatric Center, 5301 Old York Road, Philadelphia,
Pennsylvania 19141

A study was conducted to assay the erythrocyte and plasma
phospholipids of residents of the Philadelphia Geriatric
Center. The purpose of this research was to ascertain whether
an aging pattern could be defined by using the red blood cell
as a simple model. The age range of the persons studied was
70-95 years with a mean of 81.3 years. The phospholipids were
extracted and separated by thin layer chromatography. The
fatty acid composition for the various classes was analyzed
by gas liquid chromatography for plasma and erythrocytes.
The red blood cell phospholipid distribution was phosphatidyl
choline (PC) 33.3%, phosphatidyl ethanolamine (PE) 30.8%,
sphingomyelin (SM) 18.1%, and a grouping of phosphatidyl serine
(PS), phosphatidyl inositol (PI), and lysolecithin (lysoPC)
17.8%. The plasma phospholipid result was PC (61.0%),
PE (12.6%), SM (20%), and PS, PI, and LysoPC (6.2%. The fatty
acid exhibited a characteristic pattern in each class. The
effect of aging on these patterns will be discussed.

EPIDEMIOLOGICAL STUDY ON HYPERLIPIDEMIA AMONG JAPANESE

Y. GOTO, Y. NAKAMURA, E. ASANO, and H. NAKAMURA

School of Medicine, Keio University, 35 Shinanomachi,
Shinjuku-ku, Tokyo, Japan

The incidence of hyperlipidemia was assessed in two
farm villages and a fishing village of Japan according to the
classification of Fredrickson and his group with some
modification.

Total incidence of hyperlipidemia was 55.7% and 48.8% in
farm village and 65.5% in fishing village. In farm village,
Type IV was more frequent with concomitant increase of
carbohydrate intake, while in fishing village Type II was
more pronounced in frequency accompanied by high daily
cholesterol intake.

Subjects were divided into following 4 groups: (a) Diet-
control with Anabolic steroid group, (b) Anabolic steroid
group, (c) Diet-control with Placebo group, (d) Placebo group.
Every 6 month, blood and dietary examination was performed
on these subjects. In 6 months, plasma cholesterol and

triglyceride level in anabolic steroid group significantly decreased compared with placebo group.

In 18 month, the incidence of arteriosclerotic vascular disease has been examined. No such disease has been so far noted in (a) or (b) group, while in (c) group 2 cerebral thrombotic cases and in (d) group 1 cerebral thrombosis and 1 myocardial infarction has been confirmed.

COMBINED DETERMINATIONS OF LECITHIN-CHOLESTEROL-ACYL-TRANSFERASE

(LCAT) AND LIPOPROTEIN-X IN DIFFERENT FORMS OF LIVER DISEASE

H. GRETEN, H. WENGELER AND D. SEIDEL

Medical Clinic, University of Heidelberg, Bergheimer Strasse 58, 6900 Heidelberg, Germany

Indirect evidence suggests that lecithin-cholesterol-acyl-transferase (LCAT) is synthesized in the liver. There are, however, controversial reports in the literature correlating LCAT activity to various forms of liver disease. The purpose of this study was to determine LCAT activity in icteric patients which were classified not only by the convential methods, but also with respect to the presence or absence of LP-X, an abnormal plasma lipoprotein most specific to demonstrate or exclude cholestasis. With ^{14}C labelled cholesterol as substrate, our enzyme assay was (1) linear over 6 h, (2) reproducible within 1% accuracy, (3) sensitive to measure even smallest amounts of LCAT activity in plasma. LCAT was measured at different stages of the disease and the patients divided into 4 groups: I. Hepatitis with cholestasis (LP-X pos.) (14); II. Hepatitis without cholestasis (LP-X neg.) (16); III. Extrahepatic biliary obstruction (LP-X pos.) (12); IV. Chronic liver failure (LP-X neg.) (10). Compared to normal controls (15), patients from group I had low, from group II had normal, from group III had normal and from group IV had low LCAT activity. In vitro studies clearly excluded circulating inhibitors of LCAT. Additional experiments demonstrated that LCAT is released or activated by human liver. These data explain contradictary findings on LCAT activity in liver disease by different investigators and suggest that combined determinations of LCAT and LP-X may prove useful as a means to differentiate not only between obstructive and non-obstructive jaundice, but also between extrahepatic biliary obstruction and intrahepatic cholestasis.

TREATMENT OF PRIMARY HYPER-β-(TYPE II) AND HYPER-PRE-β-

LIPOPROTEINAEMIA (TYPE IV) WITH D,L-α-METHYLTHYROXINE-

ETHYLESTER (CG 635)

GRIES, F.A., MISS, H.D., CANZLER, H., KOSCHINSKY, T., VOGELBERG, K.H., and JAHNKE, K.

2 Medical Clinic, Diabetes Research Institut, University of Dusseldorf; Stadtische Ferdinand Sauerbruch Krankenanstalten, Wuppertal Elberfeld; Department of Innere Medizin, Medizinische Hochschule Hannover, Germany

Studies on the effect of CG 635 on lipoproteins in primary hyperlipoproteinaemia (HL) are presented.

37 out-patients with primary HL types II - V were tested. The study included 2 placebo-periods of 4-8 weeks and 2 CG 635 periods (2 x 20 mg per day orally) of 6-20 weeks alternately. Lipid determinations and clinical examinations were performed at least twice per period. Diet was kept constant.

In 19 of 21 patients with type II HL (mean cholesterol 391 mg/100 ml) cholesterol was lowered by CG treatment 10% (mean decrease 21% or 56 mg/100 ml). Replacement of CG 635 by placebo resulted in elevation of cholesterol in 11 of 14 patients examined. The effect on triglycerides (mean 152 mg/100 ml) was irregular and minute.

Cholesterol was also lowered 10% in 10 of 12 patients with type IV HL (mean cholesterol 346 mg/100 ml, mean decrease 23% or 69 mg/100 ml). Triglyceride concentration (mean 734 mg/100 ml) decreased 10% in 7 patients (mean decrease 44% or 251 mg/100 ml).

There were no significant changes in body weight or symptoms of calorigenic action. During treatment with CG 635 serum alkaline phosphatase and transaminases rose above normal range in 16,21,15% of the treatment periods respectively. The elevations were reversed promptly after cessation of treatment.

THE EFFECTS OF A NEW BILE ACID-SEQUESTRANT, COLESTIPOL (U-26,597A),

ON SERUM CHOLESTEROL IN A HYPERLIPIDEMIC PRISON POPULATION

KARE GUNDERSEN, M.D.

The Upjohn Company, Kalamazoo, Michigan 49001

Colestipol, a new bile acid-sequestering granular polymer made from tetraethylene pentamine and epichlorohydrin, has been studied in male hyperlipidemic prisoners for two years, and compared with placebo (avicel) and cholestyramine (Questran). Four and 5 gram doses t.i.d. compared well with 4 gram doses of cholestyramine as far as cholesterol lowering was concerned. Consistent serum cholesterol decreases of 15-20% from baseline values were seen in all active drug groups throughout the two years. A placebo effect is also seen at times, indicating a need for placebo control in such studies. Active drugs also showed significant lowering of serum cholesterol when compared to placebo. A significant cholesterol-lowering effect was seen in subjects with triglycerides well about 200 mg%. 80-90% in the three drug groups (21-23 in each) responded by a fall in cholesterol of 15% or more most of the time, while 76% of the placebo group showed no such fall. Serum triglycerides showed little change, fluctuations being due to apparent sporadic changes during the study. The polymer has no taste or smell, and side effects were minimal.

LONG-TERM EFFECT OF THE PHENOLIC ETHER Su-13437 (CIBA) ON

HYPERLIPIDEMIAS

GEORGES HARTMANN

Medizinische Universitatsklinik, Inselspital, Bern, Switzerland

29 patients (17 men, 12 women) with hyperlipidemia (11 Type II, 4 Type III, 7 Type IV, 3 Type V, 4 Type undetermined) have been treated for 12-40 months with the compound 2-methyl-2-p-(1,2,3,4-tetrahydro-1-naphthyl)-phenoxy propionic acid (Su-13437-Ciba). The doses varied from 300-600 mg/day, blood specimens were drawn at 2-6 weeks intervals. Evaluation is made by comparing results obtained from the 4th week of treatment on with pretreatment + placebo-values (the latter being interspersed after 1 year of treatment or later). The mean effect in % for the 5 groups was (incl. standard-dev.):

	Cholesterol	Triglycerides
Type II	-20.9 ± 5.7	- --
Type III	-33.1 ± 13	-57.6 ± 8.5
Type IV	-26.9 ± 13.1	-63.2 ± 11.7
Type V	-22.1 ± 2.4	-65.6 ± 3.1
Undetermined	-22.2 ± 11.4	-57.5 ± 12.6

There was no resistance to the drug, but the least effects were achieved in Type II. Intra-individual differences (means) between treatment - and control - periods are all statistically significant with p-values < 0.05 to < 0.001 for cholesterol and/or triglycerides. The only side-effects observed are transient increased transaminase-levels (3 Type II, 1 Type undetermined), which were dose-dependent and reversible.

EFFECTS OF A SINGLE ADMINISTRATION OF L-ASPARAGINASE ON SERUM LIPIDS

P. HEIMSTADT and N. ZOLLNER

Medizinische Poliklinik der Universitat Munchen, Pettenkoferstrasse 8a
8 Munchen 15, Germany

Under therapy of leukemia with L-asparaginase a decrease of serum cholesterol is observed regularly. Since there is a concomitant rise of serum transaminase the behaviour of cholesterol levels is considered to be a consequence of liver damage. Recently it was found that a single intravenous administration of L-asparaginase is followed by a drop of serum cholesterol, particularly of the ester fraction (ASTALDI). Reinvestigation and extension of this finding confirmed the cholesterol lowering effect (30-35 per cent) of a single dose of 500 u. L-asparaginase, the maximum response being obtained between the 4th and 9th day. The decrease of total cholesterol was accompanied by a proportional decrease of cholesterol esters; when the individual esters were studied there was no change in the proportions of the various fatty acids. After administration of L-asparaginase triglyceride levels rose from normal starting values to concentrations between 250 and 400

mg/100 ml reaching the maximum between the 2nd and 6th day.
Electrophoretic follow-up of lipoproteins revealed no changes.
All liver functions studied remained normal throughout the
period of observation. It would appear that L-asparaginase is
a valuable tool for producing a defined change in serum lipids.

EFFECT OF W1372 ON LIPOPROTEINS IN RATS AND SQUIRREL MONKEYS

P. HILL and J.F. DOUGLAS

Wallace Laboratories, Cranbury, New Jersey

        Male rats and Squirrel monkeys fed Purina chow were
given W1372 (N-phenylpropyl N-benzyloxy acetamide) in the diet.
(0.25% & 0.3% w/w respectively)

        W1372, previously reported to reduce atheromata in
Squirrel Monkeys (Berger et al J. Pharm. Expl. Therap. 170,
371, 1969) and serum lipids in rats (Kritchevsky & Tepper,
Arzneim--Forsch. 20, 584, 1970), reduced the low density
lipoproteins (LDL) phospholipid, triglyceride and cholesterol
as shown by dextran sulphate precipitation and ultracentrifugation.

        No inhibition of synthesis of triglyceride, phospholipid
or cholesterol occurred in the liver of treated rats as shown
by the incorporation of $U^{14}C$ glycerol, Me^3H choline and $2^{14}C$
acetate. In Squirrel Monkeys, W1372 similarily reduced the LDL-
phospholipid and cholesterol but did not alter the hepatic
synthesis of cholesterol or phospholipid. In monkeys the serum
and liver (mg/g) triglyceride was unaltered. The adrenal but not
the skin sterol content was decreased by W1372, while intestinal
cholesterol biosynthesis was unaltered.

        The reduction of atheromata may occur, in part, by
interference with the release of LDL, reducing the circulating
lipids.

THE COMBINED USE OF CLOFIBRATE AND CHOLESTYRAMINE OR DEAE

SEPHADEX IN HYPERCHOLESTEROLAEMIA

A.N. HOWARD and D.E. HYAMS

Department of Investigative Medicine, University of Cambridge
and Chesterton Hospital, Cambridge, England

        A comparison was made of the effect of DEAE Sephadex
(an anionic exchange resin) and cholestyramine ('Questran')
with and without the addition of clofibrate in normal and
type II hypercholesterolaemic patients. DEAE Sephadex
(12-15g/day) alone appeared to be as effective as cholestyramine
in lowering the plasma cholesterol by 12-15%. Clofibrate acted
synergistically with DEAE Sephadex and increased the activity
of the latter by over two-fold, such that a mean decrease in
plasma cholesterol of 35% was seen in two weeks. The

combination of clofibrate with cholestyramine was less effective
and gave a mean lowering of 20%.

THE IN VITRO EFFECTS OF CLOFIBRATE (ETHYL P-CHLOROPHENOXY-

ISOBUTYRATE, CPIB) ON LIPID SYNTHESIS IN HUMAN SKIN

S.K. HSIA, Ph.D. and JAMES E. FULTON, JR., M.D.

Departments of Dermatology and Biochemistry, P. O. Box 875,
Biscayne Annex, Miami, Florida 33152

In studying drugs affecting lipid metabolism, there is an
obvious need for a model system, ideally utilizing a human
tissue, which is active in lipid metabolism and responds to
metabolic regulations. We have found that human skin fulfills
these requirements. Small biopsy specimens of human skin are
relatively easy to obtain. These specimens synthesize in vitro
a variety of lipids, including sterols, fatty acids, sterol
esters and wax esters, glycerides, and polar lipids (Vroman
et al. J. Lipid Res. 10:507, 1969). This activity is decreased
in diabetes or after fasting, and is restored towards normal
after insulin treatment or refeeding (Hsia et al. J. Invest.
Derm. 46:443, 1966; Proc. Soc. Exptl. Biol. Med. 135:285, 1970).
Our current study showed that CPIB inhibits lipid synthesis
from acetate-1-^{14}C or glucose-U-^{14}C by human skin in vitro.
The inhibition is dose dependent, and can be partially reversed
by increased glucose concentration. The inhibition affects all
lipid classes, but is most pronounced in the sterol and the
di- and monoglyceride fractions. These experiments illustrate
the potential usefulness of human skin as a model system for
the study of control of lipid metabolism.

EXPERIMENTAL HYPERLIPOPROTEINEMIA INDUCED BY ENDOTOXIN OR FRACTURE

KARL HUTH

Giessen (West Germany) Medizinische Univ.-Klinik.

Up to now, the behaviour of blood lipids following trauma
and during shock has not been studied extensively.

Pronounced alterations of blood lipids can be induced
in rabbits by two shock models: by intravenous injections of
endotoxin, or , similarily, by unilateral or bilateral femur
fracture. Already a few minutes after the application of
endotoxin free fatty acids and free glycerol are elevated.
After 24 hours also triglycerides have risen to several times
the initial value. Electrophoresis reveals the pattern of
endogenous type IV hyperlipoproteinemia. Accelerated lipolysis
and consecutive hyperlipoproteinemia develop in the same
manner after femur fracture with pulmonary fat embolism.

Phenoxybenzamine and reserpine significantly suppress the
lipid mobilization syndrome in both shock models. In addition to

the catecholamines histamine is an important mediator of
alterations in lipid metabolism described here, since mepyramine
is an effective inhibitor of the increase in free fatty acids
and triglycerides. Serotonin and kinines seem to be of minor
importance. The proteinase inhibitor Trasylol (R) prevents
the blood lipid alterations in experimental fat embolism
following unilateral femur fracture but not following endotoxin
application.

Experimental hyperlipoproteinemia induced by endotoxin
or fracture is not necessarily correlated to severity of trauma
or mortality rate. Reserpine therapy prevents hyperlipacidemia
and hypertriglyceridemia after endotoxin, although the
mortality increases.

STIMULATION OF RAT LIVER LYSOSOMAL LIPASE BY ENDOGENOUS LIPID

AND ACIDIC PHOSPHOLIPIDS

ARNOLD KAPLAN and MASAO KARIYA

Department of Microbiology, St. Louis University School of
Medicine, 1402 South Grand Boulevard, St. Louis, Missouri 63104

Purified lysosomal triglyceride lipase from rat liver is
stimulated by endogenous lipid. The effect of the factor in
crude homogenates of rat liver was first observed as a non-
linear relationship of homogenate concentration to enzyme
activity indicative of the presence of dissociable activators.
A two step differential centrifugation procedure for the simultaneous preparation of the lipase activity in soluble form free
of interference from factor, and a microsomal fraction rich in
factor has been developed to simplify analysis of the properties
of the factor. The factor is associated with the particulate
fraction of rat liver homogenates, is non-dialysable, remains
active and insoluble after a 10 min. heat treatment at 100° in
the absence of detergent, and is active and solubilized after
10 min. of heating at 70° in detergent. It can be extracted by
and recovered from lipid solvents. Brain fractions rich in
either phosphatidyl inositide or phosphatidyl serine stimulate
lipase activity 20-fold. Phosphatidic acid stimulates the activity 6-fold. Other phospholipids are comparatively ineffective.
The factor specifically stimulates the lysosomal lipase with a
pH optima of 4 and does not alter the pH optimum. The relationship of these findings to lipotropic phenomena will be discussed.

THE HYPOLIPIDEMIC EFFECTS OF TRELOXINATE

TAKASHI KARIYA, THOMAS R. BLOHM, J. MARTIN GRISAR, ROGER A.
PARKER and JEANNE R. MARTIN

The Wm. S. Merrell Company; Division of Richardson-Merrell, Inc.
110 E. Amity Road; Cincinnati, Ohio   45215

Treloxinate (methyl 2,10-dichloro-12H-dibenzo[d,g] [1,3]
dioxocin-6-carboxylate) and its acid were found to be potent

hypolipidemic agents in rats and in hypothyroid dogs. Comparative studies in Wistar rats indicate that this compound is approximately 10 times as potent as clofibrate in lowering plasma cholesterol, and 30 times as potent in lowering plasma triglycerides.· Liver slices from rats treated with treloxinate incorporated signifi- cantly less acetate into cholesterol than slices from control rats; mevalonate incorporation into cholesterol was not affected by treloxinate treatment. Oxidation of rat lipoprotein cholesterol- $26-^{14}C$ (Whereat and Staple lipoprotein labeling) to $^{14}CO_2$ was increased by treloxinate treatment of rats. This effect was not accountable to reduction of the total plasma-liver cholesterol pool.

Hepatomegaly occurred in treated rats, similar to that occurring with clofibrate. Liver weights returned to normal promptly on cessation of treatment. No accumulation of liver lipids was observed. A rapid and sustained reduction of plasma cholesterol levels was obtained in dogs made hypercholestero- lemic by prior treatment with ^{131}I. This reduction occurred in the LDL fraction.

The possible relation of molecular conformation to hypolipidemic activity will be discussed.

UNCOUPLING EFFECT OF HYPOCHOLESTEREMIC DRUGS

S. L. KATYAL, J. SAHA and J. J. KABARA

Michigan State University, College of Osteopathic Medicine, 900 Auburn Road, Pontiac, Michigan 48057

Clofibrate or AY9944 can lower blood cholesterol. Clofibrate also brings about lowering of phospholipids and triglycerides. AY9944 was suggested to inhibit cholesterol biosynthesis by blocking 7-dehydrocholesterol 7-reductase. The mechanism of action of clofibrate -- a currently used drug for the treatment of hypercholesterolemia -- is still controversial. The purpose of this study was to investigate the effect of these drugs on certain aspects of oxidative phosphorylation. Any effect on the snythesis of ATP in liver would affect lipid biosynthesis. Both these compounds uncoupled oxidative phosphorylation, inhibited the oxidation of DPNH- linked substrates and stimulated mitochondrial ATPase activity with and without DNP or Mg^{++}. The significance of these effects in cholesterol biosynthesis will be discussed.

ON THE EFFECT OF SALICYLATE ON INCORPORATION OF ACETYL-CoA AND MALONYL-CoA INTO CHOLESTEROL AND FATTY ACIDS

A.N. KLIMOV, O.K. DOKUSOVA, L.A. PETROVA and E.D. POLIAKOVA

Laboratory of Lipid Metabolism, Institute of Experimental Medicine, Leningrad, USSR

Salicylate, at a concentration of 10^{-2}M, inhibits the incorporation of 1-^{14}C-acetyl-CoA into cholesterol and fatty acids by the supernatant fraction of rat liver homogenate, but has no effect on the incorporation of 2-^{14}C-malonyl-CoA into these compounds. The absence of the inhibitory effect of salicylate on the incorporation of malonyl-CoA into cholesterol proves that malonyl-CoA is not subjected to decarboxylation in this condition. These data allow us to conclude that the salicylic acid may be considered as an inhibitor of acetyl-CoA carboxylase. At the same time the results obtained in our work show the possibility for malonyl-CoA to be converted into sterol as it was proposed or shown by other authors earlier. Citrate has no effect on the incorporation of 1-^{14}C-acetate or 1-^{14}C-acetyl-CoA into cholesterol but stimulates the incorporation of these substrates into fatty acids. This effect of citrate is increased by the addition of Mn^{++}.

INHIBITION OF CHOLESTEROL BIOSYNTHESIS BY SOME DERIVATIVES OF

MEVALONIC ACID

A.N. KLIMOV, T.A. KLIMOVA, L.A. PETROVA and E.D. POLIAKOVA

Laboratory of Lipid Metabolism, Institute of Experimental Medicine, Leningrad, U.S.S.R.

The effect of ten aromatic acids structurally similar to mevalonic acid was studied on the biosynthesis of cholesterol in rat liver homogenate from 1-^{14}C-acetate and 2-^{14}C-mevalonate. The following acids were used: 3-p-tolyl-3,5-dioxypentanic (I), 2-phenyl-3-p-tolyl-3,5-dioxypentanic (II), 2,3-diphenyl-3,5-dioxypentanic (III), 3-p-tolyl-3-oxypentanic (IV), 3-benzyl-3-oxypentanic (V), 2-phenyl-3-p-tolyl-3-oxypentanic (VI), 2,3-diphenyl-3-oxypentanic (VII), 2-phenyl-3-benzyl-3-oxypentanic (VIII), cis (H, C_7H_7)-3-p-tolyl-5-oxy-2-pentenic (IX) and 3-p-tolyl-2-pentenic (X) acids. The most efficient inhibitors of cholesterol biosynthesis from mevalonate are acids VI, VII, and VIII, possessing aromatic radicals at positions 2 and 3, and having no hydroxyl at position 5, as well as unsaturated acids IX and X with double bond at position 2. The study of the action of some inhibitors in vivo will be discussed.

EFFECTS OF NICOTINIC ACID AND PLANT STEROLS ON CHOLESTEROL

METABOLISM IN MAN

B.J. KUDCHODKAR, L. HORLICK, and H.S. SODHI

Department of Medicine, University of Saskatchewan, Saskatoon, Saskatchewan, Canada

The effects of nicotinic acid and plant sterols ("Positol") were investigated in three subjects by cholesterol balance techniques using both radio-isotope and gas-liquid chromatographic methods. Nicotinic acid reduced plasma cholesterol concentrations by about 15% (229 $\pm$ 11 to 206 $\pm$ 13 mg/100 ml). Unlike "Positol", nicotinic acid had no effect on the absorption of dietary cholesterol (33 $\pm$ 4% before and 34 $\pm$ 5% after the treatment). Nicotinic acid caused modest increases in the fecal excretion of both neutral (370 $\pm$ 90 to 430 $\pm$ 28 mg/day) and acidic (52 $\pm$ 30 to 100 $\pm$ 14 mg/day) steroids whereas "Positol" caused a marked increase in the excretion of neutral (268 $\pm$ 26 to 358 $\pm$ 55 mg/day) and a modest increase in the excretion of acidic (146 $\pm$ 60 to 202 $\pm$ 19 mg/day) steroids.

The synthesis of cholesterol is increased by "Positol". On the other hand, the decreases in the plasma cholesterol specific activity slopes suggested that nicotinic acid caused an inhibition of synthesis of endogenous cholesterol. In all three subjects there were acute increases in the specific activity values immediately after administration of the drugs which lasted for 2 to 3 days and these could only be explained by the entry of high specific activity cholesterol from tissue pools (Pool B) into plasma in accord with the hypothesis previously suggested by us.

USE OF COMBINED BILE ACID SEQUESTRANT ADMINISTRATION AND SIMPLE-

CARBOHYDRATE RESTRICTION IN TYPE II HYPERLIPOPROTEINEMIA

PETER T. KUO

Hospital of the University of Pennsylvania, Philadelphia, Pennsylvania 19104

A bile acid sequestrant (Cholestepanine or Cholestipol) was administered to 50 patients with Types II_a and II_b hyperlipoproteinemia, after their body weight and serum lipids were stabilized on a simple-carbohydrate restrictive diet. Daily dose of 20-30 grams of either drug persistently reduced serum cholesterol in 47 patients by 24.1 - 45.2% for 15-18 months as compared with values obtained during placebo control period. In all patients there was a fall in low density lipoprotein (LDL) cholesterol. The reported triglyceride and very low density lipoprotein (VLDL) elevations with the drug administration and similar plasma lipid elevations in Type II_b patients were controlled by simple-carbohydrate calorie restriction in 47 well-motivated patients. The program may be applied to study the value of long term control of LDL and VLDL increases in the prevention of atherosclerosis.

LIPOLYTIC ACTIVITY OF SOME PHOSPHODIESTERASE INHIBITORS

F. P. KUPIECKI

Diabetes Research, The Upjohn Company, Kalamazoo, Michigan 49001

Since the discovery by Sutherland and Rall that theophylline inhibits cyclic AMP phosphodiesterase, many reports have demonstrated that theophylline stimulates lipolysis by

increasing tissue concentrations of cyclic AMP. During studies
with three lipolytic agents (I, II, III)* and theophylline, it
was observed that these four agents stimulate basal free fatty
acid (FFA) and glycerol release. However, when lipolysis is
maximally stimulated by epinephrine they further increase FFA,
but not glycerol, in tissue and medium. All four compounds
inhibited cyclic AMP phosphodiesterase. Mechanism studies
showed that glucose oxidation in adipose tissue is diminished
by theophylline or I, which is more potent than theophylline
as a phosphodiesterase inhibitor. This suggests that one
possible reason for FFA accumulation is reduced availability
of α-glycerol phosphate for reesterification.

Other studies suggested that II and III, but not I, are
lipolytic agents in vivo since they increased plasma FFA
levels in rats. Also, both compounds reduced weight gain of
rats during part of a 4-day treatment period but food
consumption was also reduced.

*   I.   2,5-bis(2-chloroethylsulfonyl)-pyrrole-3,4-dicarbonitrile,
   II.   2,4-diamino-6-butoxy-s-triazine,
  III.   2,3-dihydro-5,6-dimethyl-3-oxo-4-pyridazinecarbonitrile.

β-PYRIDYLCARBINOL-ENHANCED OXIDATION OF CHOLESTEROL FROM VARIOUS

LIPOPROTEIN FRACTIONS AND DECREASE OF PLASMA CHOLESTEROL IN RATS

H. LENGSFELD, H. GALLO-TORRES and K.F. GEY

F. Hoffmann-La Roche & Co. Ltd., 4002 Basle, Switzerland

It has previously been shown that β-pyridylcarbinol as
well as its oxidation product, i.e. nicotinic acid, increase the
oxidation of ^{14}C-cholesterol in liver homogenates (KRITCHEVSKY*)
and of plasma ^{14}C-cholesterol in intact starved rats
(LENGSFELD & GEY*). In the present experiments 26-^{14}C-
cholesterol-labelled serum and lymph were obtained from donor
rats and fractionated into chylomicrons and very low density
lipoproteins, low density lipoproteins, intermediate density
lipoproteins, and high density lipoproteins from serum as well
as chylomicrons and very low density lipoproteins from lymph.
The various labelled lipoprotein fractions or total serum or
lymph respectively were injected via tail-vein into female
albino rats which, one hour later, received either β-pyridyl-
carbinol (1 mmole/kg rat weight) or placebo by stomach intuba-
tion. The expired ^{14}CO$_2$ was taken as an indicator of cholesterol
oxidation.

The initial oxidation rate of the various lipoproteins
differed and was proportional to the ratio of free to

esterified cholesterol. β-pyridylcarbinol increased by a constant factor (nearly 2) the oxidation rates of cholesterol from all lipoprotein fractions tested. The drug-induced enhancement of cholesterol oxidation was dose-dependent between 0.1 and 4.6 mmoles/kg. The absolute increment of cholesterol oxidation was similar in rats starved for 24 hours and in animals without prestarvation, but percentagewise the enhancement was greater in starved rats (because of their lower basal oxidation rate). Simultaneous measurements of plasma cholesterol showed that the enhancement of cholesterol oxidation fairly paralleled the plasma cholesterol depression.

It is proposed that enhancement of cholesterol oxidation is a prerequisite for plasma cholesterol depression by β-pyridylcarbinol.

* in: "Metabolic Effects of Nicotinic Acid and Its Derivatives", Gey & Carlson, Eds.; Huber Publ., Bern 1971.

STRUCTURE AND FUNCTION OF LIVER MICROSOMES DURING ACTIVATION OF

THE LIPID PEROXIDATION SYSTEM AND ITS POSSIBLE ASSOCIATION WITH

CCl_4-HEPATOTOXICITY

V.V. LYACHOVICH, I.B. TSYRLOV, V.M. MISHIN and O.A. GROMOVA

Central Research Laboratory, Institute of Medicine, Krasny Prospect 52, Novosibirsk 91, U.S.S.R.

It is currently assumed that vector CCl_4-hepatotoxicity is the activation of the microsomal system of lipid peroxidation. In this connection we have investigated the structure and spectral characteristics of microsome electron carriers and the activity of enzyme systems accompanying microsome membrane alteration during $NADPH_2$- or ascorbate-induced peroxidation of lipids. A drop has been revealed in microsomal suspension absorption as well as a marked decrease in the binding of 8-anilino-1-naphthalene sulfonate to the microsome due to the destructive alteration in the phospholipid component of the membrane. A sharp decrease in b_5 and p-450 cytochrome content as well as the appearance of the absorption peak with a maximum at 420 nm has been observed. The functional abilities of the microsome enzyme systems containing cytochrome p-450, which are extremely sensitive to damage of membrane structures were found to be considerably lowered. Phenergan and EDTA, offering protective action during CCl_4-intoxication, prevented the above-mentioned changes in structure and function of liver microsomes in vitro.

Thus, activation of the lipid peroxidation reaction results in pronounced membrane structural disorganization accompanied by damage of its inherent hemoproteins and a drop in hydroxylation and detoxication activity. In the light of modern conceptions of the pathogenic role of microsomal disturbances due to CCl_4-intoxication, the presented approach may be applied in studying the problem of CCl_4-hepatotoxicity

and in the search of substances preventing necrosis and fat
degeneration of the liver.

EFFECTS OF D-TRIIODOTHYRONINE ON SERUM CHOLESTEROL AND TRIGLYCERIDES

IN HYPERCHOLESTEROLEMIA AND HYPERTRIGLYCERIDEMIA

HANS J. MEYER

First Department of Medicine, St. George's Hospital, Hamburg,
Germany

     The effects and side effects of the dextrorotatory
thyroid hormone D-triiodothyronine on euthyroid patients with
hypercholesterolemia and hypertriglyceridemia were tested.
The investigations were carried out in the form of double
placebo tests and long-term observation. (Double blind study
20 patients, long-term study 30 patients). With a daily dosage
of 1.5 mg D-triiodothyronine (3 x 1 tbl.) the patients showed
a therapeutically satisfactory reduction of the increased fat
fractions. The reduction was the clearer, the higher the
initial values had been. In the placebo phase the values rose
distinctly, often exceeding the initial values. In contrast
to L-triiodothyronine, with the application of D-triiodothyronine
there is an increase in the protein bound iodine (PBI) without
there being any clinical signs of hyperthyroidism. The T_3 and
T_4 tests showed also standard values. There were no certain
signs of a liver damage. Subjective side effects, in particular
tachycardia and agina pectoris, were not observed. This fact
is of special importance, as in most cases patients are
concerned who before have had a myocardial infarction. The
DT_3-preparation used has shown a good lipid-lowering effect,
and has distinguished itself by a very good tolerability.

THE EFFECT OF TAURINE ON BILIARY AND FECAL EXCRETION OF BILE ACIDS

DURING CHOLESTYRAMINE THERAPY.

DR. M.A. MISHKEL

McMaster Medical Unit, Hamilton General Hospital, Hamilton,
Ontario, Canada

     The concept that taurine feeding might increase the
ability of cholestyramine to bind bile acids is based on (1)
the low efficiency of the resin to bind bile acids; (2) the
greater affinity of the resin for taurine (T) than glycine (G)
conjugates of cholic acid and (3) the increase of taurine
conjugates in bile when taurine is fed to man. The practical
importance of this concept is that taurine supplementation
might increase the fecal excretion of bile acids during resin
therapy, resulting in a greater hypocholesterolemic effect.

     Four healthy normocholesterolemic males were given
cholestyramine 12g./day during 2 three-week periods and in
addition were given either active or placebo taurine 3g./day in

a cross-over "double blind" study. Cholestyramine led to the expected lowering of plasma cholesterol, an increased fecal excretion of bile acids and a marked increase of the G/T ratio of biliary aspirate. Added taurine caused the biliary G/T ratio to revert to normal, but did not increase the fecal excretion of bile acids, nor increase the hypocholesterolemic effect.

It is concluded that the addition of taurine 3g./day does not increase the fecal excretion of bile acids in normo-cholesterolemic subjects fed cholestyramine 12g./day.

EFFECTS OF SOME ACID MUCOPOLYSACCHARIDES UPON LIPID METABOLISM

IN EXPERIMENTAL ATHEROSCLEROSIS

L.M. MORRISON, M.D.: O.A. SCHJEIDE, Ph.D.: G.S. BAJWA, D.V.M., Ph.D. and B.H. ERSHOFF, Ph.D.

Institute for Arteriosclerosis Research, 9331 Venice Boulevard Culver City, California 90230

Some biologic mechanisms of action of chondroitin sulfate A (CSA), chondroitin sulfate C(CSC) and other acid mucopoly-saccharides were studied to explain the following phenomena. CSA was found to prevent experimental atherosclerosis and coronary athero and arteriosclerotic heart disease in monkeys, rats and rabbits and to strikingly reduce the incidence of acute coronary episodes in human patients with proven coronary heart disease. CSA was found to; 1) "clear" lipids and cholesterol out of human, fowl and mammalian cells in tissue and organ cultures; 2) "clear" and reduce C_{14} labelled cholesterol out of human aortas in perfusion systems; 3) prevent degeneration and aging of mitochondria and ribosomes of pathological and aging cells; 4) enhance the metabolism of cellular and tissue lipids and lipoproteins by radioactive isotope labelling; 5) prevent x-irradiation - cholesterol induced coronary and aortic athero-arteriosclerosis in rat models; 6) prevent hypervitaminosis D - cholesterol, atherogenic diet induced coronary and aortic athero-arterio-sclerosis in rat models; 7) prevent naturally occurring atherosclerosis in squirrel monkeys; 8) reduce serum lipids of monkeys with dietetically accelerated atherosclerosis; 9) induce regression of naturally occurring coronary athero and arteriosclerosis in squirrel monkeys.

CHOLESTYRAMINE AND THE EXCRETION OF FAECAL BILE ACIDS IN

HYPERBETALIPOPROTEINAEMIA IN THE HOMOZYGOUS AND HETEROZYGOUS FORMS

C.D. MOUTAFIS and N.B. MYANT

MRC Lipid Metabolism Unit, Hammersmith Hospital, Ducane Road, London W.12, England

Cholestyramine increases the output of faecal bile acids and the synthesis of cholesterol. It has been reported that in patients with hyperbetalipoproteinaemia, treatment with cholestyramine does not increase the output of bile acids to the same extent as in normal subjects, and it has been suggested that this defect is a cause of hypercholesterolaemia. We have studied the effect of cholestyramine (20 and 30 g/day) on bile acid excretion in three patients with homozygous familial hyperbetalipoproteinaemia and in three patients with the heterozygous form of the disease. Bile acid excretion, when expressed in terms of body weight, was the same in the two groups when no cholestyramine was given, but in the presence of cholestyramine it was higher in the homozygotes than in the heterozygotes. There was no change in appearance of the xanthomata or in plasma cholesterol level in the homozygous patients, but the plasma cholesterol level fell in two of the heterozygotes. Our findings suggest that homozygotes can increase bile acid output and cholesterol synthesis to a greater extent than heterozygotes on the same dose of cholestyramine, and are against the hypothesis that hyperbeta-lipoproteinaemia is due to a defect in the capacity to form bile acids.

EFFECT OF UBIQUINONE-9 ON THE EXPERIMENTAL ATHEROSCLEROSIS

H. NAKAMURA, Y. NAKAMURA, E. ASANO, Y. GOTO

School of Medicine, Keio University, 35 Shinanomachi, Shinjuku-ku, Tokyo, Japan

Cholesterol and ubiquinone are known to be biosynthesized via isopentenyl pyrophosphate. Possibility is also presented on the regulation of hepatic cholesterogenesis by ubiquinone.

The present study was conducted to assess the effect of ubiquinone-9 on the lipids of plasma and arterial wall in 1% cholesterol-fed rabbits.

Male rabbits were fed 1% cholesterol in lab chow for 3 months with or without 30 mg of ubiquinone-9 orally. Blood lipids were determined through the experimental course of feeding in both groups. Liver and arterial wall lipids were also analyzed. Incorporation of Cl4-acetate into cholesterol and the esterification of Cl4-cholesterol were also measured in liver and arterial wall.

Blood cholesterol increased after the start of feeding. The difference was not significant in both groups. Plasma triglyceride and free fatty acids also increased to the lesser degree. Lipoprotein electrophoresis on cellulose acetate revealed marked increase in beta-lipoprotein in 4 weeks. Prebeta-lipoprotein increased gradually in 6 weeks without showing sharp separation from beta-lipoprotein, namely manifesting "Broad beta type." Alpha-lipoprotein was diminished in both groups. However, it was maintained fairly rich in ubiquinone administered group.

CLINICAL EXPERIENCES WITH DH- 581 (BIPHENABID) IN THE TREATMENT

OF HYPERCHOLESTEREMIA

DAVID T. NASH, M.D.

600 E. Genesee Street, Syracuse, New York 13202

A group of 33 patients with hypercholesteremia was treated for a period of one to nine months, with an average of five and a half (5½) months, for a total of 170 patient-months. One patient had a cholesterol decrease of 33%, eight patients had a drop of 20-29%, averaging 22%, and thirteen patients had an average drop of 15%. Eight patients had less than 9% reduction, averaging 6%. There were three patients who demonstrated an elevation of cholesterol; one with 12%, and two patients averaging 5%.

There were drops of 20% in Type II hyperlipidemia, 17% in Types III and IV, and approximately 11% for the large group who could not be typed.

The average decline for all 33 patients was 12%, among the 30 patients who showed a decrease, the average was 14%.

Triglyceride values did not change significantly in any predictable way. No definite pattern of response could be ascertained in relation to lipid type.

It has not been possible to determine who will respond to DH581 prior to a therapeutic trial with the agent.

The mechanism of action of DH581 is yet to be elucidated.

EFFECTS OF CHOLESTYRAMINE ON CHOLESTEROL METABOLISM IN MAN

D.J. NAZIR, L. HORLICK, and H.S. SODHI

Department of Medicine, University of Saskatchewan, Saskatoon, Canada

In four hypercholesterolemic subjects investigated by the sterol balance techniques, cholestyramine decreased plasma cholesterol concentrations by 24 to 28% within 7 days. It was associated with a 2.4- to 6.8-fold increase in the fecal excretion of bile acids and only insignificant increases in the excretion of neutral steroids. The fecal excretions of endogenous cholesterol and its metabolites exceeded losses from the plasma cholesterol pool by 350 to 450 mg/day. A marked increase in the slope of plasma cholesterol specific activity time curves after the start of treatment suggested that the extra fecal steroids might have been derived from the increase in synthesis of endogenous cholesterol. However, it is also possible for some of the extra fecal steroids to have come from the mobilization of tissue cholesterol in response to the fall in plasma cholesterol as previously suggested by us.

Cholestyramine did not cause any change in the absorption of dietary cholesterol.

EFFECTS OF ORAL CALCIUM UPON SERUM CHOLESTEROL AND TRIGLYCERIDES

IN PATIENTS WITH HYPERLIPIDEMIA

A.G. OLSSON, L.A. CARLSON, S. FROBERG, L. ORO and S. ROSSNER

Department of Geriatrics, University of Uppsala, Uppsala, Department of Internal Medicine, Karolinska Hospital and King Gustaf V Research Institute, Stockholm, Sweden

The effect of peroral administration of 2 g calcium daily during 8 weeks on serum lipids was studied in 16 hyperlipidemic patients. The study was preceded by a 4 week placebo period. Five patients were classified as having type II A hyperlipidemia according to Fredrickson et al. as modified, 10 patients as having type IIB and 1 patient as having type IV. Body weight before the study and mean values during placebo and calcium therapy were $70.2^{\pm}2.49$ kg, $70.0^{\pm}2.54$ kg and $69.4^{\pm}2.55$ kg respectively. The difference between placebo mean value and calcium mean values was significant on the 5 percent level.

The average serum triglyceride value before treatment was $2.89^{\pm}0.383$ mmol/l, during treatment with placebo $2.45^{\pm}0.266$ mmol/l and during calcium treatment $2.70^{\pm}0.286$ mmol/l. The decrease during placebo therapy when compared to mean value before treatment was significant on the 5 percent level. No decrease in serum triglycerides could be ascribed to calcium therapy. The average serum cholesterol value before treatment was $337^{\pm}13.5$ mg per 100 ml and decreased to $321^{\pm}12.8$ mg per 100 ml during placebo treatment and to $303^{\pm}12.0$ mg per 100 ml during treatment with calcium. The decrease was significant on the 1 percent level when mean value before treatment was compared to average value during placebo therapy and significant on the 0.1 percent level when the mean value during placebo treatment was compared to mean value during calcium treatment. No correlation was noted between either total or low density lipoprotein cholesterol levels before treatment and decrease in total cholesterol levels.

DEVELOPMENTS IN STATIONARY PHASES FOR GLC ANALYSIS OF LIPIDS

D.M. OTTENSTEIN, W.R. SUPINA, D.A. BARTLEY and NICHOLAS PELICK

SUPELCO, INC., Supelco Park, Bellefonte, Pennsylvania 16823

Recent developments in stationary phases is the theme of this presentation. Gas chromatograms will be shown to illustrate their uses for lipids and long and short chain fatty acids. Some of the new phases will be characterized with respect to polarity and type and compared to ones which are currently being used. The new McReynolds constants will be discussed in the classification of the phases.

DEXTRO-THYROXINE IN TREATMENT OF LIPID DISORDERS

WILLIAM R. OWEN, M.D.

6410 Fannin, Suite 643, Houston, Texas   77025

A. Objective evidence of effect on atheromata by DT4: Over
    100 patients were studied during the past 12 years. They
    show reduced skin and tendon xanthomata, clearing of
    peripheral arterial obstruction, and reversion of exercise
    electrocardiographic abnormalities to normal as evidence
    of regression of atheromatous deposits due to dextro-
    thyroxine effect.

B. Relationship of DT4 to thyroid metabolism: A study of
    50 patients utilized T3, T4, and Free thyroxine techniques
    to detect any tendency to hypermetabolism on DT4. The
    effect on normal thyroid gland function and its recovery
    potential on omission of therapy was also studied. In
    the euthyroid patient any calorigenic effect from dextro-
    thyroxine is promptly balanced by the body's metabolic
    adjustments, and no hyperthyroid state develops. No
    depression of thyroid function occurred on omission of
    DT4 treatment despite such adjustments.

C. Patients with angina pectoris, prior myocardial infarction,
    and arrhythmia were selected especially for this group
    of 100 patients. These fragile conditions proved
    remarkably tolerant to doses up to 8 mg. daily of DT4.
    This seemed to confirm a lack of hypermetabolism from a
    dose of dextro-thyroxine sufficient to improve lipid
    abnormalities.

ACTION OF BASIC ALUMINUM CLOFIBRATE* ON HYPERLIPEMIC PATIENTS'

HEMOSTASIS

PANAK E., DAVER J., PODESTA M., EDMOND E.

Centre d'Etudes Pour l'Industrie Pharmaceutique, 195 Route
d'Espagne, 31 Toulouse (France)

During a pilot epidemiological study on atherosclerosis,
hemostasis was studied on 258 atherosclerotic patients, using:

- 4 coagulation tests (thromboplastin generation time
test, QUICK's time, thrombin time and fibrinemia).

- and 4 fibrinolysis tests (fibrin clot lysis time,
fibrin plates, JOHNSON's euglobulin lysis and FEARNLEY's diluted
clot lysis time).

Results show there is no correlation between the different
fibrinolysis tests, except for FEARNLEY's test.

In a second stage, the same investigations on coagulation
and fibrinolysis were carried out on 30 cases of hyperlipidemia,

treated during three months, in a double-blind trial, by basic
Aluminium clofibrate.

In addition to the action on serum lipids, results show:

- thromplastin generation time is decreased, as expected,
for this test is considered as an expression of platelet
activity. Furthermore, these results confirm our preliminary
in vitro study, showing a decrease in platelet aggregation
under basic Aluminium clofibrate*.

- Variations in prothrombin time are more pronounced than
normal, including increases as well as decreases. The classical
concept of diminishing the anti-vitamins K in every clofibrate
treatment has thus not been confirmed.

- Of the tests generally considered as expressing the
fibrinolytic activity, only FEARNLEY's test results are
significantly modified by Clofibrate treatment.

They are also the only ones modified in atherosclerosis.

* ATHEROLIP

THE EFFECT OF ETHANOL ON SERUM LIPIDS IN PATIENTS WITH PRIMARY

AND SECONDARY HYPERLIPOPROTEINEMIAS

J. PAPENBERG und G. SCHLIERF

Medizinische Universitats-Klinik, Bergheimer Strasse 58,
(69) Heidelberg, Germany

A standardized oral and intravenous ethanol load is
described in humans. The following parameters are measured in
serum: triglycerides, cholesterol, free fatty acids (FFA),
lactate and pyruvate. Results are:

1. Cholesterol concentrations in serum are not influenced by
ethanol.

2. Ethanol effects an elevation of the serum triglycerides up
to Delta c = 60 mg/100 ml in control persons, alcoholics and
patients with primary hyperlipoproteinemias of the types II,
III and V.

3. On the other hand patients with Type IV hyperlipoproteinemia
(if the serum triglycerides are not higher than 500 mg/100 ml)
and in patients with secondary ethanol inducible hyperlipoproteinemia show an abnormally high elevation of serum triglycerides
(delta c = 111 - 246 mg/100 ml) after ethanol.

4. In opposition to these results in patients with hyperlipoproteinemia Type IV with triglyceride concentrations as high
as 1000 mg/100 ml serum the serum triglycerides decrease after
ethanol.

5. Because of the release of catecholamines after ethanol, FFA
are elevated in serum in control persons and patients with

primary hyperlipoproteinemias of the types II and IV.   In
patients with type III hyperlipoproteinemias and in patients
with chronic alcoholism ethanol effects a decrease of serum FFA.

6. The different effects of ethanol on lipid metabolism
are discussed and related to the biochemical effects of ethanol
on the oxidation reduction status of the liver cell and on
the Microsomal Ethanol Oxidizing System.

Thus ethanol is a very potent drug in elevating serum
triglycerides and FFA and consequently lipids in the liver cell.

THE EFFECT OF ESSENTIAL PHOSPHOLIPIDS ON THE LIPID AND FATTY ACID

PATTERN OF LIPOPROTEINS IN TYPE II PATIENTS

H. PEETERS, V. BLATON, B. DECLERCQ, and D. VANDAMME

Simon Stevin Instituut voor Wetenschappelijk Onderzoek
Jerusalemstraat, 34, B-8000 BRUGGE   Belgium

Phosphatidyl choline rich in poly-unsaturated fatty acids
plays a multi anti-atherogenic role by lowering plasma cholesterol,
by increasing the stability of the lipoprotein molecule by
insuring adequate proportion of hydrophilic compounds, by
mobilising cholesterol from arteries and by preventing the
sclerogenic action of this sterol on connective tissues.   The
present investigation concerns the effect of intravenous
administration of poly-unsaturated phosphatidyl choline
(lipostabil - Nattermann) on the lipid and fatty acid distribution in plasma lipoproteins of type II patients.

From 300 male and female patients 35 type II were selected
on their lipid and lipoprotein profiles.   The patients received
intravenously a daily injection of 20 ml 5% aqueous solution
of EPL during 14 days.

Plasma lipids and the lipoprotein profiles are determined.
The ratio of PC/CE was followed and fatty acids of serum,
cholesterol esters and phosphatidyl choline are analysed,
according to an integrated way of procedure.

Total lipids and total cholesterol are decreased
respectively with an average of 70 mg% and 50 mg%.   Oleic acid
is decreased as well in total amount as in percentage (2 - 3%)
in cholesterol esters and phosphatidyl choline, while linoleic
acid shows a percentual increase ($\pm$4%) in both lipids.   The
lipoprotein profiles however are rather unchanged.

STUDIES OF THE MECHANISM OF ACTION OF CLOFIBRATE AND OTHER

RELATED HYPOCHOLESTEREMIC AGENTS

JOSEPH N. PEREIRA, GERALD A. MEARS, GERALD F. HOLLAND

Medical Research Laboratories, Pfizer Inc., Groton, Connecituct

Previous studies have demonstrated that single doses of clofibrate depress rat plasma lipid levels, increase the activity of hepatic mitochondrial α-glycerophosphate dehydrogenase (MGPD), reduce hepatic levels of α-glycerophosphate and reduce the ability of the perfused liver to synthesize and secrete triglycerides. The present study examines the means by which clofibrate stimulates the activity of MGPD. Increased synthesis of mitochondrial proteins is observed two hours after the administration of hypolipemic doses of clofibrate. Similar dose-related effects on protein synthesis are seen with the related hypolipemic agents, SaH-2348 and SU-13,437. A time course of the stimulation of protein synthesis reveals a peak at 12-15 hours and a return to baseline levels after 48 hours. Studies with the antibiotics, cycloheximide and chloramphenicol, indicate that increased synthesis of mitochondrial proteins occurs on the cytoplasmic ribosomal system. Sucrose density gradient studies demonstrate that increased synthesis of RNA precedes the induction of protein synthesis; 2-3 fold increases in RNA synthesis were observed one hour following administration of clofibrate. These findings indicate that the hypolipemic effects of clofibrate may be due to its primary effects on the synthesis of RNA and mitochondrial proteins, one of which is MGPD.

LONG TERM DH-581 IN HYPERCHOLESTEROLEMIA

POLACHEK, A.A., KATZ, H.M., and LITTMAN, M.

Veterans Administration Hospital, 800 Poly Place, Brooklyn, New York 11209

Hypercholesterolemia is frequently associated with atherosclerosis and treatment at present includes the reduction of serum cholesterol by the use of drugs. DH-581 (Probucol) is an experimental drug whose mechanism of action has not been established but it probably inhibits one of the early reactions in the biosynthesis of cholesterol. The purpose of the study was to assess: (1) the ability of DH-581 in a dose of 500 mg b.i.d. to maintain lowered serum cholesterol levels up to one year, and (2) the safety and tolerance of long term administration. Sixty-four patients were started on the study including 48 on the drug and 16 on placebo. By the end of 3 months, 8 had stopped (2 because of uncontrolled diabetes, 2 for possible toxicity, and 4 for various other reasons). Of the 56 patients who completed 3 months of treatment, 41 patients on the drug had a mean decrease in serum cholesterol of 16.4% compared to 15 patients on placebo with a mean drop of 3.2%. Ten of the patients on placebo for 3 months were started on the drug, and after 3 more months had a further decrease of 16.2% vs. their previous drop of 1.8% on placebo. Forty-five patients continued the drug with a further sustained decrease in serum cholesterol. Except for one patient with a vasomotor reaction there was no evidence of significant toxicity. One patient with xanthelasma had complete disappearance of the lesions in 9 months.

COMPOUNDS WHICH INHIBIT OR STIMULATE BRAIN CEREBROSIDE HYDROLYSIS

N.S. RADIN and R.C. ARORA

Mental Health Research Institute, University of Michigan,
Ann Arbor, Michigan 48104

Galactosyl ceramide β-galactosidase (GCG) hydrolyzes
galactocerebroside and is thus probably involved in the
metabolism of myelin. Synthetic compounds related to the
substrate and its products (ceramide and galactose) were tested
as inhibitors with partially purified GCG of rat brain. N-Acyl
amides of 3-phenyl-2-amino-1,3-propanediol acted as noncompetitive
inhibitors, apparently on a site (Site 2) other than the
substrate-active site (Site 1). The DL-erythro form of the
amine was more active than the D- or L-threo forms. (The
natural substrate has the D-erythro configuration and contains
both D-α-hydroxy and nonhydroxy fatty acids.) The optimal
chain length of the acyl group was about 10 carbon atoms and
an OH group in the α-position enhanced the inhibition. At a
concentration of 0.3 mM, the C_{10} amide inhibited 48%; the DL-
hydroxy derivative inhibited 68%. Substituents on the benzene
ring and removal of one of the OH groups on the amine reduced
the effectiveness. Galactonolactone acted as a competitive
inhibitor (63% at 0.5 mM, using 0.14 mM substrate), presumably
acting on Site 1. Cerebrosides containing short chain acids
also inhibited: N-acetyl galactosyl sphingosine at 0.3 mM
inhibited 57%. The inhibition was of the "mixed type" nature;
presumably the compound acts on Sites 1 and 2. 2-Methyl-2-
aminopropanol amides proved to stimulate GCG, rather than
inhibit. The C_{10} amide stimulated 62%.

STUDIES ON REGRESSION OF ATHEROMA.   RELEASE OF INTRACELLULAR

ARTERIAL LIPIDS

A. LAZZARINI ROBERTSON, JR., M.D., Ph.D.

Research Division, Cleveland Clinic, 2020 East 93rd Street,
Cleveland, Ohio 44106

The therapeutic use of hypocholesterolemic agents in the
treatment of clinical atherosclerosis is based on the assumption
that significant reductions of plasma cholesterol levels may
facilitate the release of arterial cell lipids and induce
regression.

The current studies followed observations in which
chlorophenoxyisobutyrate inhibited incorporation of labeled
serum cholesterol by human cell cultures but had no significant
effects on the excretion of intracellular sterols. Using time-
lapse cinematography combined with electron microscopy-cyto-
chemistry it was found that arterial intimal cells are only
able, in the early stages of lipid storage, to release intracellular sterols following incubation in normocholesterolemic
pooled sera.

Lipid laden "foam" cells, in contrast, do not release
membrane-bound intracellular lipids including cholesterol

esters. Irreversible cell changes usually ensue with eventual cell death and lysis followed by recycling of these sterols by surrounding cells.

These findings suggest that early use of pharmacological or dietary hypocholesterolemic measures may be indespensable in order to effectively induce regression of fatty lesions at arterial cell level.

THE EFFECT OF PYRIDONOLCARBAMATE (ANGININ) ON ARTERIAL WALL

METABOLISM

R. SANWALD AND H. WAGENER

Medizinische Universitatsklinik (Ludolf-Krehl), Heidelberg Bergheimerstr. 58 (Direktor: Professor Dr. G. Schettler),Germany

Pyridinolcarbamate was claimed to prevent atherosclerotic lesions. It was the purpose of the present investigation to study the effect of Anginin on in vitro metabolism of arterial wall of cholesterol fed rabbits.

The parameters studied were: weight gain, serum cholesterol, phospholipids, and triglycerides, acid mucopolysaccharide-content of aortae and specific radio sulfate incorporation rates, as well as phospholipid-content and incorporation of ^{32}P into sphingomyelin, lecithin, inositol, phosphatidylserine, phosphatidylethanolamine, and cholesterol-content of aortic tissue.

Weight gain was slightly less in the Anginin-group. Serum cholesterol, triglycerides, and phospholipids increased continuously during the experiment. After 9 weeks triglycerides were lower in the Anginin-group, whereas there was no difference in cholesterol and phospholipid levels. Both aMPS-content and its various fractions - separated by cellulose acetate electrophoresis - were unchanged. $^{35}SO_4^{--}$ incorporation into various aMPS fractions was identical in both groups. The same holds for phospholipid content and ^{32}P incorporation into the phospholipid fractions separated by thin layer chromatography. There was a suggestive decrease of cholesterol content.

These studies do not show an effect of Anginin on arterial wall metabolism. If the favourable clinical reports can be confirmed by other authors, the effect of Anginin is probably due to changes other that local changes of arterial wall metabolism.

BINDING OF LIPID COMPONENTS OF LIPOPROTEIN BY PARTIALLY PURIFIED

STEROL CARRIER PROTEIN. A HYPOTHESIS CONCERNING LIPOPROTEIN ASSEMBLY

TERENCE J. SCALLEN, H.B. SKRDLANT, and M.V. SRIKANTAIAH

Department of Biochemistry, School of Medicine, The University of New Mexico, Albuquerque, New Mexico 87106

We have previously presented evidence that a noncatalytic carrier protein (Sterol Carrier Protein or SCP)' is involved in the conversion of squalene to cholesterol by an acetone powder of rat liver microsomes (J. Biol. Chem., 246, 224, 1971). In the present report we have tested the binding of several compounds by partially purified SCP. The results show that SCP has a high affinity for cholesterol (74% bound) and its water insoluble precursors (59-78% bound), but little affinity for such steroids as testosterone or estradiol (0.9-0.3% bound). In addition, partially purified SCP shows significant binding of triglyceride (triolein, 78%), phospholipid (phosphatidyl choline, 84%), and cholesterol ester (cholesteryl oleate, 69%), all of which are known lipid components of lipoprotein. No binding by SCP could be demonstrated for glucose, glycerol, or glycerol phosphate. These observations have led us to propose the hypothesis that SCP is a protein precursor of lipoprotein, and that a sequential enzymatic assembly of the lipid components of lipoproteins may occur with biosynthetic lipid intermediates and products bound to SCP. It seems logical that the binding of drugs by SCP may be a useful in vitro technique for identifying compounds with potential effects upon lipoprotein formation.

ALCOHOLIC HYPERLIPEMIA

ROBERT SCHEIG

Department of Medicine, Yale University School of Medicine, 333 Cedar Street, New Haven, Connecticut 06510

Following a single large dose of ethanol (7.5 gm/kg body weight), non-fasted male rats consistently developed lipemic sera within 1 hour which reached its peak at 2 and fell to normal at 4 hours. Hepatic triglyceride content also increased. No defect in post-heparin lipolytic activity was demonstrable nor was there any increase in lipoprotein synthesis by liver or free fatty acid release from adipose tissue. However, by adding tracer amounts of ethanol-1-^{14}C to the ethanol feeding, 35% of the increase in plasma and liver triglycerides could be accounted for by lipid synthesis from ethanol. When liver slices were incubated with either 10mM ethanol-1-^{14}C, 4 mM glucose-1-^{14}, or 5 mM glucose-6-^{14}C, 8 times more ethanol than glucose was converted to lipid. About half the lipids formed from ethanol were triglycerides, 27% phospholipids and the rest diglycerides. Between 65-80 of the label were in the fatty acid moieties of the complex lipids of which 17% were palmitate, 5% stearate, 6% palmitoleate, 18% 8-14 carbon chain fatty acids and the rest 20-22 carbon unsaturated fatty acid. It was also shown that hepatic triglyceride synthesis from ^{14}C-palmitate was enhanced by ethanol in vivo. In summary, alcoholic hyperlipemia in rats may be due in part to hepatic lipid synthesis from ethanol.

MODIFICATION OF "CARBOHYDRATE-INDUCED" TRIGLYCERIDEMIA BY NOCTURNAL SUPPRESSION OF LIPOLYSIS - COMPARISON OF NICOTINIC ACID AND GLUCOSE

GUENTER SCHLIERF and ECKEHARD DOROW

Medizinische Universitatsklinik, Bergheimer Strasse 58, D 69 Heidelberg, West Germany

Previous studies (Schlierf and Stossberg 1969) have shown that carbohydrate induction of triglyceridemia in normal subjects occurs at night and appears to be related to a rebound rise of free fatty acids following diurnal feeding of a high-carbohydrate formula diet. The present investigation was undertaken to observe the effect on 24-hour triglyceride and free fatty acid profiles of inhibition of nocturnal lipolysis by nicotinic acid or glucose.

In 10 normal subjects, plasma triglyceride and free fatty acid levels were followed hourly for 24 hours while an isocaloric 80% carbohydrate, fat-free formula diet was given in 6 equal portions during the day (control experiment). This procedure was repeated in the same subjects, 5 of whom received additional feedings of glucose between 20^{00} and 6^{00} hours while the other 5 persons were given nicotinic acid by intravenous infusion during the same time interval. Both procedures resulted in maintained lowering of free fatty acid levels over 24 hours. Mitigation of carbohydrate-induced triglyceridemia was observed with the additional glucose. Nicotinic acid almost completely abolished the nocturnal rise of plasma triglyceride levels which in the control studies resulted in approximate doubling of triglyceride levels in 24 hours.

The significance of these finding with regard to management of endogenous hypertriglyceridemia is discussed.

COMPETITIVE EFFECT OF FATTY-ACID SOAPS ON THE SEQUESTERING OF

BILE SALTS BY CHOLESTYRAMINE

D.L. SCHNEIDER and L.M. HAGERMAN

Mead Johnson Research Center, Evansville, Indiana 47721

In vivo bile salt binding by cholestyramine is considerably less than that predicted on the basis of theoretical anion-exchange capacity of the resin. Factors which may influence binding of bile salts to the resin are concentration and type of bile salt in the intestine, active transport of bile salts in the ileum, and competition from other anions, particularly fatty-acid soaps (FAS). The competitive effect of FAS on bile salt binding was evaluated in vitro. Graded levels (0-40 mM) of FAS ($C_{8:0}$, $C_{9:0}$, $C_{10:0}$, $C_{11:0}$, $C_{12:0}$, $C_{18:1}$, and $C_{18:2}$) were dissolved in bile salt solutions (20mM) and the soap-bile salt mixture equilibrated with cholestyramine in saline at $37^{o}C$. With equimolar amounts of long-chain FAS ($\geq C_{12:0}$) and bile salts, bile salt binding was decreased by about 50%. FAS < $C_{12:0}$ were less effective and $C_{8:0}$ had virtually no effect. With or without FAS, cholestyramine preferentially bound dihydroxy bile salts over trihydroxy salts, and taurine-conjugated bile salts over the glycine conjugates. In other studies, bile salt previously bound to cholestyramine was readily displaced by subsequent addition of long-chain FAS to the medium.

EFFECT OF CLOFIBRATE IN HYPERLIPEMIC RATS

P. SEGAL, P.S. ROHEIM, and H.A. EDER

Albert Einstein College of Medicine, 1300 Morris Park Avenue,
Bronx, New York 10461

Feeding of a diet containing 60% sucrose caused an
increase in plasma triglyceride concentration and very low
density lipoproteins (VLDL). When clofibrate was administered
(0.25% w/w) in this diet for 2 to 4 days, VLDL levels in the
plasma did not change but there was an increase in the
incorporation of ^{14}C-leucine into the protein portion of VLDL.
The level of HDL and its rate of synthesis were decreased within
12 hours of administration of clofibrate. The increased
synthesis of VLDL, in the face of unchanged plasma levels,
suggested that there must be increased rate of removal of VLDL.
To assess the effect of clofibrate on turnover of VLDL, we
employed the double lable of Schimke et al. (J. Biol. Chem.
<u>244</u>: 3303, 1969) and found an increased turnover of VLDL. These
data suggest that the lowering of levels of VLDL is due to
increased rate of removal rather than to decreased synthesis
as occurs with HDL.

ALTERATIONS OF HIGH- AND VERY-LOW-DENSITY-LIPOPROTEINS IN

PATIENTS WITH LIVER DISEASE

D. SEIDEL, H. GRETEN, H. WENGELER, and H. WIELAND

Medical Clinic, University of Heidelberg, Bergheimer Strasse 58,
69 Heidelberg, Germany

It has previously been demonstrated that various liver
disorders are associated with decreased concentrations of serum
high density lipoproteins (HDL) and pre-beta-lipoproteins. Our
studies are designated to evaluate the possible mechanisms
responsible for these altered lipoprotein patterns. Evidence
will be presented that the decreased concentration of HDL is
primarily due to an impaired lipid binding capacity of apo-A,
the major protein moiety of HDL, resulting in an abnormally
high protein/lipid ratio and a lack of neutral lipids in the
HDL fraction. In contrast to normal alpha-lipoproteins, this
fraction does not stain for lipids, but shows two distinct
precipiting bands on immuno-electrophoresis and on Ouchterlony
plates. The isolated very-low-density-lipoprotein fraction
(VLDL) from patients with liver disorders revealed a protein/
lipid composition close to normal, but developed beta-mobility
on electrophoresis. Analyses of the protein moieties of this
fraction indicated a lack of apo-A, which is a compound of
normal VLDL. The data suggest that disturbed liver function
leads to the synthesis of an altered apo-A resulting (1) in a
LP-A dissociated into its two polypeptides and (2) in a VLDL
lacking apo-A. Both findings may be explained by the impaired
capacity of this apo-A to bind neutral lipids.

ISOLATION AND CHARACTERIZATION OF AN ABNORMAL PLASMA LIPOPROTEIN,

CHARACTERIZING HYPERTHYROIDISM

D. SEIDEL and H. WIELAND

Medical Clinic, University of Heidelberg, Bergheimer Strasse 58,
6900 Heidelberg, Germany

It is generally true that serum lipoproteins exhibiting
α-mobility sediment at a density 1.063 g/ml, whereas those with
β-mobility float at this density. Evidence will be presented
that in case of hyperthyroidism (25 patients) the d 1.063
bottom fraction contains not only α-lipoproteins, but also
β-lipoproteins in high concentration. This abnormal lipoprotein
(designated β-HDL) was isolated by ultracentrifugation and
polyanion precipitation. The protein-lipid-composition of
β-HDL is distinguished by a high content of protein and low
content of cholesterol, compared to normal β-lipoproteins and
the particles are smaller in size (E.M., P.A.A.). The VLDL,
LDL, and α-HDL fraction of the same patients revealed a protein-
lipid-composition close to normal and showed normal electrophoretic mobility. Immunochemical studies indicated identity
between normal β-lipoproteins and β-HDL and excluded similarity
between β-HDL and the Berg's Lp(a) lipoprotein. However, the
anti-serum prepared against β-HDL developed two strong
precipiting lines with whole plasma from normals or from
patients with hyperthyroidism. One line identical to the
β-lipoproteins stained for lipids and a second, non-identical
line with a mobility less than that of β-lipoproteins, which did
not stain for lipids. This second protein compound has not yet
been identified, apparently it does not belong to the albumin
or immuno-globulin fraction. The amino acid composition of the
second protein compound is significantly different to the known
apolipoproteins, and we found aspartic-acid to be its N-terminal
amino acid. In vitro lipid combining studies suggest that the
abnormal protein-lipid-composition of β-HDL is determined by
the protein moiety of this plasma lipoprotein. After the
successful treatment of hyperthyroidism, β-HDL is no longer
demonstrable in the patients' plasma.

REGULATION OF HEPATIC HMG-CoA REDUCTASE

DAVID J. SHAPIRO and VICTOR W. RODWELL

Department of Biochemistry, Purdue University, Lafayette,
Indiana 47907

HMG-CoA reductase (mevalonate:NADP oxidoreductase
(acylating CoA) EC 1.1.1.34) undergoes striking protein
synthesis-dependent cyclic variations with distinct activity
peaks at midnight and 1:45 am (EST). Cycloheximide prevents
both the initial (6 pm to midnight) rise in the rate of HMG-CoA
reduction and the second smaller rise from 12:30 am to 1:45 am.
A rapid 35-40% decrease in the rate of HMG-CoA reduction occurs
from midnight to 12:30 am. After 1:45 am the rate of HMG-CoA
reduction declines with a half time of 2-3 hours, reaching
basal levels in the morning.

The rate of HMG-CoA reduction decreases 20-25 fold in rats fasted 36 hours. However, the cyclic rhythm with both peaks in activity persists in rats fasted for 12-18 or 36 hours. This indicates that cyclic variations in food intake and hepatic tryptophan levels are not responsible for the cyclic rise in HMG-CoA reduction. By contrast, short-duration cholesterol feeding supresses the cyclic rise. Cholesterol and fasting may therefore regulate HMG-CoA reduction through different mechanisms. Supported by a predoctoral fellowship from the U.S. Public Health Service (D.J.S.) and a grant from the Indiana Heart Association.

EFFECT OF PHENOBARBITAL ON THE FORMATION OF BILE ACIDS FROM

CHOLESTEROL-4-^{14}C IN THE BILE-FISTULA RAT

CHARLES M. SIEGFRIED and WILLIAM H. ELLIOTT

Department of Biochemistry, St. Louis University School of Medicine, St. Louis, Missouri   63104

A comparison was made of the proportions of bile acids derived from cholesterol-4-^{14}C in bile from rats treated with phenobarbital or with saline. Treated male rats received phenobarbital sodium (85 mg/kg) intraperitoneally daily for 7 days prior to cannulation of bile ducts. After intracardial administration of the sterol, injections of the drug were continued up to 14 days. Control animals received identical volumes of saline. Bile flow of the treated animals averaged 30% higher per day over controls, although biliary ^{14}C was only slightly increased. Analysis of the acid fraction of hydrolyzed daily bile samples by glc and tlc and by separation of the acids by partition chromatography showed a) an increase in total bile acids, but no significant change in concentration over controls, b) a decreased excretion of cholic acid (10-40% below controls), whereas chenodeoxycholic acid increased to nearly twice that of controls, and c) small increased excretion of α - and β-muricholic acids. These studies show that phenobarbital stimulates and maintains an increase in the bile flow of rats with bile drainage continuous up to 14 days, demonstrate a dramatic change in the proportions of dihydroxy- to trihydroxy bile acids, and indicate that the drug affects, in vivo, the relative rates of side chain oxidation and/or 12 α-hydroxylation. (Supported by U.S.P.H.S. Grants HE-07878, 2Ti GM-446, and St. Louis University Committee on Grants.)

HYPOCHOLESTEROLEMIC AGENTS, INCREASES IN THE FECAL EXCRETION OF

CHOLESTEROL, AND THE INDIVIDUAL RESPONSES TO FALL IN PLASMA

CHOLESTEROL CONCENTRATIONS

H.S. SODHI, B.J. KUDCHODKAR, and L. HORLICK

Department of Medicine, University of Saskatchewan, Saskatoon, Saskatchewan, Canada

A number of subjects were investigated by cholesterol balance techniques to elucidate the mechanisms of action of clofibrate, nicotinic acid, plant sterols, and unsaturated fats. After taking into account the changes in the rates of endogenous synthesis, losses from the plasma pool, changes in the amounts of cholesterol secreted into the gastrointestinal tract or excreted into the feces, the amounts of cholesterol mobilized from the tissues were estimated. The estimates were also corroborated by the changes in the plasma cholesterol specific activity resulting from the mobilization of higher specific activity cholesterol from tissue pools. A review of the data indicated that increases in the fecal excretion of neutral steroids were not related to any single drug but were seen in some subjects and not in others. Increases in the fecal excretion were seen only in those subjects who showed evidence of mobilization of high specific activity cholesterol from tissue pools and an increase in the secretion of endogenous cholesterol into the intestinal lumen. Although the drugs decreased plasma cholesterol concentrations through different mechanisms, it is suggested that the increases in fecal excretion were determined by the responses of the subjects to the fall in plasma cholesterol.

STUDIES ON RELEASE OF LIPOPROTEIN LIPASE ACTIVITY FROM FAT CELLS

JAMES E. STEWART and MICHAEL C. SCHOTZ

Research, Veterans Administration Hospital (Wadsworth), Los Angeles, California 90073, and Departments of Biological Chemistry and Oral Diagnosis, UCLA Center for the Health Sciences, Los Angeles, California 90024

When fat cells prepared from rat epidydmal fat pad are incubated in Krebs-Ringer buffer containing glucose and albumin the release of lipoprotein lipase activity into the incubation medium is approximately linear for 45 min. In these cells that are releasing lipoprotein lipase activity the intracellular level of this enzyme activity remains essentially unchanged during this 45 min of incubation. During this time 3 times as much lipoprotein lipase activity was found in the medium compared to the amount of this enzyme activity measured in the cells. When protein synthesis was inhibited with cycloheximide the amount of intracellular lipoprotein lipase activity as well as the amount of this enzyme activity release was essentially unchanged. It is concluded that this process by which lipoprotein lipase activity is released from fat cells does not require protein synthesis. Furthermore, we suggest that lipoprotein lipase is activated prior to or in conjunction with release from these cells.

DIET AND DRUG-INDUCED CHANGES IN LIPOPROTEIN PATTERN MONITORED

BY MEMBRANE FILTRATION AND NEPHELOMETRY.

M.C. STONE and T.B.S. DICK

Clinical Research Unit, Leigh Infirmary, Leigh, Lancs. England

The technique of "MNC Analysis" (membrane filtration, nephelometry and serum cholesterol estimation) described by Stone and Thorp, has recently been validated by comparison with analytical ultracentrifugation and can be used to estimate quickly and inexpensively the concentrations of S_f 0-20, S_f 20-400 and S_f 400 lipoproteins in the majority of serum samples encountered in practice.

We have used this technique for the surveillance of acute and chronic changes in lipoprotein pattern induced by diet and Clofibrate, and have studied the relationship between the index patterns recorded in the stable state and the different types of "transitional" pattern.

UNUSUAL BIOCHEMICAL AND MICROBIOLOGICAL FEATURES OF STEROL

METABOLISM IN WHITE CARNEAU PIGEON

M.T. RAVI SUBBIAH, BRUCE A. KOTTKE, and WILLIAM J. MARTIN

Mayo Clinic and Mayo Foundation, 200 First Street Southwest, Rochester, Minnesota 55901

Sterol excretion and distribution were examined in spontaneously atherosclerosis-susceptible white carneau pigeons using thin-layer chromatography (TLC), argentation TLC, gas-liquid chromatography (GLC), and mass spectrometry. Unlike man and rodents, these pigeons excreted no coprostanol or coprostanone derivatives of sterols. In roosters, however, 5 - stanols accounted for 20-50% of total fecal sterols. Incubation of ^{14}C-cholesterol with pigeon feces indicated that, unlike humans, this species is unable to convert it to coprostanol. Microbiological examination indicated that pigeon feces lacked anaerobes (such as Peptostreptococcus species and Bacteroides melaninogenicus, fragilis, and incommunis) found in man, which might account for the inability to form coprostanol. The unusual amount of 5α-cholestan-3β-ol excreted in pigeon feces (on cholestanol-free diet) equaled about 20% of sterols of the cholesterol group and 13% of total 5α-stanols. Testes contained 5α-cholestan-3β-ol in the highest concentration reported in any normal animal tissue (26% of total sterols, 384 g/gm). Other pigeon tissues contained only 1-8% of this stanol; the stanol content of the rooster testes was only 2%. Fecal cultures containing ^{14}C-cholesterol indicated that this stanol could not be formed by intestinal bacteria suggesting that this stanol is of endogenous origin.

NEW ASPECTS OF HYPOGLYCIN EFFECT ON FATTY ACID METABOLISM

KAY TANAKA and KURT J. ISSELBACHER

Department of Medicine, Harvard Medical School and Gastro-intestinal Unit, Massachusetts General Hospital, Boston, Massachusetts 02114

Hypoglycin is a plant toxin which has been identified as the cause of the vomiting sickness of Jamaica. Methylenecyclopropyl-acetic acid (MCPA), a metabolite of hypoglycin, inhibits β -oxidation of long chain fatty acids by forming unmetabolizable esters with carnitine and CoA. It was previously thought that this compound did not inhibit oxidation of short chain fatty acids in general. In recent studies, however, we have shown that hypoglycin specifically inhibited isovaleryl CoA dehydrogenase and glutaryl CoA dehydrogenase. As a result, when a single dose (15 mg) of hypoglycin was given to rats, serum levels of isovalerate elevated to 500 x normal. Large amounts of N-isovaleryl-glycine (12 mg) and glutarate (95 mg) were also excreted in the urine in 48 hours. Since isovalerate is neurotoxic, elevations of serum isovalerate may explain, in part, the mechanism of disturbed central nervous function in the vomiting sickness of Jamaica.

In addition, after hypoglycin, five unknown compounds were also found in urine in large amounts. They were identified as cis-4-decene-1,10-dioate (51 mg), cis-cis-4,7(8)-decadience-1,10-dioate (8 mg), cis-4-octene-1,8-dioate (24 mg), adipate (17 mg) and N-MCPA-glycine (8.5 mg). For the first time, these compounds were identified from natural sources.

USE AND ASSESSMENT OF SOLUBLE POLYBASIC COMPOUNDS AS

HYPOCHOLESTEROLAEMIC AGENTS

G.R. THOMPSON, J.D. CAMERON, T.J. PETERS and C.N.C. DREY

Department of Medicine, Royal Postgraduate Medical School, London, and Department of Chemistry and Polymer Technology, Polytechnic of the South Bank, London, England

Non-polar lipids, such as cholesterol, must undergo solubilisation in mixed (bile salt-polar lipid) micelles within the intestinal lumen prior to absorption. We have previously shown that the polybasic antibiotic neomycin interferes with this process by precipitating cholesterol from micellar solutions, both in vitro (1) and in the human small intestine (2). This effect is due to interaction between fatty acid and bile acid anions and the amino groups of neomycin. We have also obtained evidence in germ-free pigs that this mechanism, which provides an explanation for the hypocholesterolaemic action of neomycin, is exerted independently of the drug's antibiotic effects or mucosal toxicity.

Recently, by quantitating the precipitation of labelled cholesterol in vitro, we have assessed the micelle-precipitating properties of two other polybasic but non-antibiotic compounds, poly-D-lysine (PDL) and polyethyleneimine (PEI). At pH 6.5 the relative efficacy of equal concentrations of neomycin, PDL and PEI was 1.0:1.3:2.0. In contrast to neomycin both the polymers largely retained their precipitating ability at pH 8.5. Preliminary results suggest that PEI has a hypocholesterolaemic action in young pigs and its effect on faecal steroid excretion is now being measured. The identification and use of such soluble, polybasic compounds may provide a new approach to the therapeutic control of cholesterol absorption in man.

References:

1) Thompson, G.R., MacMahon, M. & Claes, P. (1970) Europ. J. clin. Invest. 1, 40.

2) Thompson, G.R., Barrowman, J., Gutierrez, L. & Dowling, R.H. (1971) J. Clin. Invest. 50, 319.

LINOLEAMIDES: ENZYMATIC HYDROLYSIS AND CHOLESTEROL-LOWERING

ACTIVITY

K. TOKI, H. NAKATANI

Medical Research Department, Pharmaceuticals Division, SUMITOMO CHEMICAL CO., LTD., 40, 2-chome, Doshomachi, Higashi-ku, Osaka, Japan

It was reported that d-isomer of α-methylbenzyl linoleamide (melinamide) showed greater cholesterol-lowering activity than l-isomer.

Studying the metabolism of the linoleamide using carboxy ^{14}C-labeled compounds in rats revealed that respiratory $^{14}CO_2$ after oral administration of l-isomer was significantly greater than that of d- or dl-isomer and the rate of urinary excretion of ^{14}C activity in rats given d-isomer was higher than that of l- or dl-isomer.

Though the amide linkage of the linoleamide was not hydrolyzed by simulated gastric and intestinal fluids nor by treatment with alkali and acid, it was hydrolyzed by rat liver homogenates at pH 7.4 and the enzyme activity was also found in the small intestine and kidneys. The rate of hydrolysis of these isomers in vitro was markedly different in the order of l-, dl- and d-isomer, which was reverse to the order of cholesterol-lowering potency.

From above results and other studies on structure-activity relationship, it could be thought that cholesterol-lowering potency of linoleamides depends on the metabolic pattern to some extent.

INCORPORATION OF PALMITATE AND L-ALPHA-GLYCEROPHOSPHATE INTO

LIPIDS BY LUNG SUBCELLULAR FRACTIONS DERIVED FROM HAMSTERS

E.G. TOMBROPOULOS

Biology Department, Battelle-Northwest, P.O. Box 999, Richland, Washington 99352

In previous studies on the origin and synthesis of lung lipid surfactant we have shown that lung tissue is capable of synthesizing long chain fatty acids. The mitochondrial fraction was the most active when acetate was used as a precursor. In this report we will describe results from experiments in which the incorporation of ^{14}C and ^3H into lipids from $(1-^{14}C)$ and $(9,10-^3H)$ palmitate was examined and compared with the incorporation of ^{14}C from $(U,L-^{14}C)-L$-alpha-glycerophosphate. It was found that 1) Mitochondrial and microsomal lung fractions are able to incorporate the above components into lipids and that the microsomal fraction is the most active fraction. 2)The rate of palmitate incorporation is biphasic, and that of L-alpha-glycerophosphate is linear during the 40 min incubation period. If the incorporation of $(^{14}C)-L$-alpha-glycerophosphate is taken as an indicator of de novo synthesis, the synthesis of lecithin is much slower than that of phosphatidylethanolamine or triglycerides. When lung fractions were incubated with $(U,L-^{14}C)-L$-alpha-glycerophosphate and $(9,10-^3H)$ palmitate the ratio of $^{14}C/^3H$ indicated that 1) triglycerides and phosphatidylethanolamine are synthesized mainly by the diglyceride pathway, and 2) the major part of palmitate incorporation into lecithin is by exchange reaction.

CONTROLLED COMPARISON OF Sul3,437 AND CLOFIBRATE IN TYPE II

HYPERLIPOPROTEINAEMIA

A.S. TRUSWELL, G. WATERMEYER AND J.I. MANN

Department of Medicine, University of Cape Town Medical School, Observatory, Cape Town, South Africa

Sul3,437 (Su) was given (300 mg daily) for 12 weeks to 11 reliable out-patients with primary Type II. Fasting serum lipids were measured 2-weekly and in control periods before and after. Following this each patient was given clofibrate (clo) (1.5 g daily). Repeat courses of Su or Clo were given to 5 patients.

Serum cholesterol fell more on Su in 6/11 (in 5 of whom the effect of clo was poor or nil). Both drugs were equally effective in 3/11. In a 10th patient cholesterol did not fall on Su but was moderately decreased on clo. The last patient had a large cholesterol reduction on Su and even more on clo. Individual responses were very consistent in 5 repeat courses. Overall mean cholesterol changes were -14% on Su and -9.6% on clo.

Serum Triglyceride (TG) changes averaged -27.5% on Su and -15.7% on clo. Tgs were lower on Su in 7/11. Preferences between Su and clo coincided for cholesterol and TG in 8/11. Transient SGOT elevations occurred on Su in 2/11, in clo in 2/11 and on both drugs in 2/11.

Conclusions: Su was a 1½ times stronger lipid-lowering agent but there were consistent individual exceptions.

THE EFFECT OF DL-ETHIONINE ON THE INCOPORATION OF ^{14}C-GLYCEROL

INTO LIVER GLYCERIDES AND PHOSPHOLIPIDS IN RATS IN VIVO

VAVRECKA, M.

The British Industrial Biological Research Association,
Carshalton, Surrey, England

The role of glyceride and phospholipid synthesis in the
development of ethionine fatty liver was studied by measuring
the incorporation of ^{14}C-glycerol into liver lipids in rats
which received ethionine (1 g/kg s.c.) 6 hours previously.
^{14}C-glycerol (5-10 uCi) was injected i.v. 10 minutes before
the liver was removed. In starved female rats, ethionine
increased the incorporation of glycerol into total glycerides
and phospholipids 3.6 times and 1.4 times respectively and the
total liver triglycerides 2.6 times. Lecithin and phosphatidylethanolamine were the main phospholipid fractions containing
labelled glycerol. When glucose was administered orally to
starved female rats, the increased incorporation of glycerol
into glycerides and the triglycerides accumulation were prevented,
while the phospholipid labelling was unaffected. This same
result was obtained when ethionine was administered to ad
libitum fed female rats.

No increase in glycerol incorporation into glycerides and
phospholipids, nor triglyceride accumulation in liver were
found in ethionine treated starved male rats.

The increase in glycerol incorporation into liver glycerides
was interpreted as indication of increased triglyceride synthesis,
as it was always accompanied by increase in liver triglycerides
and plasma free fatty acids. The small increase in phospholipid
labelling can be explained by increased specific activity of
α-glycerophosphate due to diminished pool size.

The results support the view, that the differences in
fat accumulation in ethionine treated male, female, starved and
fed animal could be accounted for by the differences in the
rate of triglyceride synthesis in liver.

EFFECT OF CLOFIBRATE ON FAT MOBILIZING LIPOLYSIS AND CYCLIC AMP

LEVELS IN ADIPOSE TISSUE

G. WALLDIUS, R.W. BUTCHER and L.A. CARLSON

Department of Geriatrics, Box 641, S-751 27 Uppsala, Sweden
Department of Biochemistry, University of Massachusetts Medical
School, Worcester, Massachusetts 01604, U.S.A.

Clofibrate effectively lowers plasma triglycerides (TG) in
man and animals. The mechanism for this action is not known.
As inhibition of mobilization of FFA (free fatty acids) from
adipose tissue may lower plasma TG we wanted to see if clofibrate
could act through such a mechanism. Isolated rat and human

adipose tissue was incubated in vitro. Glycerol release and
cyclic AMP levels were determined.

In rat fat a significant inhibition of basal lipolysis
was seen with doses from 133 µg/ml. Lipolysis stimulated with
catecholamines was inhibited both in rat and human fat.
Stimulation of lipolysis with catecholamines and ACTH in adipose
tissue from rats caused marked increases in the content of
cyclic AMP, which were reduced about 80 percent by addition of
2000 µg/ml of clofibrate.

As other hypolipidemic drugs, such as nicotinic acid,
also lower the adipose tissue content of cAMP, it is possible
that one primary site of action for such drugs may be on
mechanisms regulating the content of cAMP in adipose tissue.

Supported by grants from the Swedish Medical Research
Foundation (19x-204-08) and from U.S. Public Health Service
(AM 13904).

CEREBROSPINAL FLUID STEROL PATTERNS IN PATIENTS TREATED FOR

MALIGNANT BRAIN TUMORS

JOSEPH F. WEISS, JOSEPH RANSOHOFF and HERBERT J. KAYDEN

Department of Neurosurgery and Medicine, New York University
Medical Center, 550 First Avenue, New York, New York 10016

Desmosterol is present in malignant brain tumors and
occasionally can be detected in the cerebrospinal fluid (CSF)
of patients with brain tumors. The CSF desmosterol level is
usually raised in these patients after a short period of
triparanol administration.

Sterol levels were measured in the CSF of 7 control
patients and in 45 patients with proven malignant gliomas, and
the levels were correlated with the biological activity of the
tumors. Cholesterol and desmosterol concentrations were
determined at various stages: initially; after triparanol
administration for 5 days; after surgery, chemotherapy, or a
combination of treatments. Cholesterol levels were higher in
the CSF of patients with gliomas than in control patients.
After triparanol administration, the CSF desmosterol level was
increased to > 0.1 µg/ml in about 60% of the patients with
gliomas. Surgical treatment was carried out in most patients,
and in addition, approximately one-half of the group received
chemotherapy, usually BCNU (1,3-bis-(2-chloroethyl)-1-nitrosourea).
In this small series of patients, the response of the tumors
to therapy could not be correlated conclusively with the
sterol patterns after triparanol augmentation.

INFLUENCE OF PORTO-CAVAL SHUNT OPERATION ON SPECIFIC ACTIVITY (SA)

OF FREE CHOLESTEROL (FC), ESTERIFIED CHOLESTEROL (EC) AND PLASMA

LIPID CONCENTRATIONS

A. WEIZEL

Medizinische Universitats-Klinik, Berheimerstrasse 58,
69 Heidelberg, Germany

A 49 year old male patient with liver cirrhosis was
injected with 50 μC 4-14C-cholesterol 10 days prior to a porto-
caval shunt operation. No bleeding occured during the time of
the study, no blood was given during the operation. Between
9 and 10 determinations of FC-SA, CE-SA, as well as total
cholesterol (TC), FC, CE, Triglyceride (TG), and phospholipid
(PL) concentrations were performed before and after the operation.
TC values fell from a pre-operative average of 157-11 mg% to
105-11 mg% postop. Most of this decrease was due to a fall in
CE concentration (97 -9 mg% vs. 59-9 mg%), FC concentrations
fell only from 60-4 mg% to 47-4 mg%. There was a moderate
decrease of PL (222 -14 mg% - 171 - 33 mg%), and almost no
change in TG concentration (71-10 mg% vs. 62 mg%). The operation
did not alter the slope of the SA curves of either FC or CE,
the crossover took place 3 days after the injection. The results
suggest that there was no major influence of the operation on
FC synthesis, the capability to esterify FC however was greatly
reduced after the procedure.

EFFECT OF CHOLESTYRAMINE ON CHOLESTEROL AND MEVALONATE BIOSYNTHESIS

LAWRENCE W. WHITE, M.D.

Department of Pharmacology, Case Western Reserve University,
Cleveland, Ohio 44106

Oral administration of cholestyramine is associated with
interruption of enterohepatic circulation of bile salts,
reduced plasma cholesterol concentration, and increased
hepatic cholesterol biosynthesis. To localize the biochemical
step at which compensatory augmentation of cholesterol
synthesis is regulated, liver slices and cell-free fractions
were prepared from control rats and rats fed 3% cholestyramine
for 3 days. In slices, incorporation of acetate-C^{14} (Ac-C^{14})
into cholesterol and mevalonate (MVA) increased by 355% and
225% respectively. In fractionated liver homogenates, incorporation of Ac-C^{14}, Ac-CoA-C^{14}, and 3-hydroxy-3-methylglutaryl-
CoA-C^{14} (HMG-CoA) into MVA increased 17, 35, and 19 fold,
indicating a marked increase in HMG-CoA reductase activity.
Incorporation of Ac-C^{14} and Ac-CoA-C^{14} into HMG increased by
468% and 34%, indicating increased Ac activation and HMG-CoA
condensing enzyme activity. These data indicate that cholesty-
ramine-enhanced excretion of cholesterol results in increased
activity at two key pre-MVA steps.

In an attempt to suppress the compensatory increase in cholesterol synthesis, the effect of clofibrate, known to inhibit HMG-CoA reductase, was examined. While clofibrate alone reduced synthesis in rat liver slices, augmented cholesterol synthesis in slices from cholestyramine-fed animals was not attenuated by co-administration of clofibrate, further indicating the importance of HMG-CoA condensing enzyme in regulation of cholesterol synthesis.

THE EFFECT OF FENFLURAMINE ON LIPOGENESIS IN HUMAN ADIPOSE TISSUE

WILSON, J.P.D. and GALTON, D.J.

Department of Medicine, Royal Postgraduate Medical School, Ducane Road, London W. 12, U.K.

Fenfluramine and other drugs were tested for their ability to inhibit lipogenesis in human adipose tissue. Only fenfluramine was found to inhibit the incorporation of T-palmitate and ^{14}C-glucose into neutral lipid in intact tissue. This effect was observed at drug concentration above 1mM. Fenfluramine inhibited lipogenesis in broken-cell preparations of adipose tissue at concentrations of 1 mM and above. The N-benzoyloxyethyl derivative of fenfluramine was also found to inhibit lipogenesis in this preparation, significant inhibition occurring at 0.4 mM. During inhibition of lipogenesis in homogenates of adipose tissue by fenfluramine, radioactivity accumulated in long-chain acyl-CoA which suggests that the drug may interfere with acylation of glycerol phosphate. Evidence that fenfluramine may have a similar effect in vivo was considered but results were not statistically significant.

RESPONSE OF THE GERIATRIC PATIENT TO A HYPOLIPIDEMIC AGENT

A. WOLDOW

Philadelphia Geriatric Center, 5301 Old York Road, Philadelphia, Pennsylvania 19141

Preliminary investigation of the incidence of hyper-lipidemia among elderly residents over 70 years of age residing in the Philadelphia Geriatric Center, revealed an elevation of blood cholesterol and/or triglycerides in approximately one-third of the residents studied. In an effort to reduce the above mentioned hyperlipidemia, a double-blind study was designed using an experimental Ciba hypolipidemic agent (SU-1343-tetralin phenoxy isobutyric acid), involving 36 patients. Sixteen patients recieved the drug for one to six months duration, the remaining 20 were controls.

Of the 16 subjects who received the drug, eleven showed, before treatment, elevated cholesterol levels and eleven showed elevated triglyceride levels - either alone or in combination, with a consistent lipid electrophoretic pattern.

At the end of six months, the study was stopped because of a report of tumors produced in experimental rats with massive doses administered over 18 months.

The results of this contracted study show the following: Five out of six cases with combined elevated cholesterol (above 300 mg) and elevated triglycerides (above 150 mgm), showed significant decreases in both fractions, the sixth showed a reduction in triglyceride level only. Four out of five cases showing only cholesterol elevations, showed a significant response. All of the five cases showing only triglyceride elevations responsed to treatment. Side effects were minimal - one case showing a diffuse maculo-papular rash and another G.I. symptoms. In one instance a transient SGOT elevation was noted.

These results show, therefore, a definite drug effect in a geriatric population.

DRUG-INDUCED LIPIDOSES: NIEMANN-PICK-LIKE SYNDROME CAUSED BY

4,4'-DIETHYLAMINOETHOXYHEXESTROL

AKIRA YAMAMOTO, SUSUMU ADACHI, KATSUNORI ISHIKAWA, TERUO KITANI, TERUSHI NASU, YOSHITAKE SHINJI, KO-ICHI SEKI and MITSUO NISHIKAWA

The Second Department of Internal Medicine, Osaka University Medical School, Fukushima-ku, Osaka, 553 Japan

A type of foam cell syndrome accompanying hyperlipidemia and hepatosplenomegaly has been reported in Japan (1). A coronary vasodilator, 4,4'-diethylaminoethoxyhexestrol, was found to be the cause of this syndrome (2). Weight loss, subfever, marked increase of blood sedimentation rate, positive CRP test and an increase in serum alkaline phosphatase activity were noticed in almost all the cases. Leucocytes showed marked vacuolization changes. Intracellular inclusions with concentrically laminated structure were present in almost all the tissues. There was an increase in total phospholipids in the liver and some other tissues with an accumulation of phosphatidylinositol and lysobisphosphatidic acid. Free cholesterol was increased and desmosterol was detected at a concentration between 3-10% of the total sterol in the liver, spleen, bile and blood serum.

Accumulation of the drug in the liver and some other tissues was detected on TLC of total lipids. In rats, the accumulation of the drug itself was much less than in human cases, while another unidentified spot appeared on TLC.

Storage of lysobisphosphatidic acid was reported in Niemann-Pick disease (3). Similarities in symptoms and pathological changes in drug-induced lipidosis and in Niemann-Pick disease may shed light on the biological significance of the peculiar glycerophospholipid, lysobisphosphatidic acid.

References: 1) Yamamoto et al.: Lipids 5, 566, 1970.
            2) Yamamoto et al.: J. Biochem. (Tokyo) 69, 613, 1971.
            3) Rouser et al.: Lipids 3, 287, 1968.

BIOCHEMICAL AND CLINICAL EFFECTS OF PYRIDYL CARBINOL, A

CHOLESTEROL LOWERING DRUG.   RESULTS OF A FIVE YEARS FOLLOW-UP

NEPOMUK ZOLLNER AND GUNTHER WOLFRAM

Medizinische Poliklinik der Universitat Munchen, 8000 Munchen 15, Pettenkoferstrasse 8a, West Germany

Seventy-seven patients with hypercholesterolemia (more than 330 mg/100 ml) had been treated with β-pyridyl-carbinol (average daily dose 1.2 grams) during the years of 1964 to 1966; plasma cholesterol had been normalized or lowered significantly in 76 percent of them.   In 1969, 49 patients could be reevaluated.   In all patients who had continued therapy the cholesterol lowering effect of the drug was sustained.   There were no side effects attributable to the drug.   In patients originally treated successfully who interrupted therapy cholesterol levels rose again.   Under continuous therapy with pyridyl carbinol xanthoma disappeared.   Intermittent claudication disappeared in five out of six, angina pectoris in seven out of eight cases.   Among the cases who had interrupted therapy only two had lost angina pectoris while there were three new cases and one case of a coronary reinfarction.   Intermittent cluadication had disappeared or become much better in five out of eleven and had reappeared or become worse in additional three cases.   Two cases interrupting therapy had died of their obliterating vascular disease.

Pyridyl carbinol exerts a considerable and sustained hypocholesterolemic effect in the majority of patients with hypercholesterolemia while side effects are negligible. Concomitantly the prognosis of clinical disease of coronaries and peripheral arteries would appear to be much improved.

AUTHOR INDEX

(Underscored numbers indicate complete papers in this volume.)

SUBJECT INDEX